Take Control
of Your Health
and
Escape the Sickness Industry

Ninth Edition

Elaine Hollingsworth
Director
Hippocrates Health Centre of Australia

www.doctorsaredangerous.com

ISBN: 0646402978

Published by
Empowerment Press International
PO Box 1400
Mudgeeraba
Queensland 4213
Australia
Phone: (07) 5530 2939
Fax: (07) 5569 0884
E-mail: sales@doctorsaredangerous.com

The recommendations in this book are based on the research and personal experiences of the author. Because we are all different, readers are strongly urged to check with qualified health professionals before implementing any suggestions made in this book.

There is always a possibility of risk where matters of health are concerned; therefore, readers should not use this book unless willing to assume that risk. It is a sign of wisdom to seek second, or third, opinions when making important decisions regarding health.

By The Same Author
ZULMA (Warner Books)

Author's Note

It is customary for writers and publishers to have their work scrutinised by lawyers prior to publication in order to preclude the possibility of lawsuits from companies who feel affronted by statements and evidence presented which are critical of their products, commercial practices and ethics. I have chosen not to do so. Instead, I have gone to extreme lengths to ensure the accuracy of my statements and the veracity of my evidence. Any offence and distress caused to organisations and companies criticised in this book is entirely intentional. They deserve it. It is the least I can do in defence of the millions of their victims who have suffered much more than distress as a result of their disgraceful, self-interested conduct.

In particular, should any of those I have singled out for dishonourable mention feel that my attack is unwarranted in their case, I would welcome the opportunity to debate the issue with them in court and in public. I can assure them that there is now a massive and growing worldwide audience of victims and their relatives who would be very interested to hear their defences. If they have any.

Elaine Hollingsworth

The most dangerous man to any government is the man who is able to think things out for himself, without regard to the prevailing superstitions and taboos. Almost inevitably he comes to the conclusion that the government he lives under is dishonest, insane, and intolerable.

H. L. Mencken

Contents

Contents

Acknowledgements

Throughout this book I make unflattering references to orthodox medicine (which holds natural healing in contempt and even acts to suppress it), and to those scientists who knowingly obscure data to enable pharmaceutical companies to earn billions of dollars from dangerous drugs. This, however, is not a blanket condemnation of everyone in these professions.

Even though my website is called, with intentional irony, "doctorsaredangerous.com", I do not for one moment deny that there have been, and still are, many courageous physicians and scientists with the independence to think for themselves, stand up against entrenched ideas and prejudices, and truly embrace the Hippocratic ethos. Such men and women have taught me a great deal and I respect their courage. And I acknowledge with admiration those professionals who devote their skills to repairing physical damage resulting from accidents, disease and genetic abnormalities, and the doctors and nurses who selflessly and voluntarily expose themselves to pain, hardship and danger in order to help sufferers in remote and disadvantaged regions of our world.

I shall forever be grateful to my friend, doctor and teacher, the late Henry Bieler, MD, who helped thousands of his patients regain their health through natural methods. He lost his hospital privileges because of this, but it didn't really matter, because he taught his patients how to avoid hospitals. I am indebted to the late Ann Wigmore, founder of Hippocrates Health Centre of Boston, who taught me so much, and reached millions through her books.

Most of all, my thanks go to such enlightened pioneers as Raymond Peat, MA, PhD, endocrine physiologist and prolific author; the late John R. Lee, MD, whose work on progesterone has helped millions of women; clinical nutritionist Krispin Sullivan; Lipid Chemist Mary Enig, PhD and her associate, nutrition expert Sally Fallon of the Weston A Price Foundation; and Dr Barry Durrant-Peatfield, a British physician who truly exemplifies the patient-friendly, common sense principles of Hippocrates. Without the extensive research and generous help given by these and many other caring health professionals who took the time to talk with me, this book could not have been written.

Elaine Hollingsworth
Hippocrates Health Centre
Queensland
Australia

Introduction

Fasten your seatbelt, and hang on – this is going to be a bumpy read! You are going to be exposed to ideas that refute the propaganda the 'experts' have been spewing for decades. *They have used us as dupes and guinea pigs.*

The food industry and the drug manufacturers have been unconscionable in their zeal to earn hundreds of billions of dollars, aided and abetted by scientists who have been handsomely paid to fudge, and even falsify, test results. I promise you that not one of the biochemists, physicians and scientists quoted in this book is in the employ of multinational corporations. They are dedicated men and women whose conclusions are based upon sound science, not upon the propaganda, the power and the coercion of the legal drug industry. Because they are free to speak their minds, they are the only scientists I trust. Their opinions rarely find their way into the establishment media which is, like much of the world, under multinational domination.

But you and I are not under multinational domination. At least not completely, and not yet. We are still free to refuse to be poisoned by their dangerous drugs. We are still free to refuse to eat their health-destroying 'foods'. We are still free to avoid their staph-filled hospitals by living according to the laws of nature. We are still free, at least some of us, to think for ourselves and remain uninfluenced by their persuasive television and glossy magazine ads. We are still free to question physicians who learned all they know in medical schools that are financed by the companies that manufacture the drugs that are killing us.

I'm angry! I guess you noticed that. My anger and disgust drove me to write this book, and I hope it will inspire you, and many like you, to join our crusade. For those of you who are tempted to dismiss what I write, just remember what a wise man said years ago: "Contempt, prior to complete investigation, will enslave a man to ignorance."

Elaine Hollingsworth

Preface to the Ninth Edition

Sadly, in the five years that have passed since the preceding Introduction to this book was written, little has changed. Food and drug manufacturers are still releasing dangerous products onto the market; our trusted watchdogs and regulatory authorities are still turning a blind eye to blatantly biased and 'doctored' research and testing; men, women, children and babies are still suffering unnecessary pain, even death, as a direct result.

People still pursue unhealthy eating and drinking habits, either through ignorance, through the influence of slick advertisements or, even worse, on the 'recommendations' of those so-called health professionals who are perhaps more concerned with the state of their bank balance than that of their patients' health, or are afraid to question what they are told by those who have a vested interest in maintaining the *status quo*.

But it's not all bad. I have been encouraged by the thousands of readers who have indeed been inspired to join our crusade, especially those who have taken the trouble to write to me to say that they were helped by this book. Many tell me they have found relief from long-endured conditions, merely by taking my advice to make a small change to their diet, or by quitting a product that they had been assured was 'safe', but which actually made them sick. Even some doctors have told me that, as a result of reading this book and investigating the medical and scientific sources from which I quote, they have re-evaluated some of their long-held beliefs and looked more seriously to alternative treatments.

This latest edition has been updated and contains some new material. I am grateful to the many true health professionals and other concerned individuals who have contributed new information that I have been able to add here for the benefit of readers. I hope you will 'Read in Good Health!'

Elaine Hollingsworth

Foreword

This book once again proves Elaine Hollingsworth is a rare human being. She effortlessly cuts through the hype of the powerful pharmaceutical and food processing monoliths whose sole aim is huge profits, and certainly not the health of their clients.

Elaine teaches self-responsibility – the greatest weapon in improving your health. If everyone followed her advice, the country's medical waiting rooms and hospitals would soon be very empty.

I congratulate the reader for making the effort to seek out the health knowledge contained in this meticulously researched book. This knowledge is not easily available; not from the medical industry, and certainly not from the popular media.

Elaine compels us to keep questioning the directions of the medical, pharmaceutical, food manufacturing and agricultural industries. We need to force these bodies and government authorities to justify themselves, because very few major indicators of community health are improving.

Each year we are becoming more obese, have far more chronic diseases, are more stressed by everyday pressures, and take more and more prescription drugs. Not one of these trends indicates our health is getting better. Yet national expenditures on health just keep climbing.

I urge you to keep on questioning everything to do with your own health – especially the "experts". Take full responsibility for your own health, until you become satisfied with all aspects of your own health directions. This book provides a light to follow.

Karen Coates
MBBS, Dip. Obs. RACOG, MACNEM

Burying Their Mistakes...

More than 500,000 Australians were victims of medical mistakes last year – and 11,000 people died as a result.

An estimated 80,000 were admitted to hospitals because they were either given the wrong medication or they took the wrong doses of drugs.

The head of the Australian Council for Safety and Quality in Health Care, Professor Bruce Barraclough, confirmed about 3 percent of hospital admissions, representing half a million patients, were the result of "adverse events" in the health system.

These medical and hospital errors cost about $4billion a year.

*From the **Sunday Mail**, Brisbane, July 14, 2002*

Think that's bad? Every year the injuries and deaths increase dramatically, and the cancer statistics are chilling: one in two men will be diagnosed with cancer, and one in three women. So, please pay attention to the revelations in this book and avoid the Sickness Industry!

For ethical reasons, we cannot give health advice by telephone, email, fax or post. Natural practitioners are listed, by area, on www.acnem.org. Some know what they are doing, but others are influenced by multinational propaganda, so caution is advised.

1

That "Mystery Illness"

... it's *not* all in your head!

I have some really *bad* health news for you; and some that's really *good*. First, the *Bad News*:

There is a medical problem that affects an estimated 40 percent of people in the developed world. It can cause symptoms that vary wildly – from exhaustion to killer heart disease, and everything in between. The majority of physicians haven't a clue; they don't know how to diagnose it, they don't know about the 64 diseases it causes, and they don't know a safe and effective way to reverse it. All but the most progressive doctors leave their patients in limbo. And now for the *Good News*:

You can diagnose yourself, and it won't cost you a penny. Even better, if you have been suffering briefly, or for a lifetime, with one or more of the 64 documented illnesses caused by this problem, one tiny, safe drug can make the difference between feeling full of life and just dragging around. Those two words, "safe" and "drug" do not appear together in any other sentence in this book, and with good reason. Generally there are none. However, in this case I make an exception because the drug I am about to endorse comes from a natural source, and it is a lifesaver for those who need it.

For want of this tiny pill, people can suffer for years from exhaustion, allergies, chronic viral illnesses, severe light sensitivity, menstrual problems, constipation, cold extremities, infertility, inability to lose weight, headaches, migraines, diabetes, dreadful skin diseases and anaemia. Even fibromyalgia, Meniere's Disease and weak muscles can result due to this condition. If depression is the form this illness takes, it can sometimes be so severe that if left undiagnosed (and frequently it is) victims are institutionalised, and often destroyed by psychotropic drugs. Even Alzheimer's Disease and arthritis can be the result of mis-diagnosis of this common, easily-remedied illness.

If your cholesterol is extremely high for no apparent reason, and if your physician is paying attention, lack of this crucial substance should be considered before any other measures are taken. Tragically, millions of people are taking deadly statin drugs to lower cholesterol, because doctors (heavily influenced by the pharmaceuticals) don't even consider the correct way to diagnose this common problem. Don't allow yourself to be one of them.

What is this lifesaving substance? It's _natural thyroid hormone_, and your health can be compromised if you are _only a tiny fraction under 'normal'_.

Has the following happened to you? You are feeling awful, with one or more of the above symptoms, and you go a doctor for help. You complain of your symptoms and leave, clutching a prescription to take to a laboratory so they can test you for everything under the sun. And why not? Medicare or private insurance pays for it. When you return to the doctor, hoping to learn some painless, simple way to feel well again, you are told that all of your results are "normal". If you remonstrate, the doctor may suggest a psychiatrist, which, if you have any gumption, should get your back up. Trust me, it is _not_ all in your head and, like millions of sufferers who have gone undiagnosed, you need _medical_, not _mental_ help.

Unrelenting Propaganda

Don't get me wrong – I am not saying that all of our woes can be traced to a lack of sufficient thyroid hormones. What I am saying is that this _must_ be ruled out if you have any unexplained physical problems. And it _cannot_ be ruled out by a blood test, because these tests are hopeless, and have been known to be inaccurate for as long as they have been used.

Thyroid illnesses have been in epidemic proportion for many years and for many reasons. Pollution, especially tobacco smoke, plastics, and the dangerous chemicals in our water, damage thyroid glands. Thanks to unrelenting propaganda, people are freaked out about cholesterol, not realizing that our bodies cannot make thyroid hormones, and other important hormones, without this misunderstood substance. Oestrogen, taken by so many women, suppresses the thyroid gland, and the sodium fluoride many local authorities are forcing us to drink in our water supply is known as a potent inhibitor of the thyroid. Stress damages all of our glands and the thyroid is no exception.

If you have been taking huge doses of vitamin C or PABA, there is strong evidence that they can inhibit the gland, as can aspirin and many other medications. Junk food junkies, vegans and strict vegetarians run the risk of damaging their thyroids, due to lack of necessary nutrients in their diets. Reliance on heavy grain consumption, common with vegetarians, as well as most people these days, suppresses the thyroid. If you were born or live inland, the lack of iodine in the air or water will, sooner or later, cause your thyroid to struggle.

Last, but far from least, eating lots of soy is a one-way trip to life-threatening thyroid illnesses (see **Chapter 9**, *Soy - the Abominable Bean*).

So, you can see that it is small wonder nearly half our population is suffering from mild or extreme symptoms of thyroid insufficiency. What is to be done about it? First, test yourself this way:

Shake down a thermometer at night and place it next to your bed. First thing in the morning, before getting out of bed, put the thermometer snugly in your armpit. Leave it there for ten minutes, without getting out of bed. Read it immediately and make a note of the result. Repeat on three consecutive mornings, and, for best results, not during menstruation. If your temperature is consistently 36.4° to 36.8° Celsius or 97.8° to 98.2° Fahrenheit, you have a well-functioning thyroid gland. If below, you need to take urgent measures to bring it up to speed.

The Barnes Basal Temperature Test

Your first job will be to find a physician willing to accept this time-honoured test and not relegate you to the rat-bag category. Actually, it will be the doctor who belongs with the rat-bags, as this test has been in the **Physicians' Desk Reference** (the reference book all American doctors use) for many years, and is known as the *Barnes Basal Temperature Test*. Long before blood testing for thyroid conditions was used, this was *the* test doctors used, in conjunction with the symptoms reported by patients. If your physician doesn't know who Broda Barnes, MD, was he should; this man was the number-one researcher and acknowledged authority on the thyroid gland for fifty years. As Stephen E Langer, MD, author of a superb book on the thyroid, **Solved - The Riddle Of Illness**, said in his Acknowledgments, "I know of no one else in the world who has done so much as a medical doctor, writer, lecturer and talk show guest to alert millions to the often hidden causes of illness, as well as to simple ways to stay well for life."

Many prestigious medical journals have printed papers on this test and I find it extraordinary that doctors are not taught about it in medical schools. After all, it is logical when you consider that if the metabolism is low, the temperature is also low. As Dr Langer says, "More than a hundred years of research has established a definite relationship between sub-normal temperature, no matter how slight, and hypothyrodism."

If you have found a physician who is willing to prescribe thyroid medication on the basis of this test, as well as symptomatology, congratulations – you have passed the first hurdle. Next is to convince your physician to prescribe the right kind of drug. This can be tricky, because most of them are wedded to the synthetics. After all, they were taught this way in their medical schools, which are financed by the companies who are making billions selling synthetic thyroid hormones. Unfortunately for our thyroid health, these synthetics contain only what is known as T4.

A healthy thyroid gland, however, produces not only T4, but T3, reverse T3, three kinds of T2, T1, T0 and calcitonin. An underactive thyroid gland cannot be brought back to health if all of the nine thyroid hormones it requires are not supplied. Dr Barnes, and all of the enlightened physicians who have followed him, think that nature knows best what is needed for the body, and man, with all his synthetic chemicals, can only guess and throw a monkey wrench into the works.

Armour thyroid, and the other porcine, desiccated thyroid hormone medications, come closest to providing these exact hormones that your body would make if it could. They contain all nine of them, naturally; they are not added.

Calcitonin

Calcitonin is the hormone produced by the parathyroid gland. It removes calcium from the blood and deposits it in your bones, where it is needed. As mentioned above, the natural thyroid medications contain calcitonin. The synthetics do not, and this is one of the reasons they cause osteoporosis. The studies that were done proving oral thyroid causes osteoporosis were all done on *Synthroid*, not natural, porcine desiccated thyroid hormone.

Chances are your physician will argue that the T4 in the synthetics is easily converted to T3, because after all, don't the pharmaceuticals say so? They do, indeed, but unfortunately for patients, conversion is capricious, and dependent upon excellent nutrition, a healthy liver, a stress-free life, ample selenium, vitamin A, the adrenal hormone cortisol, magnesium, the B vitamins and the 'good' fats. And if your body can't convert it, due to lack of any of these factors, tough luck, or so the pharmaceutical companies and physicians seem to think.

This is what will happen if your physician refuses to switch you over to natural medication: because your thyroid gland is only being treated 'halfway', your tissues will develop T4 resistance, and they will lose the ability to convert T4 into T3. Your cell receptor sites will shut down and cease to function, leaving you damaged, possibly permanently. The longer your thyroid gland remains untreated, the harder it will be to respond to the right medication, when and if you get it.

Some of your tissues will be just fine, and you may even notice improvements in wellbeing when you first take the synthetics. Your blood serum levels will probably rise on them, leading your physician to an "I told you so" reaction. But this rise is just T4, and because he or she is a slave to blood serum laboratory results, in spite of overwhelming evidence that they don't work, you may be condemned to a lifetime of suffering, and be at extreme risk of the long-term effects of hypothyroidism, as listed above. Your body will remain 'hungry' for T3, and your physician's neglect will deprive you of the full spectrum thyroid hormones you desperately need. If this happens, you will spend the rest of your life in a state of cellular hypothyroidism, in spite of the blood tests your pharmaceutically-orientated physician believes in.

Don't let this happen to you – 'physician-shop' until you find one who has done the research. Chances are, this open-mindedness will not occur with an endocrinologist, as many are more hide-bound than GPs.

If your physician refuses to cooperate, refer him or her to *The New England Journal of Medicine (1999; 340: 424-429, 469-470)*. This report describes greater improvements in mood, energy and brain function when patients receive treatment with desiccated thyroid hormone, rather than Synthroid.

If this doesn't impress, British medical journal, *The Lancet*, reported that synthetics may accelerate neurological aging and create nutritional deficiency states. The *Journal of the American Medical Association* reported a lowered bone density and low TSH levels in patients taking synthetics, but not with natural tablets.

Even the National Organization Of Women, the Grey Panthers seniors' organization, and the Stop Patient Abuse Now coalition, have gotten into the act. They have joined forces, calling for a class action suit against Synthroid, demanding that it be withdrawn from the market. When will our doctors get the message!

This is what Dr Robert Jay Rowen has to say about thyroid medication, in his *Second Opinion Newsletter:*

> "I've never liked Synthroid or any of the L-thyroxin products for treating thyroid problems, because I've rarely seen good results with them in my patients. In fact, many of my patients have complained about terrible reactions with the drug. Instead of these conventional medications, I've long relied upon desiccated thyroid products, such as *Armour* or *Westhroid*.
>
> "Now the Food and Drug Administration (FDA) is finally seeing what I've known for years and has announced it will prohibit marketing of non-approved L-thyroxin products, which includes Synthroid. This comes about after numerous complaints from users and subsequent findings that the product has been poorly standardised.
>
> "Recent studies suggest that all L-thyroxin products, even those with approved standardisations, may be inferior to the methods I've employed for years... If you're taking Synthroid, it's likely from a pharmaceutically-manipulated physician. I suggest you contact a doctor who understands how to use desiccated thyroid products and give them a try. You'll be amazed at how well these products work. To find a doctor in your area [*in the US*], contact the International College of Integrative Medicine at www.glccm.org ."

Natural thyroid preparations have been used for more than 100 years. The synthetics have been available only since 1959. During those years the makers have orchestrated a misinformation campaign demonising the natural, and extolling the virtues of the synthetic. Many doctors have been taken in by this PR campaign. Now, finally, due to a successful lawsuit brought against Synthroid for misleading marketing, natural thyroid is regaining the reputation for reliability it enjoyed for so many years.

Nowadays, most doctors order the Thyroid Stimulating Hormone test (TSH) when trying to diagnose a patient's thyroid health. This is done in spite of the huge body of literature, by many thousands of doctors, discrediting TSH. But this is the test that is taught in modern medical schools. It is used in combination with synthetic thyroid medication, the way the pharmaceuticals want it used, and everyone is happy except the victims of this (dare I say it?) conspiracy. Chronic Fatigue Syndrome and Fibromyalgia, 'incurable' and debilitating illnesses, arrived in our midst in alarming numbers not long after this deadly duo was foisted upon patients. *This is no coincidence*, and it is now well known among thinking health professionals that these two dreadful afflictions are caused, at least in part, by improper treatment of thyroid disease, and the adrenal insufficiency that often goes hand-in-glove with hypothyroidism.

It is well worth any effort it takes to persuade your physician to prescribe natural thyroid. As thyroid expert Dr Howard Hagglund says, "I find the natural thyroid gives an even, smooth ride to the equilibration of the thyroid patient. I find that it is very forgiving and will often stand two or three days of forgetting to take the dose."

Low Dose First

Experts I've consulted recommend starting therapy at an extremely low dose (¼ grain), twice a day, increasing gradually every week or two, until the optimal therapeutic dosage is reached. They say it's best to take it on an empty stomach, first thing in the morning, and again before lunch. As Dr Hagglund says, "This is an extremely helpful way to present thyroid to the body. The T_3 will not last longer than four hours and there is no reason to be taking all of your daily T_3 in the morning. Spread it around. The noon dose will carry the patient through the three o'clock let down of the cortisone level in the blood." It can take four to six weeks at the optimal dose to feel the full benefits. A bit of trial and error may be necessary, and it is possible that the basal temperature may not come up to normal until after a year of therapy. Each case is different, and it is wise to proceed carefully, with the help of your doctor.

The prominent American endocrine physiologist, Oregon University's Dr Raymond Peat, MA, PhD, agrees, saying, "When a large amount is taken at one time, the liver is likely to convert much of it to the inactive, reverse-T_3 form, in a normal defensive response."

Your physician may refuse to prescribe desiccated thyroid because it contains T₃ and he has been told by the synthetics makers that it's dangerous. If this happens, remind him that if he is healthy he has T₃ in his body because it is necessary, and it is not harming him. And, if he found a way to remove his natural T₃, he would become seriously ill. The only people who need to be concerned about the oral T₃ in desiccated thyroid are cardiac patients, and they shouldn't be deprived if their thyroids are underactive, because they need it for survival. But it must be given in tiny doses, throughout the day, with a physician monitoring.

You might also remind your physician, even though he should already know, that if he does not provide you with natural thyroid, you will never feel up to par and your body will slowly die. And, very important, *your risk of osteoporosis will be great if you are given, or continue to take, synthetic thyroid medication*. This has been firmly established, and reported in many medical journals, and all of the scientists I respect concur.

Vitamin A plays a key role in thyroid health, and those with low function often have symptoms that indicate malabsorption of this vitamin, such as *milia*, night blindness, etc. In these cases, no amount of carrot juice guzzling will be of the slightest use, as the carotenes in plant foods are not converted into vitamin A in those with low thyroid function. Only animal sources of this vitamin, such as liver, egg yolks, cream and butter, can be utilised in those with underactive thyroids.

Natural Remedies

There are natural remedies you can try before resorting to medication. The Peruvian root vegetable *Maca*, about which you can read in **Resources** and in **Chapter 11**, *The Menopause*, is, for example, known to help support the thyroid. Having all mercury amalgam 'silver' fillings removed from your mouth is paramount; thyroid restoration is impossible while mercury fumes are being released each time you eat or drink. Shunning all soy products, including lecithin, is also essential, as soy suppresses the thyroid gland and, when taken to excess, can destroy it (see **Chapter 9**).

Eliminating all grains from the diet can sometimes restore function. Cabbage, turnips, cauliflower, mustard greens and kale contain *progoitrin*, which inhibits thyroid function. And watch out for millet, Brussels sprouts, walnuts, peanuts, radishes and oestrogen, as they also suppress thyroid, as do all of the widely-advertised polyunsaturated oils.

According to Dr Peat, "It is now known that polyunsaturated fats interfere with thyroid hormone in just about every conceivable way." Dr Peat has done groundbreaking research on these oils, and recommends coconut oil to promote thyroid production.

Dr Earl Conroy, a thyroid expert from New Zealand, developed a thyroid regeneration protocol that he has been successfully employing for four years to restore proper functioning to *hypo*thyroids (under-active) and *hyper*thyroids (over-active). *He has found that even with the serious Graves Disease and Hashimoto's Thyroiditis it is rarely necessary to even consider surgery or radioactive iodine treatments. These conventional medical interventions are so damaging that, once they have been employed, it is not possible to restore function.*

Serendipitously, Dr Conroy flew from New Zealand to spend time attending the Hippocrates Health Centre program. He wanted to know what he could learn in order to help his patients in New Zealand. During his stay we spent lots of time talking about that pesky thyroid gland. He explained how his protocol works, and I had the opportunity to observe three women who have used Dr Conroy's natural methods; two have been able to discontinue their medication. One was overjoyed to find that the disfiguring and uncomfortable lump in her throat (from a swollen thyroid gland), that restricted her breathing, had disappeared. Unlike conventional drugs, this restorative program can be discontinued as soon as normal function has occurred. Dr Conroy mails his economical and effective protocol all over the world and his contact details are listed in **Resources**.

If natural methods are inconvenient, or if your gland is in need of immediate resuscitation, it is reassuring to know that, at last, desiccated thyroid is available in Australia. I do not have proof, but I suspect that the ban we had on this product for decades was due to drug company chicanery. Thanks, I have been told, to consumer complaints, the law has been changed and some pharmacies now stock it. Armour is not available, but Westhroid and Nature-Throid are, and they are the natural, desiccated, product. Westhroid is bound with cornstarch, which is allergenic for some, whereas Nature-Throid is bound with microcrystalline cellulose, making it suitable for those with allergies.

Natural Hormone Products

Jerry Loizou, of Australian Bio-Identical Hormone Laboratories, has agreed to formulate a line of hypoallergenic, 100% natural hormone products. He stocks both of the above thyroids and, for my readers and anyone else who enquires, he makes up the Nature-Throid in vegetable capsules (I don't approve of the animal – gelatin – capsules due to the poisons) and no preservatives. It is necessary to request "the thyroid that Elaine likes." Jerry is in Southport, Queensland, on the Gold Coast, but will ship throughout Australia (see **Resources**). A prescription from a registered Australian doctor is necessary, which must specify "desiccated thyroid".

Several people have complained to me that some compounding chemists in Australia have apparently hopped on the porcine thyroid bandwagon and are selling capsules which do not 'work', or actually cause health problems. They have told me that, after switching from Armour Thyroid (for the sake of convenience) to go on a so-called porcine product formulated by an Australian pharmacist, they went steadily downhill and only recovered after switching back to Armour.

I rang Will Tomkins, a compounding chemist in Niagara, New York, to see if he could make sense of this problem. He couldn't, but did say that Armour Thyroid has the most stringent quality controls and the best assays. He also said that there is a "narrow window of therapy", and that sometimes merely switching brands can cause problems, even among natural thyroid medications.

There was no time to have these faulty capsules analyzed before this book had to go to the printer. All I can do is warn people to be extremely cautious. I can say with confidence, and from experience, that the above-mentioned porcine capsules formulated by Jerry Loizou are effective.

For American readers, Armour thyroid is available in all pharmacies. For those of you who live in rural areas, Will Tomkins, from Pine Pharmacy in Niagara Falls, will ship anywhere (details in **Resources**). A prescription from any country will be honoured, and again, be sure your doctor specifies "desiccated thyroid".

Armour thyroid comes measured in what are known as 'grains'. Each grain, in case your physician needs to know, contains 9mcg of T_3 and 38 mcg of T_4, as well as the full spectrum of thyroid hormones. Some experts suggest taking the dosage well before meals for maximum absorption.

Dedicated vegans will have reservations regarding natural thyroid, as it is *porcine,* being a meat industry by-product derived from the thyroid glands of pigs. Almost 200 years ago, physicians used the actual glands to save the lives of severely deficient patients. Fortunately they learned to dry, powder and encapsulate the glands. Not a pretty thought, and any sufferers whose ethical beliefs preclude the use of animal-sourced products will have to make their own judgement regarding the relative values of taking the remedy or denying themselves an effective treatment for their condition. Desiccated thyroid is not 'live' the way some glandulars are, and does not carry a contamination risk.

Always Tired?

Thyroid illnesses are serious, prevalent and frequently undiagnosed. These few pages can barely skim the surface, but if you are concerned, you will find some informative websites and superb books listed in **Resources** that I can thoroughly recommend for those of you who just can't figure out why you are always tired – and want to learn why.

Finding your appropriate dose is tricky, and is really up to you; blood tests mean little and it's how you *feel* that counts. According to thyroid expert, Dr. David Derry, taking the conventional porcine dose of 60 - 120mg daily is too low in many cases, and is likely to actually turn your thyroid gland's output off, lowering its natural levels even farther. This explains why some patients feel worse when they start medication. Dr. Derry has learned that dosage often needs to be between 180 - 300mg per day before improvement is seen. But remember to work your way up slowly, depending upon what your body tells you.

Some health professionals recommend painting a 50-cent piece sized spot of Lugol's Solution (called Aqueous Iodine Solution, or APF in Australia) on the skin. If the yellowish stain disappears in fewer than 24 hours, it is an indication of iodine deficiency. Most then recommend taking 2 - 3 drops of this solution in a glass of water that has apple juice or lemon in it. Dr. David Brownstein, leading thyroid expert, highly recommends that people take at least 5 drops of Lugol's Solution (or APF) as above, and not to exceed 50mg per day, which is 8 drops. According to Dr. Derry, it is best to divide the dose and take it morning and evening. Iodine, taken this way, is excellent for detoxification.

> ### *Words Of Wisdom From America's Leading Thyroid Treatment Hospital*
> Fear of cancer of the thyroid has encouraged the unnecessary surgical removal of many benign nodules of the gland. About one third of all thyroid nodules are cystic lesions, and the great majority of these cysts – 95% – can be treated by aspiration... At present, my colleagues and I at the Cleveland Clinic do not operate on patients with thyroiditis, Graves disease, or clearly benign adenomas or cysts of the thyroid unless they are big nodular goitres with obstructive symptoms. Malignancy is really the only indication for thyroidectomy, and malignant lesions can be differentiated by cytologic examination of specimens removed by aspiration biopsy... It is now well established that neither total thyroidectomy nor radical neck dissection is often necessary in the treatment of papillary thyroid cancer. Morbidity can be avoided if total thyroidectomy is done only when there is gross evidence of cancer bilaterally or bilateral involvement of lymph nodes... All patients are given suppressive doses of desiccated thyroid as a prophylactic measure... Our peak year for thyroid surgery at the Cleveland Clinic was 1927, when 2,700 operations were done... Now, since we no longer remove thyroid adenomas surgically, the number is down to about 50 a year.

See **Resources** for a new, accurate blood spot test for thyroid function. To locate a doctor who understands the importance of natural, porcine thyroid, go to the internet and key in Mary Shomon. Then follow the prompts to Top Docs. She lists doctors world-wide. Give preference to a doctor who is listed as practicing alternative, integrated, complimentary or holistic medicine, as not all on Mary's list are willing to buck Big Pharma by prescribing Armour Thyroid or hydrocortisone, even to patients who obviously, and desperately, need it.

2

Adrenal Insufficiency
... the Thyroid Connection

It would be reassuring if I could tell you that taking desiccated thyroid, if it is indicated, will be the answer to your health concerns. In some instances it may be, but for many hypothyroids, getting well can be much more complex. If your temperature is dramatically low, and if it is raised to normal after a few months of thyroid therapy, and if you're feeling great, you can be pretty sure that this health problem is solved. Perhaps not forever, but for quite some time, depending upon your stress levels and diet. You will, however, need to keep an eye on your progress by observing symptoms and monitoring your morning temperature. If it drops, and if you start feeling tired again, and if minor illnesses are hard to shake off, some re-thinking is in order.

There are, unfortunately, people whose temperatures don't rise, no matter how much thyroid hormone they take. They may feel better, due to the hormone, but they do not feel fabulous, or have the validation of a raised temperature. This is a symptom that something else is amiss, and the problem may be the adrenals, those crucial little glands that are located above each kidney. They bear the brunt of our stress, both chronic and acute, and we all suffer stress, unless we are vegetables.

Adrenal glands produce adrenal hormones. One of these hormones is cortisol, which our adrenals demand when they are faced with stress. No matter how peaceful your surroundings may be, simply coping with 21st Century life is stressful, and this explains why adrenal insufficiency is so common. Simply put, stress sometimes uses up more cortisol than our glands can produce. Carried to the extreme, the total loss of adrenal cortex function produces *Addison's Disease*, a condition made famous by the late President John F. Kennedy. This disease, although rare, is well documented in every medical textbook, and physicians understand it well. Their tests are able to diagnose and treat this extreme form of adrenal dysfunction, which is potentially fatal. What the textbooks fail to mention, and for which conventional endocrinologists and physicians seldom test correctly, is a milder form of adrenal stress, which is extremely common.

Bodyguards

Symptoms of this milder form can manifest in many ways; a lifetime of allergies and exhaustion, joint and muscle pain, headaches, Crohn's Disease, asthma, ulcerative colitis, rheumatoid arthritis, bone demineralisation, chronic fatigue, frequent infections, acne, infertility, hypoglycemia, hay fever, autoimmune disorders, low blood pressure (under 120/80), breathing difficulties, sleep apnoea, skin problems *and the inability to conquer thyroid disease*. A physician is likely to treat you for one or more of the above with a drug that will mask the symptoms, and make you worse in time. What is needed in this case is a test for adrenal function, not a drug. If the glands prove to be under stress, they need to be rested so they can go to work on your health problems, as nature intended. Think of your adrenals as your bodyguards – they stand between you and ill health.

Some of us are born with low adrenal function, and this can be a curse, because it often leads to a life of delicate health. Take a look at your earlobes. Are they small, and close to your head? One of my teachers, famous American physician and author, Henry Bieler, explained to me that the Chinese have taught for many thousands of years that this is a sign of low adrenal function. This observation is as valid today as it was during Buddha's time, when he warned men never to marry small-lobed women because they wouldn't be strong enough to work long hours in the fields and produce many heirs. Dr Bieler told me that during his over fifty years of practice he never saw it fail – all of his small-lobed patients had delicate constitutions. More information on adrenals will be found in the section, *Check the Short and Curlies!*, in **Chapter 20**, *Legal Drugs*.

But don't despair if your lobes are tiny. This does not mean that you are going to drop dead tomorrow. It means that you had better take good care of yourself, and live by the rules in this book. If you do, you can easily live longer, and with better health, than your meaty-lobed friends if they abuse themselves with junk food, tobacco, drugs (legal and illegal) and alcohol.

If your earlobes are chunky and hang like pendulums, consider yourself fortunate, because you are a naturally robust person, born with strong adrenal function. They may not be aesthetically pleasing, but those hanging lobes will ensure that your health is strong and you can enjoy a long life. But don't be complacent – abuse your good genetic luck and you will eventually be subject to the ills of your tiny-lobed friends.

What do the adrenals have to do with the thyroid? Plenty. If taking desiccated thyroid, in an appropriate dose for your condition, does not make you feel on top of the world, you will need to address your adrenal function. Actually, your doctor should have done this *before* giving you a thyroid prescription, because many patients feel much worse when taking thyroid hormones while in adrenal stress.

As prominent British adrenal expert, Dr Barry Durrant-Peatfield, MB, BSc, LRCP, MRCS, says, "Thyroid supplementation may, at worst, precipitate the adrenal problem; but what usually happens, is that the thyroid replacement may either not apparently work at all, or the patient may have thyroid overdose symptoms on quite a low level of replacement. Hence, where low adrenal reserve is suspected, it is possibly dangerous, and certainly ill advised, to treat the patient without supplementation of the adrenals."

Borders On Malpractice

This is where I get really cross with the specialists and GPs. The literature and drug inserts are full of admonitions such as those in the Armour Thyroid packs, which state categorically that the product "... *should not be taken by patients with uncorrected cortisol deficiency... May increase symptoms of adrenal insufficiency.*" Indeed. And it borders on malpractice that so many physicians don't mention this precaution when handing out prescriptions. Many don't know, but now *you* know, and you can take steps to learn the condition of your incredibly important adrenal function. If it is low, no matter how much desiccated thyroid you take, it will not be able to convert T_4 into T_3 and it will not make it into your cells and tissues. Worse, it will further suppress your adrenals. These glands need each other; all of our glands work together.

What you need is the appropriate test, and this may lead to another tussle with your physician, because there are several adrenal tests, and only one is worthwhile. The adrenocorticotropic hormone (ACTH) test and the all-day urine test are inaccurate. The test you want is the all-day cortisol test, and it involves spitting into four tubes, at four well-spaced intervals throughout the day. These multiple samples make it possible to map the diurnal curve of free cortisol in the body, relative to the DHEA level. This gives a clearer picture of adrenal function.

In Australia, Analytical Reference Laboratories (ARL) of Melbourne will mail boxes to patients, with all the necessary supplies and instructions, and once you have completed your part, they send a courier to pick up the box. This test has to be arranged through your doctor, who will give you a prescription form. ARL can be contacted by emailing info@arlaus.com.au, or by phoning 1 300 554 480. In the US, Great Smokies Diagnostic Laboratory in North Carolina (800 522 4762) runs this test, and I assume labs in New Zealand, the UK and continental Europe do them as well.

The next hurdle will be over interpretation of the test results. Wouldn't it be wonderful if you could simply go to a doctor, complain about your symptoms, and say, "Fix me!?" Unfortunately, unless you have an amazing doctor, it usually doesn't work out that way, and if you don't do most of the research yourself, chances are you will remain feeling under par, possibly permanently.

Your doctor may look at your all-day cortisol test and see that you are in the bottom of the 'normal' range all day, and say, "That's fine, you're normal". Before you have a chance to say, "Yes, but I still feel terrible!", you are out of the office so the next patient can come in. This is known as the "bum's rush", and it's not good enough. Bottom is just the way it sounds, and do you want to feel 'bottom' for the rest of your life? What you want is to be right smack in the middle range throughout the day and night. If you are not, you need to take steps, because this is where you will feel your best, and where your thyroid, helped by your adrenals, will start perking again. You don't want too little cortisol and you don't want too much.

Cortisol is so important for so many functions, that when the body requires large amounts, it 'cannibalises' our sex hormones to create it. This leaves us with low progesterone, in comparison to oestrogen or testosterone, creating oestrogen and/or testosterone dominance. Both are associated with irritability and even violence. Further, in women, oestrogen dominance can lead to increased risk of uterine and breast cancer, PMS, fibroids and heavy menstrual periods and clots. Progesterone is needed to check the conversion of testosterone into dihydrotestosterone (DHT) which in men can lead to low testosterone, high DHT, prostatic enlargement, low libido and balding. We need our progesterone desperately, and any health abnormality that removes it from our bodies must be identified and rectified.

When you have your cortisol test, it could come back showing a *yo-yo* function. This indicates underlying *hypo*function that is interrupted by episodic *hyper*function. The Great Smokies Laboratory states that this is significant and is seen in adrenal fatigue, so a yo-yo result needs to be addressed as urgently as a rock bottom result. Whether it's bottom, or yo-yo, you need help. But you may not be able to get help, understanding or sympathy from a conventional endocrinologist, or even from your family doctor. As is so often the case, you may have to depend upon yourself and be your own doctor. Once you have established that your adrenals are exhausted, there is a non-medical solution: raw desiccated glandulars, made from the glands from organically raised New Zealand and Argentine animals. These glandulars have both critics and supporters, and it is up to individuals to make up their own minds. Some think there is a danger of contamination from raw glands, others insist that they are safe and effective. Dr Barry Durrant-Peatfield told me that he always uses glandulars before trying drugs, and that 60-70% of his patients do extremely well on them. (See Appendix, page 345 for details on the Adrenal Cortex solution.)

Those with adrenal insufficiency need to give their glands an opportunity for a profound rest. It's easier said than done but, depending upon the severity of the cortisol lack, taking a long holiday in a peaceful place can be of great help. But rest needs to be combined with hormonal and nutritional support. That means a superb diet - in other words, strictly following the rules in this book.

Diet is Crucial

You will need to eat a protein-containing meal shortly after rising, (organic beef, lamb or chicken, eggs, nuts) because if you do not, your cortisol levels will rise and may overshoot the normal range, leading to yo-yo levels. Then, during the rest of the day, never go longer than five hours between nourishing, protein-containing meals. In extreme cases it might be necessary to eat small meals five times a day. Waiting too long to eat can lead to exhaustion and anxiety in those with adrenal /thyroid problems. Research has shown that the worst stress of all for the adrenals is hypoglycaemia. For some, merely eating concentrated protein every 4-5 hours can banish adrenal weakness and the symptoms this produces.

Heavy grain consumption, so trendy in the past two decades, is another cause of our epidemic of thyroid/adrenal illnesses. The ill-conceived 'carb loading' many coaches prescribe and athletes embrace, has led to glycogen depletion and severe derangements in cortisol rhythm. You will be amazed by improvements in wellbeing by quitting all grains and eating lots of vegetables, fruit and complete proteins. Refer to **Chapter 16**, *Against the Grain*, for details.

Taking the *natural* hormones, progesterone and pregnenolone, because they act in the body as precursors of cortisol, can support the adrenals sufficiently to bring them back, provided they are not too far-gone. The B vitamins, with particular emphasis on pantothenic acid (B5) and the rose hip vitamin C I recommend, can also help with this problem, as can Maca, a potent natural glandular and hormonal aid (see **Resources** and **In Other Words...**).

It is impossible to overemphasise the importance of rest and, especially, sound sleep, while re-building the adrenals. It is best to go to bed no later than 10pm, and to share your bed with a good book, rather than with a stressful partner. Difficult people are toxic to your glands and if you have someone like this in your life, do your utmost to get him/her out. Meditation can be a great help and excellent instruction books are available in libraries.

Those of you with inadequate glycogen stores to provide your body with energy throughout the night may suffer from interrupted sleep. Since protein replenishes glycogen, a bedtime snack of a concentrated protein may be needed for a while, until the glycogen stores in the liver are sufficient to sustain the brain throughout the night.

Exercise is also important. Start slowly, if exhausted, and work up. Our bodies are meant to be used, and they fall apart if sedentary.

Clued-up physicians and naturopaths have protocols that can rest and rejuvenate glands. Natural therapies are, of course, preferable. In extreme cases, however, especially when hypothyroidism was neglected, or treated for years with damaging synthetics, more heroic measures may be warranted.

Heroic Measures

But what are these "heroic measures"? In a word: *hydrocortisone*, if diet and a tranquil life and raw adrenals don't "work". Please don't panic. I know what you're thinking and you're right – this drug has earned a terrible reputation in the past 50 years, and with good reason. Initially, however, it was touted as a "miracle medicine," and the doctors who discovered what it could achieve were awarded the Nobel Prize because victims of arthritis, lupus, scleroderma, allergies, bronchial asthma, hay fever and eczema experienced great relief when they took it. Even patients with certain cancers went into remission.

Tragically, dosages were dangerously high, and dreadful side effects, such as severe osteoporosis, atherosclerosis, blood sugar abnormalities, weight gain and a characteristic 'moon face' appeared. The medical profession panicked and, instead of investigating proper dosages, this extraordinary natural hormone fell into such disfavour that its huge benefits have been largely ignored by physicians.

Well-publicised steroid abuse by body-builders, who tended to take it in huge doses, further damaged the reputation of this important hormone, but it has now been firmly established that these terrible side effects only occur when hydrocortisone is used *in excess of replacement doses*.

Persuade Your Doctor

Once you have established, through the correct test, that your cortisol levels are low or yo-yo, the next step will be to persuade your doctor to prescribe hydrocortisone, or at least do some research which will enable him or her to save your health as well as the health of many other patients. Or, find a doctor who will. There are several books, and many scientific reports, dealing with this subject. *The Safe Uses Of Cortisol*, by William McK. Jefferies, MD, FACP, (see *Resources*) is comprehensive, and should be sufficient for any physician who is willing to learn. Dr Jefferies, whose credentials are impeccable, has demonstrated the safety of his program in over one thousand patient years of experience. During that time, over 200 babies were born to his patients, who had been taking small doses of cortisol during their pregnancies. As Dr Jefferies says in his book, "There is no evidence that patients who have taken physiologic dosages for over forty years have experienced any harmful effects, nor that children born to women taking physiologic dosages have any increased incidence of congenital defects or other difficulties."

Dr Jefferies, who pioneered the use of sub-replacement doses of hydrocortisone, found that 10-20mg per day does not lead to the negative side effects of the larger doses, nor does it cause the adrenals to cease their own production of this crucial hormone. Dr Jefferies says that "...chronic allergic disorders might be related to mild adrenal-corticol deficiency, either primary in the adrenal glands or secondary to deficient stimulation by adrenocorticotropic hormone (ACTH) from the pituitary gland... Mild adrenocortical deficiency, a diagnosis that is not mentioned in medical textbooks, is very probably a factor in the development of many, if not all, allergic and autoimmune disorders... Cortisol is a normal hormone, the only hormone that is absolutely essential for life, so *it must be safe in proper physiologic amounts!*" If your doctor still baulks, point him or her in the direction of Dr Jefferies' book.

Clear Indications

Another book, *The Great Thyroid Scandal and How to Survive It*, by the previously-quoted Dr Barry Durrant-Peatfield, is an eye-opener. If reading the information in his book (and in mine) isn't sufficient to persuade your physician to order the cortisol test, or if you live in a remote area where testing is impractical, Dr Durrant-Peatfield says that your history and certain signs should be a clear indication of adrenal exhaustion. For example, according to this acknowledged expert, "... the blood pressure is usually quite low, often very strikingly so. The difference between the lying (or sitting) blood pressure, and the standing one, may be very important. Normally, it rises when the patient stands. In low adrenal reserve, it either does not change at all, or lowers further. The pupil reflex is low, or unstable, or even reversed, to bright light. Reflexes may be abnormal, especially the Achilles reflex – in the heel. The heart sound is characteristically altered."

If you are fortunate enough to have an old-fashioned physician, who will diagnose by these indications, one who understands "hands on" medicine, you may be able to forego testing and save time and money. But testing may be necessary if these indications are absent. Merely having hypothyroidism that isn't banished by taking porcine thyroid medication, or suffering from unexplained exhaustion, or having illnesses that hang on interminably, are indications that adrenals are stressed.

The experts I've studied say that hydrocortisone needs to be taken every four hours during the day, and it needs to be taken with meals, or at least with a few bites of food. Dr Jefferies says "... if the patient has sufficient adrenal reserve, the bedtime dosage may be decreased or omitted entirely without difficulty." Each patient should judge this for himself or herself. In total, usually no more than 20mg per day, divided into four doses, should be taken. When used properly, in tiny, *sub-replacement doses* (4mg to 5mg each) four times during the day, this natural hormone lives up to its earlier reputation as a "miracle medicine". Timing may be according to your schedule, starting with breakfast, and proceeding at four-hour intervals. My observations indicate that, in those with long-term weakness, skipping the evening dose can negate the good effects. And remember, spacing is important, as it maintains a steady cortisol supply.

Clear indications of low adrenal reserve are long-term illnesses, such as chronic fatigue syndrome and the other illnesses mentioned earlier, and/or the inability to recover quickly from ailments that are mild in most people. The purpose of our adrenals is to come to our rescue when illness strikes. Healthy people suffer mild common cold symptoms, while those with adrenal fatigue can be bedded for weeks, because their poor adrenals don't have the strength to fight back. This rule applies to all illnesses, including life-threatening ones, so if you have the symptoms of low adrenal function, you will be well advised to move heaven and earth to turn your adrenals into the Rottweilers they were meant to be.

Desperate Need

People with low adrenal reserve have a desperate need for extra cortisol if they are faced with any stress, whether emotional or physical. Many people who have died from pneumonia would have recovered with ease had their physicians understood the need for additional cortisol during the critical stages of their illness.

Dr Jefferies cautions, however, that when cortisol is given in pneumonia, while patients may feel well quickly, the pathologic effect of the bacteria in the lungs persists, and can progress if antibiotic therapy is not started. This is one of the rare instances where I would recommend antibiotics; their use should be curtailed, except in life-threatening illnesses, such as pneumonia. Take them for every little thing, and they won't be able to save you when you *really* need them.

Even infectious mononucleosis, notoriously difficult to treat, and usually of long duration, succumbs quickly to large doses of hydrocortisone given until recovery. Chappel reported on 111 cases of amazing recovery within a few days. (*Chappel MR: Infectious mononucleosis.* **Southwest Med** *43: 253-255, 1962*). This treatment eliminates the long period of recuperation and disability usually associated with this serious illness. It is a crime that this treatment has been known for decades, yet seldom used.

According to Dr Jefferies, when people with low adrenal reserve are treated with cortisone during common respiratory infections, accompanied by malaise and fever, no increased complications occur. He advises against antibiotic use in these instances, unless a bacterial infection is present, in order to avoid antibiotic resistance if future infections should occur. He also says, and this is important for your physician to understand, that physiologic doses are safe and beneficial, but that when cortisone is given people with acute infections, dosages are critical. He recommends dosages of 20mg, four times daily until symptoms subside (which can take as little as two days) then tapering off over a four-day period. These large doses, continued long-term, can cause problems of *hypercortisolism*. Knowledge is important here; please do your best to persuade your doctor to get the two books I recommend.

Dr Durrant-Peatfield agrees with Dr Jefferies that influenza, treated with 'emergency' doses, as described above, will clear in one or two days, which is a real bonanza for people who ordinarily lie in bed for days or weeks, aching and feverish. He also says that jet lag, not as serious, but a misery nonetheless, can be conquered by small doses, even in those who do not have severe adrenal weakness.

Downsides

There is a downside to most therapies, and cortisol is no exception. While this hormone causes dramatic improvements in many, there are reports of abdominal cramps in patients who have irritable bowel syndrome. Curing this common problem before starting therapy is the obvious, but often overlooked, solution. Think about it – your bowels wouldn't *be* irritable if you were not irritating them with poor food and drink choices. Strict adherence to a perfect diet is what they want, and they will cure themselves if you will just give them a chance. But then, I'm a well known food nag. Of course, it is possible to be hypersensitive to anything, and careful observation and caution are advised.

Another downside is the way cortisol increases the appetite, sometimes causing picky, unenthusiastic eaters to wolf down twice their usual portions, and to hunt frantically for more. Prudence is indicated here – we don't want to acquire strong adrenals at the expense of our waistlines and general health.

I can't point to any scientific evidence to explain this immediate reaction to replacing absent or depleted cortisol, but common sense leads me to the conclusion that low adrenal function causes malabsorption of nutrients, and that the body, by creating ravenous appetites, is making up for lost time. Fortunately, people have reported to me that their appetites, after two or three weeks of therapy, settle down to a normal enjoyment of food, but not excessive hunger.

Another interesting aspect of supplementing missing cortisol is that once the adrenals are functioning, many health problems start sorting themselves out. For example, people who have had to take hydrochloric acid, due to lack of necessary stomach acid for digestion (see **Chapter 3**, *Stomach Acid*), find that they can cut down or quit acid supplementation entirely. This was mysterious to me until I had the great good fortune while working on this chapter to speak by telephone with Dr Barry Durrant-Peatfield in England.

As mentioned earlier, he is the author of **The Great Thyroid Scandal And How To Survive It**. This book is a superb how-to-get-well-in-spite-of-your-doctor manual. It is charmingly written and infused with truth and humanity. Finding him took effort, but after contacting and explaining to his assistant that I was researching the thyroid/adrenal connection and needed help, we were soon connected. Dr Durrant-Peatfield (or Barry, as he quickly asked me to call him) is as warm and sincere about his work as his book indicates. We spoke at length and he patiently answered my long list of questions.

The first was about hydrochloric acid. His answer was simple, and explains all of the other improvements in health that go with well-functioning adrenals. In his expert opinion, metabolism is always low in the face of low adrenal function. Cortisol brings the metabolism up, and takes everything else up with it. Ergo, the whole body starts functioning well and the stomach regains its ability to manufacture its own hydrochloric acid.

Easy To Understand

I also asked Dr Durrant-Peatfield for permission to quote at length from his book, which he graciously granted. His easy-to-understand writing style is explained in his *Author's Note*, where he says, "I have written in the manner I always used in my clinics: that is, that the patient was just as bright as I was, and perfectly able to work things out given the knowledge. To give you this knowledge, without clouding it with references within the text or blinding you with science, is I hope what I have been able to do." Indeed you have, Barry, and your book is a must-read for everyone who has been struggling for years to re-build their health.

Would that all physicians were as helpful and open with their patients. It has been my experience that endocrinologists are by far the most recalcitrant group of medical practitioners. "Infuriating" is one of the kindest words I, and many of the people who pass through Hippocrates Health Centre, use to describe them. Most will denigrate patients who dare to suggest that their health hasn't improved on Synthroid and would prefer to take porcine thyroid hormone. Despite the overwhelming body of contrary evidence, they continue to insist that synthetics are better. Furthermore, few would even consider following the directions on thyroid medication packages to check and correct adrenal function prior to prescribing thyroid drugs. This is malpractice!

In his book, Dr Durrant-Peatfield expresses this problem well: "Their ignorance is only equalled by their arrogance, and their wilful refusal to listen to their patients is equalled only by their total refusal to listen also to the voice of commonsense. You will soon know more than they do, and may well be able to successfully largely treat yourself." Predictably, the British medical establishment doesn't have a good word to say about Dr Barry Durrant-Peatfield!

Not Dangerous

Another area of my concern regards treatment for long-standing adrenal insufficiency. Many people, especially those who were born with sluggish adrenals, or who acquired this weakness in youth, may be obliged to take low doses of cortisone for life. In fact, many are not able to live normal lives without it (fortunately, it is inexpensive). I asked Dr Durrant-Peatfield about this and he assured me of the safety of long-term, or even permanent, supplementation with cortisone, as long as it is low-dose. "Patients should not reduce on principle", he told me, but should monitor their reactions, temperature, feelings of well-being, etc., to guide them in their decision." This opinion is shared by Dr Jefferies, who agrees that some patients may have to take cortisone indefinitely. He writes that therapy restores normal function, rather than altering it, and that low doses do not create any excessive steroid level in the blood, nor affect the normal diurnal variation.

Rest And Rejuvenation

Some patients who have not been subjected to years of medical neglect or mistreatment are able to discontinue hydrocortisone once their glands have had an opportunity to rest and rejuvenate. Treatment can take just weeks, or perhaps up to three months, and then patients can cut down gradually, taking smaller and smaller doses.

Those who have been on thyroid hormones for a short time, or even decades, will find that, as their adrenals improve (and it can happen quickly), special care will need to be given to the amount of thyroid hormone taken. Dr Durrant-Peatfield says it may be possible to cut down or even discontinue this hormone if signs, such as consistently normal temperature and wellbeing, indicate.

I mentioned to him that my gut feeling is that many people who have been taking thyroid hormone for years didn't need it. They needed adrenal support so their thyroids could function on their own. He agrees.

Some patients, and their physicians, are concerned that cortisone will suppress the adrenals. Dr Durrant-Peatfield told me that it will not, at all. "In any event," he says, "the adrenal activity is curtailed anyway, making the options quite clear. Suppression occurs in the super-pharmacological doses [*used during illnesses*]. Even then, the adrenals are able to recover, if the primary illness is dealt with, and the dose reduced gradually."

In 1920 it was estimated that hypothyroidism affected a mere ten percent of the population. Estimates vary widely, but some scientists claim it now affects nearly 80 percent – a figure borne out by our experiences at Hippocrates.

Dr Durrant-Peatfield explains this great surge in his book. "One good reason is that hypothyroid children at the turn of the 20th Century did not live to pass on their faulty genes... Now, of course, medical science saves them. As they grow up, they are attracted to low thyroid partners (who, like themselves, would rather sit around than rush about) and so pass on the low thyroid genes. Two or three generations of this... and where are you?"

Hypothyroidism is the most common, but not the only, form of thyroid illness. There is also the problem of overactive thyroid glands. Dr Durrant-Peatfield describes the symptoms, which are quite obvious, and writes, "Clearly, the diagnosis in general isn't difficult to make. The rub comes in the treatment. First, you may not have to do very much. Mild degrees of thyroid over-activity can occur on a self-limiting basis, and may sometimes be left to run their own course, with an informed patient monitoring how they are, and seeking equally well-informed advice if things are not going right. The body has a remarkable ability to heal itself, and should be given the chance to do so... Over-intervention is the curse of modern medicine in almost any illness you can imagine; we should take to heart that sometimes a policy of 'masterly inactivity' is much better for the patient and may even spare his life."

Amen. Watchful waiting, combined with strict dietary measures, can often banish frightening symptoms. Please take careful note of the dietary suggestions in this book. Chances are, your health problems have been caused by semi-poisonous manufactured foods.

Hundreds of women, through the years, have come to the health centre with horror stories of thyroid surgery and treatment with radioactive iodine, which Dr Durrant-Peatfield says "... concentrates in the thyroid tissue and 'nukes' it." Then, of course, there is the ever-popular surgery. "The problem with these two solutions lies in their permanency; it cannot be undone ... and can only be a matter of guesswork. More often than not, the amount destroyed or removed is not right to begin with, and obviously, cannot allow for changes in thyroid function which will occur with the passage of time." As for the radioactive iodine, "Of course it goes elsewhere in the body, especially the breast... But they won't tell you that... Growths or cysts in the thyroid must be treated by surgical removal or a drainage procedure; and a much enlarged thyroid which interferes with breathing or swallowing leaves no option. But partial thyroidectomy to reduce the amount of thyroid hormone-forming tissue is a popular, if in some eyes, barbaric procedure. My view is that as a procedure it should be the last resort only; and not, as is so often and regrettably the case, almost the first option."

My strong recommendation, whatever your thyroid problem, is to send for a copy of Dr Durrant-Peatfield's book (see **Resources**). Your physician may even be willing to read it, but not all are open to being educated by their patients. As the author writes, "You would then be read a lecture about wicked and evil thyroid doctors – of whom I'm the worst evidently – who have taken it upon themselves to treat patients (thus taking advantage of their emotional state); hypochondriacal illness; getting into bad ways – such as thinking for yourself and standing your ground; or, infinitely worse, treating yourself, thereby placing yourself in the terrible danger of getting better."

Dr Durrant-Peatfield says that the initial approach to hydrocortisone should be cautious, and that 2.5mg is an excellent starting point. "The reason it is so low to start with is the fact that patients ill for some time, and perhaps receiving synthetic thyroxine, may have substantially high levels of T4 and T3 which the system cannot use. The adrenal support may kick in quite quickly, causing the T4 – T3 conversion and receptor uptake to start working quite abruptly. This may cause a sudden overdose situation to occur. With small starter doses of adrenal support, the risk of this is avoided. The first two or three days of 2.5mg of hydrocortisone given in the morning soon after waking, will be monitored by the patient for any adverse symptoms, checking pulse two or three times a day and of course the morning basal temperature."

When making important decisions regarding our health, I believe it is essential to stick as closely to nature as possible. But if natural methods don't correct the problem, the guidance of a qualified physician is needed, because this subject is vastly complex and must be approached with great care. It is not, unfortunately, always as simple as popping a few hydrocortisone pills. Because this medication is metabolised through the liver, care must be taken in patients with problem livers. Side effects, such as water retention (as in puffy eyelids), slight stomach pains, headaches, a yucky feeling and mild dizziness can occur in some. Most of these side effects disappear in time.

When the patient does not respond well to hydrocortisone, there are many factors to consider. For example, failure to produce adequate cortisol can be due to inadequate secretion of ACTH by the pituitary. Further, DHEA should be tested and the level corrected, if necessary.

The potassium/sodium balance needs to be addressed as well. If these minerals are out of balance, the adrenal hormone, aldosterone, must be checked and regulated. Aldosterone has the important function of maintaining fluid levels in the body, as well as the right proportions of electrolytes. To quote from a lecture Dr Durrant-Peatfield gave at a UK Thyroid Conference, "These electrolytes are sodium and potassium – aldosterone works by controlling the kidney output of these two minerals." So, if a patient experiences side effects from taking hydrocortisone, the physician needs to make sure that the patient's aldosterone level is not too high and not too low.

As Dr Durrant-Peatfield said in his lecture, too low aldosterone leads to "... loss of sodium and water, and contributes in part to the dizziness on standing that is the cardinal symptom of low adrenal reserve and adrenal insufficiency. And, of course, the patient will suffer from some degree of dehydration. Too high aldosterone causes a reduction in circulating potassium... This causes depression, confusion, hallucinations, anxiety, irritability, muscle weakness and extreme fatigue. How important it is, then, to check sodium and potassium levels during treatment of adrenal insufficiency, especially if progress is disappointing. One to three grams daily of potassium will reverse this."

Some patients do beautifully on *Hysone 4* alone, which is identical to naturally-occurring cortisol. Others may respond better if *Florinef* (Fludrocortisone Acetate) is added. If wellbeing is not restored within two weeks, Florinef may be increased, but not to exceed 50mcg, three times daily, according to Dr Durrant-Peatfield. People have reported great results on four evenly-spaced Hysone 4 tablets daily. Others say that four in the morning, and two in the afternoon work better. When I rang Dr Durrant-Peatfield about this discrepancy, he told me that larger doses are sometimes necessary for people, due to poor or erratic breakdown of the cortisol during digestion, much of which can get "lost". Others have reported spectacular improvements in wellbeing for the first month on low-dose Hysone 4 alone, followed by a sudden drop in energy levels. In these instances, increasing the dose brought back energy quickly. It is necessary to work out dosages for each individual, with the help of a physician.

Adrenal insufficiency, according to Thomas A Wilson, MD, Director of Pediatric Endocrinology, State University of New York, can come from "… a mere two weeks' exposure to pharmacological doses of glucorticoids." He means doses way above replacement levels, but agrees with doctors Durrant-Peatfield and Jefferies that sub-replacement doses are safe and effective. Dr Wilson says, "In developed countries, the most common cause of adrenal insufficiency is autoimmune destruction of the adrenal cortex." To avoid this calamity, ban junk food from your life and follow the other rules in this book, which is dedicated to teaching people to use natural methods to allow their bodies to heal themselves as nature intended. In extreme cases, however, we may need to nudge nature a bit and use man-made substances briefly. Adrenal exhaustion, when natural methods fail, is one of those times. Cortisol may need to be replaced until the adrenals have a chance to rest and recuperate.

Sometimes, especially in those people who were born with low adrenal function, cortisol may need to be replaced, in low doses, for life. Dr Durrant-Peatfield assures me this is perfectly safe and, as people know who have been rescued from atrophied adrenals by cortisone, it can be a miracle cure. I strongly advise delicate people, who are prone to extremely slow recovery from pneumonia, to always have a supply of 20mg Hydrocortisone on hand. If judicially used only when needed it can be a lifesaver.

One last thought; please remember that babies and older children who are exposed to second hand smoke are likely to end up not just with lung problems, but with serious adrenal insufficiency as well. Parents who sit idly by, permitting or committing this form of child abuse, belong in jail. (See page 345 for information on Raw Adrenals.)

3

Stomach Acid

Forget the clever ads – it's acid you need, not an antacid!

The health enthusiasts have been saying it for decades – "You are what you eat." The problem is that they are *wrong*! You are not what you *eat* – you are what you *absorb*, and the best diet on Earth will not sustain health if an important ingredient is missing – **stomach acid**. That's right, acid. In this case, it's hydrochloric acid (*HCl*). You cannot absorb nutrients that are vital for health if this essential part of your digestive system is destroyed by antacids, or if you were born with a tendency to low stomach acid, or if your stomach has been damaged by junk food, drink, tobacco, stress and antibiotics.

If you fall for the propaganda of the drug companies, you are being conned into believing that 'excess acid' must be neutralised. This is a blatant, self-serving lie! A seven-billion-US-dollar lie, to be exact; that is the amount the drug companies earn every year selling their profoundly damaging antacids and acid-suppressing drugs. Each year the profits soar; drugs for stomach and upper digestive system problems are the largest-selling medicines in the United States.

The professional journal, **Orthopaedic Surgeon**, said this: "Antacids, drugs which so many people take frequently, are so dangerous that they would have been removed from the market if the drug cartels were not so strong. It has been known for decades that they deplete the bones of between 130 and 300mg of calcium each time they are consumed. They contain aluminium, and also contribute to Alzheimer's Disease."

Nature didn't put acid into our stomachs so the drug companies could earn billions suppressing it. Nature put it there for a compelling reason; it is absolutely necessary for health. Our stomach acid is so strong that it can reduce the toughest steak into meat soup in about an hour. Imagine what happens to that steak when it hits an acid-deficient stomach – indigestion, malabsorption, and sometimes unpleasant and anti-social symptoms such as bloating, burning, gas and belching. Not because of too much acid, but because of too little. Because there are few warning symptoms, malabsorption can occur over many years, leading to slow starvation. This results in crumbling bones, degenerative diseases, acute and chronic infections caused by germs that are easily killed by normal stomach acid, and cancer.

Yes, even cancer, and it's logical when you think about it. When your stomach has normal acid levels it is able to kill invading micro-organisms and break down dangerous food additives. But, if your stomach lacks this vital element, additives can turn into cancer-causing nitrosamines.

Hypochlorhydria (Low Stomach Acid)

My first encounter with stomach acid taught me a lesson I shall never forget. It saved my life. I lived in Europe during the 1960s and, after six months of injudicious pasta-gorging in Italy, I became exhausted. I dragged myself to London and collapsed. A doctor was brought in, and when he took my pulse he told me it was *ten*! Then he asked who my next of kin was, and I knew I was in deep trouble. Tests were done, and the diagnosis was pernicious anaemia. Then, I had to take B-complex and iron injections and eat lots of red meat for two months — and saw zero improvement.

Finally, presumably because he was afraid I'd die on him, my doctor drove me to a Harley Street specialist. (I was too weak to get there on my own, but can you imagine a doctor doing that today?) The first thing this old-school physician said was, "Have you tried hydrochloric acid?"

I had not exhibited the classic symptoms of *hypochlorhydria*, though I do remember asking my doctor when I was 16 why my fingernails peeled, I squinted badly in sunlight and had night blindness. He would have known if he had taken the time to crack a basic medical text. He didn't, though, and merely suggested that I learn to live with it. These, and other health problems I had, were clear signs of need for additional acid, and this man could have saved me years of problems which culminated in a close encounter with death. Virtually all physicians are making the same mistake today.

The Harley Street specialist understood immediately. He prescribed a potent form of hydrochloric acid drops. These had to be diluted and sipped through a glass straw, to avoid tooth enamel damage. The potion had to be drunk prior to each meal, and after two weeks I was fighting fit. I have taken HCl ever since.

More than forty years have flown by since then, and HCl has been widely available in pharmacies and health food stores in capsules and tablets for a long time. Most contain pepsin, which is also needed for proper digestion. It is not, unfortunately, easy to find a health professional who understands our desperate need for this misunderstood acid.

In 1970, a progressive doctor friend in Los Angeles told me that hydrochloric acid in the stomach is so valuable that every antacid preparation should be prohibited by law. He also told me something that has proved extremely valuable to the people I've advised during the many intervening years; doctors in those days often wouldn't prescribe HCl without first inserting a tube in the nose, and then down into the stomach to test the acid there. When I expressed horror he laughed and said this procedure was not necessary, that the easiest way to determine if supplementation is needed is by taking a tablet with a meal. If you don't need HCl, there will be a slight burning in the stomach, which is easily neutralised by drinking plenty of water.

There are now other tests. A hair mineral analysis, which measures macro and trace minerals, is an option. If five or more minerals are deficient, particularly those known to be poorly absorbed in low acid states (calcium, zinc and iron), low stomach acid is indicated. Another test consists of a chemical analysis of the stool, with a search for undigested proteins. A well-trained iridologist can also diagnose lack of stomach acid.

> ### *The Acid Test*
>
> The *pH* system is a scale for measuring the acidity or alkalinity of a given environment (in this case, your stomach). The scale goes from zero to 14. Seven is neutral. Below seven is acid. Above seven is alkaline. Normally, the acid level in your stomach is about 2 or 3.

The Heidelberg capsule is recommended by some physicians. This is a tiny pH sensor and a radio transmitter compressed into the size of a large vitamin capsule. It is swallowed, tethered to a long thread, and removed from the stomach once the results have been relayed by radio signal to a receiver. This is expensive and far from appealing. It does not take into consideration the hourly changes in the pH of the stomach, and can vary from day to day. Expensive and possibly useless.

Then there is the '*try-it-and-if-you-don't-burn-you-need-it*' method. It's quick, it's cheap and the result is immediate. It is not, however, scientific, although (as noted earlier) a physician told me it was accurate and safe.

<u>Warning</u>: This test must not be attempted by anyone who has a peptic ulcer, or who is using any kind of anti-inflammatory medication. This includes aspirin, ibuprofen (e.g. Advil, Motrin), corticosteroids, (e.g. Prednisone), indocin, butazolidin, or any other NSAIDs (*Non-Steroidal Anti-Inflammatory Drugs*)**.**

Wise people shun NSAIDs anyway, considering that, as Dr Joseph Mercola reported on his website, www.mercola.com, "In 1993, of 140,000 hospital admissions for osteoarthritis, 25,000 deaths were directly attributed to high dosage or prolonged use of NSAIDs."

If you are taking any drugs, check with your physician before experimenting with HCl. There are so many dangerous drugs being prescribed, with new ones coming along all the time, and I may have omitted some that are dangerous with HCl. Please remember that any anti-inflammatory medications can cause stomach bleeding and ulcers. Combining them with HCl increases this risk.

Those fortunate people who have strong adrenal function will probably not need acid supplementation. Those on hydrocortisone, even in sub-replacement doses, should **not** use hydrochloric acid (see *Chapter Two*, *Adrenal Insufficiency*).

In all the years that I have been involved with natural health, I have not encountered anyone who didn't benefit from taking supplemental acid. So many things trigger this lack – the unrelenting stress most of us live with, junk food, antibiotics, smoking or exposure to second hand smoke, heavy consumption of grains, age, extremely alkaline diets, etc. Yet, most people are unaware of stomach acid, except when television commercials blare out warnings about 'excess acid'.

Monitoring dosage of HCl can be tricky. Results, of course, are a good guide, although not considered scientific. If bloating, gas, etc., have been problems these should abate quickly. If you have longitudinal lines on pale, soft fingernails, with supplementation the lines should slowly fade, and the nails should strengthen and become pink. Lifeless hair and skin problems should also improve over time, as should a general sense of wellbeing.

In cases of long-term underproduction of stomach acid, a return to health may not be as simple as popping a few pills.   In these cases a knowledgeable health professional is needed to do some detective work: are you low in copper, high in zinc? Is there some other imbalance in your body? Are your B vitamins and/or your enzymes hopelessly depleted?   Nutritionist Judy Kitchen's extraordinary three-part series*, Hypochlorhydria: A Review*, published in the *Townsend Letter for Doctors and Patients, Oct, Nov, Dec 2001,* can be ordered from the website *www.townsendletter.com* and would be of great assistance in intractable cases. It is always nice to know *why* your body is not manufacturing its own acid. Once that is understood, measures to correct any imbalance can be taken.

For decades, I have felt like a voice in the wilderness. But now, finally, two prominent American doctors, Jonathan Wright, MD, and Lane Lenard, PhD, have written a superb book, *Why Stomach Acid Is Good For You*, which should be on the desk of every health professional who cares about his or her patients. I highly recommend it for those of you who think you may have *'acid indigestion'*, and have been taking drugs to suppress it.   It outlines, in careful detail, exactly what to do in order to heal your stomach from the damage these dreadful drugs have done to it. Once healed, you can take what you need – HCl – to ensure that you will regain your health and start absorbing the nutrients you desperately need.

Appalling Junk

Many people are born with low stomach acid, or develop it in childhood. Of course, in a perfect world children would have an abundant supply of HCl. But observe the average supermarket trolley – most are stuffed with appalling junk, dangerous soy products, and the worst kind of oils. Small wonder our kids have malabsorption, due to lack of stomach acid, plus all the other illnesses caused by the amazingly unhealthy junk their poor little bodies have to metabolise! Small wonder they have asthma, recurring infections of all kinds, anaemia, parasites, coeliac (celiac) disease, and miserable skin conditions. Doctors Wright and Lenard explain in their book how the children who are brought to their Tahoma Clinic in Kent, Washington, get over these dreadful afflictions by improving their diets and supplementing their HCl.

A distraught mother told me that her four-year-old son had had diarrhoea since he was born, and had never had a normal bowel movement. The many doctors who examined the boy, and gave him drugs, were of no use and she was eventually advised to see a specialist to have a camera inserted into the child's anus. This examination would be followed, no doubt, by a painful, damaging and unnecessary operation. When I enquired about his other symptoms, she told me that he was anaemic and had *giardia*. I knew immediately what the problem was – lack of HCl. It's hard to comprehend how the doctors could have missed what every first year med student should know! The first suspect when anaemia is diagnosed should be the acid level, and the first thing to look for when parasites are suspected is, you guessed it – HCl. Because I'm not a doctor and can't take the responsibility of prescribing, especially for a child, I suggested an old-fashioned, safe remedy – a spoonful of apple cider vinegar in a glass of water half-an-hour prior to meals. It worked, and the boy is now normal for the first time in his life. But for a little apple cider vinegar, this defenceless child might have been irreparably damaged by unnecessary medical procedures. Later, when the mother told the doctor that her boy was now well because of this remedy, he said, "Oh, don't be ridiculous!" (Do *not* give HCl to a child who is too young to tell you if his or her tummy gets warm from it).

In another instance, a miner from West Australia rang to thank me for this remedy, which he read in the Fifth Edition of this book. He said that for 20 years he had complained to doctors about symptoms after eating, and none had been the slightest help. The last one told him he should be glad he was still alive! Because he was in the outback, he couldn't get to a store, but tried the vinegar, and for the first time in 20 years his symptoms were gone! These are commonplace stories, and the help I can offer people is not because I'm a genius, but because the doctors tend to ignore nature and commonsense.

Apple Cider Vinegar

When HCl supplementation is not feasible, a tablespoon of apple cider vinegar in a glass of water, 30 minutes before meals, will often relieve some, or even all, symptoms. As doctors Wright and Lenard say, "This is supported by the common practice in some cultures of treating gastric discomfort with lemon juice or vinegar. Unfortunately, even though symptoms may be improved, actual nutrient digestion and assimilation are not improved nearly as much as with HCl replacement."

To me, this is an excellent way to decide whether or not you need to take HCl. I recommend being cautious with lemon juice, as it can erode tooth enamel. Further, both lemon juice and vinegar can exacerbate *candida albicans*.

Both Judy Kitchen and doctors Wright and Lenard recommend starting with one capsule of betaine HCl with pepsin, after the first few bites of food. If no problems are noted, increase the dose to two capsules in the early part of the meal. Then, provided there is no burning in the stomach, increase again after a few more days, spreading the additional capsules throughout the meal. Amounts of HCl in tablets vary from country to country. Correct dosage, of course, depends on the amount each pill contains. In Australia the amount of acid permitted in each pill is ridiculously low – only 600mg. According to Dr Wright, adults need "… at least 40 to 90 grains," and each grain contains only 65mg of betaine hydrochloride. This means that, in order to get between 40 and 90 grains,

> ### *More on GERD*
>
> If you have it, don't call it 'acid indigestion'. Better, call it 'lack of acid indigestion'.
>
> This is how it works: When you eat, if your HCl is low, your stomach will hold food longer, and whatever HCl is present will mix in with the food. Your stomach will churn, but because it doesn't have enough acid, instead of emptying its contents into your small intestine, some of the food will regurgitate into your oesophagus. Then, because your throat is not protected against acid with the same mucosal barrier as your stomach, your throat will burn. Thus the term 'heartburn'. If you treat this burning with antacids, the burning will stop, but you will perpetuate the problem until you are a candidate for an operation. To avoid this fate, provide your stomach with what it desperately needs – hydrochloric acid with pepsin, as well as acidophilus and digestive enzymes. But don't do this unless you carefully acquaint yourself with the contraindications (ulcers, NSAIDs). And give some thought to cutting out sugar and grains, which probably caused the problem originally.

it would be necessary to take between four and ten pills, if they contain only 600mg each. Judicious experimentation is therefore necessary before finding your dose. If, for example, it takes five capsules to achieve the warming, drop back to four capsules with each meal of the same size. Eventually, once the stomach has 'righted' itself, fewer will be needed. Further testing is advisable to keep the dose appropriate. If you cannot get the capsules, tablets are available.

For those who are subject to urinary tract infections (UTI), be aware that overdosing with HCl can irritate the bladder.

Has your heart specialist warned you that, as Jonathan V Wright says in *Repairing Your Heart and Arteries*, "Low production of hydrochloric acid and pepsin in the stomach is associated with hardened arteries, high cholesterol, high triglycerides, high blood pressure, and even obesity – which can spell trouble for your heart"? Probably not; he and his colleagues are too busy handing out statin drug prescriptions and performing bypasses to think of such simple, inexpensive remedies.

And what about your internist? Has he mentioned that the western world's near-epidemic of parasites is due, in large part, to acid-suppressing drugs? If not, educate yourself by heeding what doctors Wright and Lenard say in their excellent book, that low stomach acid leaves us prey to "… salmonella, cholera, dysentery, typhoid and tuberculosis, not to mention garden-variety heartburn, diarrhoea, constipation, bloating, flatulence or other common symptoms of dyspepsia."

As these pioneering doctors state, "...there is no doubt that acid suppression promotes bacterial overgrowth and that bacterial overgrowth promotes production of carcinogenic nitrosamine compounds. There is also no doubt that acid-suppressing drugs increase the progression and severity of atrophic gastritis in people with H. pylori infection, and that atrophic gastritis is a major risk factor for gastric carcinoma." That's cancer.

What about those who say, "Yes, but I've got reflux and/or GERD and have to take acid-suppressing drugs"? I say, "*Wrong*!" Even though the acid-suppressing drugs may reduce symptoms, they are like throwing petrol on a fire, and will eventually create severe diseases.

Reflux (where acid flows back into the oesophagus) and/or the more serious Gastro-Esophageal Reflux Disease (GERD) are not caused by *too much* acid, but by *too little*. And, if your physician has prescribed any of the proton pump inhibitors or H_2 blockers such as Prilosec, Prevacid, Zantac, Pepcid, and Tagamet, they probably won't kill you outright, but please bear in mind that Propulsid did just that, until it was forced off the market.

Further, if your physician has taken the acid-suppression option, instead of telling you how to heal your stomach naturally, you need to find a physician who has not been hopelessly indoctrinated by the pharmaceutical conglomerates. He or she should have warned you that these are some of the most deadly drugs you can take. Prilosec, for example, virtually eliminates acid in the stomach around the clock. This means that necessary assimilation does not take place, and you will slowly starve.

If you have been advised to have surgery for this easily-corrected condition, ponder what Dr Joseph Mercola had to say in *Men's Journal*, *December 2002*: "A surgical solution should have no role in the management of this purely physiological problem, and future generations will realise how foolish our current medical model has been by trying to treat a primarily biochemical problem with surgery."

We have observed amazing recoveries from this condition at Hippocrates Health Centre, merely with our detoxifying diet. There is no question that *poor diet* creates this condition. It is, therefore, *good diet* that cures it. It is as simple as that; but somehow this self-evident truth has not trickled down into the average doctor's surgery. Here is what you can do to alleviate this condition yourself:

- Quit poisoning your body with junk food
- Shun sugar
- Eliminate all grains until healed, and possibly permanently
- Take acidophilus
- Take digestive enzymes
- Obtain vitamin D from the sun, food or supplements
- Drink plenty of pure water
- Eliminate stress as much as possible
- Once your stomach is healed, start taking HCl as directed above (See **Resources** for the best HCl capsule we have found).

Be aware, however, that self-diagnosis is unwise. A physician well-trained in gastroenterology is called for. Yes, I realise this is not easy, but there must be *someone* who can help, and we are starting a Registry, so please let us know if you find a knowledgeable physician we can recommend. Failing that, Wright and Lenard's **Stomach Acid Is Good For You** is a superb guide to getting well.

For those of you who wonder how it can be possible that physicians do not appear to know about this simple remedy, consider this:

The pharmaceutical industry:

- ❑ earns more than US $7billion per year selling antacids and acid-blocking drugs
- ❑ finances and controls the medical schools
- ❑ has a stranglehold on regulatory agencies, such as the United States Food and Drug Administration (FDA).

Need I say more?

WARNING!
Please see The Appendix for important information before using large doses of HCl.

4

Excitotoxins
Deadly chemicals your Government is happy for you to eat and drink
Section 1.01

Thanks to the power and tenacity of multinationals, and the scandalous neglect and complicity of Western governments, we have deadly chemical additives in most of our manufactured foods; and, no, I am not referring to preservatives, which, while sometimes hazardous, at least serve a necessary purpose. What I am much more concerned about are what are known as **Excitotoxins** – *chemicals that stimulate the neurons in the brain to excessive firing, which then totally fatigues and sometimes kills them, leading to serious diseases.*

Excitotoxins – The Taste That Kills, by US neurosurgeon Russell Blaylock, MD, (see **Resources**) is a superbly researched scientific study of these substances. After reading his book, those who desire to protect their families will never touch another product that could contain any excitotoxin.

As Dr Blaylock writes, "There are quite possibly thousands of people walking around in a perfectly normal state of health, who have a weakness for one of the inherited neurodegenerative diseases. High levels of MSG, or one of the other excitotoxins, could tip the scales and precipitate the full-blown disease – which is an excellent reason to avoid all excitotoxin food additives."

Unfortunately, this requires constant vigilance and the only sure way is to stay clear of all commercially-manufactured and processed food.

Excitotoxins are basic components of the most widely-used artificial taste-enhancers permitted to be included in manufactured and processed food and drinks: *monosodium glutamate* (MSG) *hydrolyzed vegetable protein* (HVP) and *aspartame*. The following list was compiled using data from 10 scientific reports and books, showing that among them this group of additives has been amply documented to cause, contribute to, or aggravate the following illnesses:

- Parkinson's Disease
- Cancer
- Seizures
- Vertigo
- Migraines
- Liver disease
- AIDS
- Dementia
- Brain tumours
- Endocrine disorders
- Multiple Sclerosis
- Neurological disorders
- Chronic Fatigue Syndrome
- Infections
- Birth defects
- Neuropsychiatric disorders
- Fibromyalgia
- Episodic violence
- Epilepsy
- Obesity (certain types)
- Lymphoma
- Alzheimer's disease
- Depression
- Abnormal neural development
- Blindness
- Children's learning disorders
- Epstein Barr Syndrome
- Lyme Disease
- Borreliosis
- Headaches
- Hepathic encephalopathy
- Insomnia
- PMS
- Confusion
- Memory loss
- Nausea
- Asthma
- Bloating
- Diabetes
- Weight gain
- Amyotrophic Lateral Sclerosis (ALS)
- In short, just about everything!

The *June-July 2000* issue of **Nexus Magazine** contained an excellent article by Dr Blaylock. He wrote, "It should be appreciated that the effects of excitotoxin food additives generally are not dramatic. Some individuals may be especially sensitive and develop severe symptoms and even die suddenly from cardiac irritability, but in most instances the effects are subtle and develop over a long period of time." To complicate this health hazard, combinations must be considered. According to lipid chemist Mary Enig, PhD, of the Weston A Price Foundation, "Excitotoxins, plus modern vegetable oils, equals an epidemic of MS."

As Dr Blaylock rightly says, not everyone who ingests these excitotoxins becomes ill immediately. Life would be simpler and we would be much healthier if that happened. Governments would be forced to ban any substance that caused dire symptoms the moment it was consumed. Unfortunately, excitotoxins are usually slow-acting and by the time symptoms appear, connecting them with particular foods is not even considered, or possible. Further, those blessed with strong immune systems are able to detoxify and eliminate these poisons for years. But not, of course, forever and eventually even the hardiest will succumb. Some people are exceedingly vulnerable, and if you are in that category, tough luck. At least, that is the attitude of the food manufacturers, hired-gun scientists and governments.

Let's examine these poisons in detail.

Monosodium Glutamate (MSG)

The infamous MSG was the first excitotoxin to be unleashed on the public. Most of us know about the 'Chinese Restaurant Syndrome', which is one instance of an excitotoxin causing almost immediate symptoms. A lady who attended Hippocrates Health Centre told me that a tiny amount of MSG accidentally ingested in a restaurant caused her to vomit for 24 hours!

I have seen friends become deathly ill after a Chinese meal, and when doctors were called in they warned them never to consume MSG again. Easier said than done, if you eat anything out of a packet, can or bottle. And reading labels is not a guarantee of safety, because the US government permits manufacturers to omit this unpopular additive from their labels unless the product contains 100% MSG! And, of course, most countries import a great deal of manufactured food from the US.

Further, any manufactured food you buy which lists many ingredients will almost certainly contain MSG, even though it is not itself listed. For example, a soup can which lists tomatoes as one of the ingredients does not have to disclose what is in those tomatoes. They could contain something to which you are allergic, and you would find out the hard way.

When MSG was first introduced to the US, I asked my doctor, and teacher, Henry Bieler, MD, author of the best-selling *Food Is Your Best Medicine*, if MSG was safe. He gave me an emphatic *"No!"* and said that in an experiment on rats he discovered that the additive caused their intestines to turn bright red!

Following is a list of hidden sources of MSG, adapted from Dr Blaylock's book, *Excitotoxins – The Taste That Kills*.

Additives that always contain MSG	
• Plant Protein Extract	• Calcium and Sodium Caseinate
• Monosodium Glutamate	• Yeast Extract
• Hydrolyzed Vegetable Protein	• Textured Protein
• Hydrolyzed Plant Protein	• Autolyzed Yeast
	• Hydrolyzed Oat Flour

- Malt Extract
- Malt Flavouring
- Bouillon Broth
- Stock Flavouring
- Spices
- Natural Flavouring
- Natural Beef or Chicken Flavouring
- Seasoning

Additives that __may__ contain MSG or excitotoxins

- Carrageenan
- Enzymes
- Whey Protein Concentrate
- Soy Protein Concentrate
- Soy Protein Isolate

Over the past few years I have conducted a tiny experiment of my own. When passing Chinese restaurants I have asked if they have MSG in their food. All assured me that they did not. Then I took the question a bit farther and told them that I am allergic and could become violently ill or even die if exposed to it. With the spectre of lawsuits looming, the tune always changed and they said that, while they did not add MSG, many of the products they use for flavouring do contain it. This was an eye opener for me and I hope for you, too.

Hydrolyzed Vegetable Protein (HVP)

As yet another example of why we can't trust anyone, a prominent health advocate, in her best-selling book, highly recommended a certain seasoning, claiming it to be delicious and safe. Because it's hard to find a safe seasoning, I went to a health store to investigate and, I hoped, buy some. Imagine my disappointment when I read the label and discovered that hydrolyzed vegetable protein (HVP) is second on the ingredient list. This means that most of this seasoning is made from an excitotoxin additive which none of us should touch. Like so many writing on natural health today, this trusted author did not do careful homework.

HVP became a much-used additive due to the huge amount of adverse reports regarding the danger of the enormous money-spinner, MSG. Once sales dropped, a substitute was needed and soon found – 'hydrolyzed vegetable protein'. It sounds fine, doesn't it? Vegetables, protein, how bad can it be?

Very bad, indeed, according to Dr Blaylock and other scientists. Dr Blaylock states that HVP contains MSG in disguised form, and is even deadlier! But, since it was not labelled 'MSG', uninformed people accepted it. It was even added to baby food for years, and is still in it, in disguised forms. According to Dr Blaylock, this neurotoxin (nervous system poison) causes developmental brain defects that produce behavioural problems and learning difficulties in children, and can contribute to violent behaviour later in life. Hard as it is to accept, governments know about this (they have been warned over and over by prestigious scientists) and have continued to protect the enormously powerful and wealthy multinational companies which manufacture and promote these excitotoxins.

More from Dr Blaylock: "HVP contains several known carcinogens. Incredibly, the FDA does not regulate the amount of carcinogens allowed in hydrolyzed vegetable protein, or the amount of hydrolyzed vegetable protein allowed to be added to food products. This substance poses an even greater danger than MSG itself."

Most Annoying

In June 1999, I first learned the term 'excitotoxins' by reading a review of Dr Blaylock's book in an American health journal. In thumbing through that journal, I saw that Dr Bernard Jensen was an Honorary Board Member. This struck me as a conflict, as the first, and therefore major, ingredient listed in *Bernard Jensen's Vegetable Seasoning* is hydrolyzed vegetable protein, the very same dreaded HVP that the review condemned. Of course, I immediately sent off a fax to the editor of the journal, pointing this out. What I got in return was most annoying, yet humorous as well. It was a long fax from the company that now produces this product. Here are some extracts from the fax I received from their company president, Gary Olsen:

> "... My wife, Cynthia Olson, is a Clinical Nutritionist and would absolutely never authorise hydrolyzed vegetable protein to be used in any products made for Bernard Jensen International's consumers.

> "In the future, perhaps the best course for you would be to address us at Bernard Jensen International with your concerns, before sending a potentially harmful letter that contains inaccurate and erroneous information to the general public. Your letter can be considered as liable and having the propensity to incur repercussions for Bernard Jensens International, as well as Dr Bernard Jensen that would be very unfair at his age."

Well, at my age I consider being almost duped into consuming HVP very unfair also. I wonder what Mr Olson had in mind – suing me from across the Pacific for telling the truth about his product? I still have the label specifying the ingredient Mrs Olsen "would absolutely never authorise." My readers will not be surprised to learn that I have not recanted – and that I have heard nothing further from Jensen's.

This is yet another example of our need to protect ourselves. On the off-chance that you are not already convinced to shun HVP, here is Dr Blaylock's description of the manufacturing process: "This mixture is made from 'junk' vegetables that are unfit for sale... The extraction process of hydrolysis involves boiling these vegetables in a vat of acid. This is followed by a process of neutralisation with caustic soda. The resulting product is a brown sludge that collects on the top. This is scraped off and allowed to dry. The end product is a brown powder that is high in three known excitotoxins – glutamate, aspartate, and cystolic acid. It is then added by the food industry to everything from canned tuna to baby food."

Aspartame

The original authorization for the use of the deadly neurotoxin Aspartame in commercial foods and beverages is one of the greatest public health scandals of the 20th Century! That its use is still sanctioned despite massive evidence from all over the world that it goes on killing and permanently disabling millions of people is absolutely criminal, and due entirely to the massive power and influence which its original maker, the Monsanto Corporation, and various other multinationals are able to exert over politicians, government regulators and the media. So successful have they been that aspartame is known to be contained in well over 6,000 products – food, supplements, chewing gum, drugs, children's aspirin and even *"Flintstone"* vitamins!

Twenty years ago, Woodrow C. Monte, PhD, Professor of Food Science at the University of Arizona, warned in the **Journal Of Applied Nutrition,** *Volume 36, Number 1, 1984,*

> "Aspartame (L-asparty-L-phenylalanine methyl ester), a new sweetener marketed under the trade name NutraSweet, releases into the human bloodstream one molecule of methanol for each molecule of aspartame consumed.

> "This new methanol source is being added to foods that have considerably reduced caloric content and, thus, may be consumed in large amounts. Generally, none of these foods could be considered dietary methanol sources prior to addition of aspartame. When diet sodas and soft drinks, sweetened with aspartame, are used to replace fluid loss during exercise and physical exertion in hot climates, the intake of methanol can exceed 250 mg/day or 32 times the Environmental Protection Agency's recommended limit of consumption for this cumulative toxin."

In this chapter I shall try to confine my remarks to the medical evidence of aspartame's inherent dangers. To appreciate the full extent of the corruption, fraud and commercial skullduggery which surrounds the approval and use of this deadly toxin, I recommend that you visit the websites www.dorway.com www.aspartame.com, and Bettym19@mindspring.com, where you will see a massive amount of irrefutable evidence which, were it not for the industrial/political influence of the manufacturers involved, would result in the banning of the stuff and the prosecution of the corporations, authorities and politicians who continue to profit from its continued use while the health of millions of people is being compromised.

However, it is worth mentioning here that after years of lobbying by anti-aspartame pressure groups headed by the indefatigable American activist Betty Martini and her *Mission Possible* movement, the European Parliament – alone among Western governments – has voted to re-examine the safety of aspartame. Announcing the investigation early in 2003, a statement from the Parliament said, "…the use of aspartame increases the exposure to its metabolites methanol/formaldehyde and phenylalanine and is reported to provoke, among other effects, headaches, nausea and allergic reactions, especially in the case of vulnerable persons. Its widespread use should therefore be re-evaluated by the Commission and the relevant scientific committees, taking into account all available data and respecting the precautionary principle. A historical evaluation is required as there seems to be evidence that original studies did not prove the safety of aspartame."

The final sentence is an understatement; the original studies proved it had the potential to kill and disable, but, as evidenced by FDA documents reproduced on www.dorway.com, were 'doctored' to secure FDA approval! Let's hope that our European cousins are more honest and courageous than US, Australian and New Zealand governments have been and will ultimately outlaw this 'approved' substance that serves only to bolster the coffers of multinational chemical corporations.

Many Names

The generic aspartame, besides being used as a sweetener in virtually all diet foods and sodas and numerous commercial foods and drinks, is also marketed to consumers as a sugar substitute under many different names such as *NutraSweet, Equal, Spoonful* and *Crystal Light.* As a result, it is arguably the most deadly excitotoxin of all, being consumed in enormous quantities by young, vulnerable people and by those of all ages who are trying to combat health and weight problems – the very same problems aspartame is likely to cause or contribute to.

Aspartame, Equal, Nutrasweet, etc., are not always listed on food labels. These extremely dangerous additives can also be

Inside Hollywood

There has been much speculation about the cause of the Parkinson's Disease suffered by actor Michael J Fox, but the star's addiction to *Diet Pepsi* (which contains aspartame) is no secret.

One cast member who worked with Fox said he drank at least 12 cans a day. I have no way of knowing if that is true, since I have not spoken personally with him. I do know, however, from my own Hollywood days, that whenever a celebrity endorses a product, he or she is provided with an unlimited supply, and if there is a movie or TV show involved, cases are sent each week.

Given Michael's long-standing commercial endorsement of Diet Pepsi, it's hardly surprising that not only is he himself now a victim of the neurological disease, but that several crew members who worked with him have also been reported as suffering the same terrible affliction.

PepsiCo, Monsanto and their partners-in-crime have a lot to answer for.

referred to as 'Additive 951' and must be guarded against. Remember, there is *no* safe artificial sweetener, no matter what fancy new name the manufacturers coin in order to disguise their poison. You might like to try *Stevia*, a safe herbal sweetener. Some like it, some don't, but at least it won't kill you.

Over the years I have collected a huge amount of credible medical and scientific information on aspartame, together with hundreds of heart-wrenching letters from victims of this deadly poison. There is far too much to include here, but a visit to the internet sites previously mentioned, www.dorway.com and www.aspartame.com, will reveal just how much incontrovertible and impeccable scientific and medical evidence is being ignored by regulatory authorities and suppressed by manufacturers. Even the National Medical Library in Bethesda, Maryland, lists 167 citations for studies under the heading 'adverse effects of aspartame'. So many well-credentialed authorities have published books and papers proving the dangers of aspartame, that it is hard to decide whom to quote, as their evidence would fill a library.

Let's start with a very well researched article by Dr William Campbell Douglas in his ***Second Opinion*** newsletter:

Aspartame - It's Got to Go

Right up there with the fluoride and mercury-in your-fillings scandals is the aspartame mass poisoning of the world. From Kenya to Kokomo and from Kyoto to Khartoum, the world is swimming in this highly toxic chemical – over 90 countries are selling it as NutraSweet, Equal, or Spoonful. Over half of all Americans now consume it on a regular basis.

At an environmental meeting in 1997, the keynote address was given by an official from the Environmental Protection Agency (EPA) in which he said (paraphrased): "There is an epidemic of multiple sclerosis and systemic lupus, and we do not understand what toxin is causing this to be rampant across the United States."

It's interesting that he said "what toxin." I've never heard a bureaucrat even suggest that it may be from a toxin – a slip of the tongue?

When the temperature of aspartame exceeds 86° F, the wood alcohol (methanol) in aspartame converts to formaldehyde and then to formic acid, which in turn causes metabolic acidosis. (Formic acid is the poison found in the sting of fire ants.) The methanol toxicity mimics multiple sclerosis. Thus, people are diagnosed as having multiple sclerosis when, in fact, they are often suffering from aspartame toxicity. If they had been taken off aspartame, their symptoms would, in many cases, have disappeared.

Systemic lupus erythematosis has become almost as common as multiple sclerosis and the major culprits appear to be Diet Coke and Diet Pepsi. The systemic lupus appears to be triggered by aspartame. The victim usually does not know the aspartame is the culprit and continues the Coke and Pepsi, thus aggravating the lupus to such a degree that it can be life-threatening.

Chronic methanol toxicity from Diet Coke and Diet Pepsi, usually diagnosed as something else, has similar symptoms as lupus and MS. It is usually found that the patient drinks three to four 12oz cans (or more) of Diet Coke or Diet Pepsi per day.

When patients are taken off aspartame, those with systemic lupus may improve, but they will not be cured. The damage has been done and the disease cannot be reversed. However, in 'MS' cases, the results are often dramatic, bordering on the sensational. In reality, the 'MS' is often chronic methanol toxicity and the symptoms may disappear completely with removal of aspartame from the diet.

An 'MS' case suffering from blindness is almost certainly a case of chronic methanol toxicity secondary to aspartame poisoning. Ask doctors in a country where bootleg whiskey is common, such as Russia, what is the most dramatic symptom of acute methanol toxicity from the bad hooch they drink and they will tell you it's blindness.

The symptoms of "aspartame disease," – chronic methyl alcohol toxicity – are amazingly varied, including: blindness, tinnitus, numbness in the extremities, muscle spasms, slurred speech, blurred vision, joint pain, headaches, anxiety, vertigo, and memory loss. So you can see how easily the patient can be misdiagnosed as MS, Alzheimer's disease, brain tumour, or just plain neurosis, early in the course of the toxicity.

Brain tumours have increased dramatically, and there is solid evidence to indict aspartame in the genesis of the modern epidemic of brain cancer. Furthermore, the formation of brain cancer was dose-related – the higher the dose, the more cancer.

I was astonished to find out that the first experiments done to test the safety of aspartame disclosed a high incidence of brain tumours in the animals fed what would become known to the world as NutraSweet. The study was done by the very company that was going to sell Monsanto Corp's brainchild, if you will pardon the double entendre. The G.D. Searle Co. found there was a 3.75 percent incidence of brain tumours in the rats fed aspartame and zero percent in the control rats – astrocytomas are rare in rats. It's so rare that this incidence represents a 25 times higher incidence than would be expected in rats.

Equally incriminating, the study was discontinued after only 76 weeks. Since the number of tumours continued to increase, some damage control was needed. What would any well-paid investigator do? – stop the study and declare that all the tumours were "spontaneous!" The FDA went along with the studies, which they knew to be badly flawed to the point of fraud and gross incompetence – and approved NutraSweet. Dr Russell L. Blaylock, author of the seminal book, *Excitotoxins - The Taste That Kills,* called this action "a monumental crime."

Dr H.J. Roberts, diabetes specialist and world expert on aspartame poisoning, has also written a book entitled *Defense Against Alzheimer's Disease*. Dr Roberts tells how aspartame poisoning is escalating Alzheimer's Disease. Hospice nurses are reporting that women are being admitted at 30 years of age with Alzheimer's Disease.

There are 92 documented symptoms of aspartame, from coma to death. The majority of them are neurological, because aspartame destroys the nervous system. H.J. Roberts, MD, says: "Consuming aspartame at the time of conception can cause birth defects." And Dr Louis Elsas, a Professor of Genetics, at Emory University, testified before Congress that phenylalanine, a breakdown product of aspartame metabolism, concentrates in the placenta, causing mental retardation in the baby.

Ant Poison

If you have any NutraSweet powder left over, use it to poison ants. It's more effective than Orkin and much cheaper.

A great deal more is now known as to exactly how Monsanto/Searle obtained FDA sanction for this poison to be legally introduced into our diet. It is a shocking tale of corporate greed and official corruption involving, among others, none other than the Prince of Darkness, Donald Rumsfeld, the present US Secretary of Defense. Details and documentary proof are published on both www.dorway.com and www.aspartame.com.

As James Bowen, MD, in *Aspartame Murders Infants*, published on www.dorway.com, says: "At every point in the fertility process aspartame destroys, beginning with the gleam in Mom and Pop's eyes: it ruins female sexual response and induces male sexual dysfunction. Beyond this, aspartame disrupts fetal development by aborting it or inducing defects. And if a live child is born, aspartame may have heinously damaged the DNA of the baby, cursing future generations."

The manufacturer and the FDA have steadfastly refused to put a warning on aspartame even though they have full knowledge of how it can destroy the foetus or trigger birth defects. Louis Elsas, MD, Professor of Pediatric Genetics at Emory University, testified before Congress on this issue. His testimony can also be read at www.dorway.com, along with Dr Roberts' position paper admitting that even a man consuming aspartame at conception can cause birth defects in his own child.

The following quotes are from a long article in *Flying Safely,* May 1992, a journal for professional aircraft pilots:

> "In pregnancy the effects of Aspartame can be passed directly on to the fetus, even in very small doses. Some people have suffered Aspartame-related disorders with doses as small as that carried in a single stick of chewing gum. This could mean a pilot who drinks diet sodas is more susceptible to flicker vertigo or to flicker-induced epileptic activity. It also means that all pilots are potential victims of sudden memory loss, dizziness during instrument flight and gradual loss of vision. A pilot's hot-line was set up and over 500 pilots responded, some speaking of grand mal seizures in the cockpit of commercial airline flights. Many pilots lost their medical certifications to fly, and their careers ...

> "...Monsanto reaps one billion dollars a year from the Aspartame toxic bonanza... This can buy a lot of bureaucrats! Does FDA mean Fatal Drugs Allowed? ... The NutraSweet Company and sister Searle are owned by Monsanto, which discovered Aspartame while testing an ulcer drug... If you're taking other medicine, consider possible reactions you may have.

> "In 1969 Searle approached Dr Harry Waisman to study the effects of Aspartame on primates. Seven monkeys were fed the chemical in milk. One died after 300 days, 5 others had Grand Mal seizures. Searle deleted these findings when they submitted his study to the FDA! ... The best way to understand NutraSweet is to think of it as a minute nerve gas that eradicates brain and nerve function.... Aspartame makes you crave carbohydrates and so you gain weight. The formaldehyde stores in the fat cells,

particularly on the hips and thighs... NutraSweet, Equal, Spoonful are the deadliest toxins in our society because of their ubiquitous presence in thousands of foods, even children's medicines, Kool Aid and Jello, and on every restaurant table. We're dosed with millions of pounds every year! This warning should be on every Aspartame product: CHEMICAL POISON: KEEP OUT OF REACH OF HUMANS! GENOCIDAL!"

H J Roberts, MD, recently published a monumental book (over 1000 pages) on aspartame-related illnesses. As Director of the Palm Beach Institute for Medical Research in Florida, he has spent over three decades researching the diverse effects of aspartame and has published many papers and articles. In his latest book, *Aspartame Disease, An Ignored Epidemic,* he says that the physical effects can be inflicted on all systems, organs and tissues, and the mental effects can result in psychological, behavioural, and psychiatric problems. According to Dr Roberts, numerous reactions to aspartame frequently are undiagnosed. Or, they are misdiagnosed and wrongly attributed to such serious health conditions as fibromyalgia, arthritis, lupus, multiple sclerosis, or Alzheimer's disease, among others.

Dr Roberts offers diagnostic guidance to doctors, saying that every evaluation of difficult allergic, dermatologic, gastrointestinal, or metabolic problems should include queries about aspartame consumption. "Diabetes accompanied by visual, neurological, or bowel problems should not be assumed to be complications of retinopathy or neuropathy until aspartame use is ruled out," he says.

Insidiously Addictive

The most insidious thing about aspartame is that it is addictive. In one of Dr Roberts' many scientific papers he wrote that aspartame reactors in his study found it "difficult or impossible to discontinue aspartame because of severe withdrawal effects." His case histories, of people with life-threatening illnesses due to aspartame, and their pathetic inability to "kick" the habit, are extraordinary. He has repeatedly urged the government to "declare aspartame an imminent health hazard" and remove it from the market. He has, needless to say, been unsuccessful. So far, the manufacturers have won the day, despite incontrovertible medical evidence on its addictive properties and involvement in at least 92 documented illnesses and conditions.

Dr Roberts also wrote about the dangers of aspartame in chewing gum: "Chewing aspartame gum poses a unique threat, as evidenced by the dramatic development of generalised symptoms in some aspartame reactors... The chemical may be absorbed through the mucosa of the mouth, and via a simple diffusion from the oropharynx, directly into the brain."

So, in 1999 my blood boiled (something it does frequently) when I read a story in the *Gold Coast Bulletin* in which they reported that *Wrigley's* was donating their sugar-free diet gum (which, of course, contains aspartame) to a school on the Coast. The idea was that the young children would chew the gum after eating in order to remove sugar from their teeth (apparently they didn't think of *not giving* the children sugar, a known cavity-producer, instead).

This marketing ploy is being repeated in other schools in Australia and I presume in other countries as well. I immediately rang the school principal, warning her about the danger, and was treated like a ratbag for my pains. So, I wrote an impassioned Letter to the Editor, which was fortunately printed. Sure enough, a mother rang to thank me, saying that her daughter became ill shortly after this outrageous practice was started. She was so ill that it was necessary to keep her out of school for several days. This lady then complained to the principal and warned that she would sue if her child were given any more neurotoxins.

Some scientists assert that aspartame in chewing gum poses a greater risk than in even the deadly 'diet' drinks. Small wonder; it acts like nitroglycerine under the tongue and goes straight to the brain. The younger the child, the more dangerous the effect.

When will the authorities learn? Or even listen to reason? I flirted with the idea of carrying a picket sign in front of the school, but gave it up as too time-consuming. If you feel that companies that knowingly poison children, and schools that cooperate, have forfeited all rights to respect, please write letters of protest. If your child is given sugar-free gum in school, I suggest photocopying this information and threatening a lawsuit if they continue this dangerous practice.

New Threat

Unfortunately for our health, Monsanto's patent on aspartame has run out. This means any processor can use this product, which will be showing up in even more foods. As soon as I learned about this development, I rang Mary Stoddard in Texas. Mary is the head of the non-profit Aspartame Consumer Safety Network (see **Resources**), and is doing an extraordinary job of educating and advising people who have been poisoned by this family of artificial sweeteners.

She told me something sinister; in order to keep the billions flowing in, Monsanto has developed a new artificial sweetener that they have patented. It is called *Neotame* and, according to Mary, who is in constant touch with the scientists who are fighting the use of these products, Neotame is ten times more potent than aspartame, and much more dangerous.

Monsanto opted to trial this artificial sweetener overseas, before applying to the US Food and Drug Administration for official approval in the US. It is Mary's opinion, and mine too, that they prefer to use other countries as guinea pigs before chancing problems in the US. And guess which countries they chose?

You guessed it – Australia and New Zealand, where the regulatory agencies once more rolled over and played dead for Monsanto, one of the richest companies in the world, just as they did over the company's reckless promotion of genetically modified seeds.

So, be warned about Neotame. In addition, be alert to the following on labels: 'Phenylketonurics: Contains Phenylalanine', as well as *Acesulfame-k* and *Sucralose* (sold as *Splenda*). Sucralose has a chlorinated base like DDT and can cause auto-immune disease, and acesulfame-k (the *k* is the chemical code for potassium) triggered cancer and leukaemia in original studies. The European Parliament has called for a review of sucralose and aspartame-acesulfame salt use within three years as well. Avoid all these non-food sweeteners like the plague if you value your life.

With all the negative press regarding artificial sweeteners, it is at first glance inexplicable that the American Diabetes Association wholeheartedly recommends diet foods and drinks containing aspartame. That is, until you dig under the surface and discover that this association is funded by Monsanto. I assume that the Australian version of that association has a similar connection. Or, to give them the benefit of the doubt, they may be merely influenced by their American cousin in their recommendations.

Ironically, diabetes organizations recommend these 'diet' products to people who desperately need to lose weight, when it has been amply documented that the formaldehyde in aspartame stores in fat cells, particularly on the hips and thighs, and is then difficult, sometimes impossible, to dislodge.

There has been a great deal of industry pressure on doctors who have warned of the dangers. For example, Dr James Bowen wrote, "I have come across first-hand reports of a doctor who had her medical degree revoked because she spoke on the aspartame issue. Even I have been threatened by insiders from the political camp of aspartame, that they will get my degree revoked... Yet the government defends staunchly the marketing of aspartame, which as a formaldehyde poison, is probably 500 times as potent as straight formaldehyde, causing aggravated formaldehyde poisoning in its victims... The amount you would get from a can of pop greatly exceeds what you would get from inhaled air, even by the old, more lenient standard."

And he should know; apart from his research and medical practice bringing him in contact with many aspartame victims, Dr Bowen is himself a sufferer from Lou Gehrig's disease, which he attributes to his consumption of aspartame in cold drinks supplied to desert troops by the manufacturers when he was an army medical officer.

At Hippocrates we have had a statistically significant amount of reports from students who have suffered vertigo when suddenly rising from a sitting or lying position. This is due to a lapse of delivery of blood to the brain, and the students could all trace it back to the use of aspartame, HVP or MSG, which they said they did not ordinarily ingest, but had a Chinese dinner or 'cheated' on their diets and thought that 'just this once' it wouldn't hurt to indulge. It does!

But Wait - There's More!

The multinational food industry, which has an unrivalled reputation for shamelessness, has disguised processed free glutamic acid (MSG) in the food ingredient 'citric acid'. It sounds benign, doesn't it? Believe me, it is not, as it has the same effect on excitotoxin-susceptible people as does MSG, HVP and aspartame.

Citric acid, which is widely used, is not produced, as one might imagine, from citrus fruit, but from the fermentation of crude sugars. During processing, the remaining protein is hydrolyzed, and this creates processed free glutamic acid. When combined with protein in the diet, even more of this dangerous neurotoxin is produced.

The widely-used amino acid, *cysteine*, is an excitotoxin. It is sometimes used in supplements as well, so please check labels.

As if all this were not bad enough, the US Food and Drug Administration (FDA) has approved an antimicrobial spray called *Sanova* for use on meat, vegetables and fruit. They are now trying to get approval to use it on all processed foods! Labelling is not required. I have not as yet been able to ascertain if this product is going to be permitted in Australia, but if experience is any guide, it will be. Australia, to our detriment, is a hand-maiden of the US, and our politicians slavishly copy all the bad things they do.

According to Dr Blaylock, soy, which is another of my pet hates, naturally contains glutamate and glutamine, which are excitotoxins. Further, soymilk often has HVP added to improve the flavour. Kombu, miso and soy sauce all contain HVP. Dr Blaylock says that a natural food distributor sent a flyer trying to allay consumer fears of MSG by saying that HVP is a natural source of "bound glutamate", and not dangerous. "This is not true," says Dr Blaylock.

Dr Blaylock says that there are ways to neutralise some of the harmful effects of excitotoxins: anti-oxidant vitamins and minerals, the branched chained amino acids, zinc and magnesium glyconate and magnesium lactate (but **not** magnesium aspartate, which is an excitotoxin) offer some protection. This does not mean you have a licence to consume these deadly toxins. Please inspect your home and bravely rid it of all products that list HVP, MSG, aspartame, and any other artificial sweeteners. Then, think carefully about manufactured foods that don't list these chemicals, but are vague about exact ingredients. I suggest that you box the whole shameful mess and send them off to your health minister and tell him or her to eat them as punishment for allowing them in our food supply.

Betty Martini, America's high-profile, dedicated anti-aspartame crusader, told me that she and many prominent physicians have written the Multiple Sclerosis Society frequently, alerting them to the proven connection between MS and aspartame. They have never answered, nor acted on this information, which could have saved countless lives. When in doubt, look to the funding, and like most "health" societies, they are funded by the very industry that is causing this dreadful disease. As Betty said in an email to me, "When those responsible to solve the problem, ARE the problem, it is a sad commentary on greed and lack of concern for humanity. How can anyone set aside professional ethics to allow an MS holocaust, when simply alerting those with MS to avoid aspartame and other excitotoxins, could save the lives of thousands?"

At a MS Society walk-a-thon, the Society gave out free Diet Cokes, and tried to prevent Betty's activists from giving the walkers information that could save lives. Betty called out to the crowd, saying, "The MS Society does not want you to have this life-saving information on a product triggering this disease." Many took copies, and Betty received calls later from those who had been helped by quitting diet drinks.

Good News

Aspartame activists in the US have taken a spectacular action, and we hope it will trickle down to Australia and other countries eventually. Years ago, a law was passed to break the mafia stranglehold, and it was very successful. Many of the most reprehensible men in US organised crime were jailed because of this law, called RICO (Racketeer Influenced and Corrupt Organisations). Now, a RICO complaint has been filed, charging the defendants with manufacturing and marketing a deadly neurotoxin unfit for human consumption, while they assured the public that aspartame-contaminated products were safe and healthful, even for children and pregnant women. Present Secretary of Defence Donald Rumsfeld is mentioned throughout the lawsuit.

Class action damages asked are US$350,000,000. Many household company names are defendants and Dr. Robert Moser, past CEO of NutraSweet, is cited for misrepresenting facts to public and commercial users, with full knowledge of the deceptions. Organised crime does huge damage to individuals and to the economy, of course, but this damage has been a fleabite compared to the genocide and poisoning of billions of people practiced by industry, and sanctioned by governments. These men deserve the gallows.

The RICO suit is encouraging, and more will follow. World-wide lawsuits will fly one day, when enough people have been killed and maimed so class actions appear profitable to the legal profession. But don't hold your breath that Monsanto or any other multinational will be punished. These Captains of Industry are way ahead of us mere mortals, and are already arranging for others to take the falls. Corporate swindlers/poisoners rarely end up in jails, no matter how richly deserved, due to their vast wealth and bribes to legislators.

For proof, look to the asbestos outrage/scandal. For seventy years that I know of, the huge US asbestos miner and fabricator, Johns Manville, knew their product was killing people, yet they managed, with money and government connivance, to hide the evidence and stonewall lawsuits. When class actions were finally instigated, they did what any other multinational would do --- they skipped the country, taking all their money, and leaving behind a legacy of death and suffering. The Australian company, James Hardie, is now very much in the news for similar, although not quite as blatant, behaviour.

Because of the enormous publicity the asbestos poisonings have received, people appear to have the idea that something like this could never happen again. But they are wrong, and one day it will be clear to everyone that there are things in our lives that are infinitely worse than asbestos, all of which are explained in this book. These things will destroy health in the "civilized" world, and bring health services to their knees. Populations will be miserable, governments, as usual, will be useless, and the multinationals will join the asbestos killers in offshore havens.

Our best defence is to boycott all of the products these companies produce. They are committing crimes against humanity.

Still On The Fence?

Consider the following quotes from aspartame expert and activist, American physician, Dr James Bowen:

- The intact aspartame molecule is an alcohol poison about twenty thousand times as toxic as most alcoholic beverage alcohols.

- Aspartame manufacturing plants around the world now protect their employees with face masks and full body protective garments lest their employees come into any contact with the dust! This all started with the death of an employee named Krossic who first passed out from the inhaled dust's toxic effects... His death occurred even after all were made to wear face masks so they couldn't breathe the dust. Krossic absorbed enough through the skin that he died from a toxic cardiomyopathy. The post mortem exam revealed an "alcoholic cardiomyopathy". Jim Krossic was a teetotaller who used NO beverage alcohol!

- Aspartame ingested by the mother before and during conception is horribly damaging to the fetus, causing fetal loss, deformity, fetal alcohol syndrome and many other horrible problems.

- The maternal transmission of damaged MtDNA can occur for the rest of a woman's reproductive years, and may directly affect both her children and grandchildren, as well as becoming a persistently transmitted genetic woman's problem. The mother, therefore, does not necessarily have to have been drinking aspartame when she got pregnant, nor while carrying the baby. SINCE THE FEMALE IS BORN WITH ALL THE EGGS SHE WILL EVER HAVE ALREADY PRESENT IN HER OVARIES, IT MAY WELL BE THE NUTRASWEET HER MOTHER DRANK WHICH IS THE SOURCE OF HER OFFSPRING'S PROBLEM.

Warning: If you want normal grandchildren, teach your daughters to be more afraid of artificial sweeteners than they are of poisonous snakes.

5

Processed Foods
A convenient way to shorten your life

It's hard to know where to start when dealing with this infuriating and frightening subject. A section in a book can only skim the surface; to really understand the complexity and dangers of food additives one must be a biochemist or, at the very least, read several thick, intimidating, hard-to-understand tomes.

If you eat processed food you can be sure it will be filled with potent chemicals that the human system never encountered prior to the advent of the test tube.

Our body computers simply don't know how to deal with these chemicals, and are thrown into confusion by them. This confusion can lead to dividing of cells, and we all know what that means. As respected cancer researcher, Dr William E. Smith, said, "The growing custom of introducing an endless series of biologically foreign molecules into the human organism for various commercial advantages is not unlike throwing a collection of nuts and bolts into the most delicate machinery known."

Virtually everything you eat has been chemicalised somewhere along the line; your body, if you use processed foods, will have to deal with emulsifiers, preservatives, dyes, artificial flavours, humectants, drying agents, artificial sweeteners, bleaches, neutralisers, disinfectants, thickeners, antifoaming and anticaking agents, alkalisers, deodorants, extenders, gasses, conditioners, hydrogenators, hydrolisers, maturers, sulfites, sulphur dioxide, fumigants, antifungal preservatives, stabilisers, texturisers, antibiotics, steroids, and even irradiation. And you thought you were eating *food*!

The scope of this book does not permit a detailed list of the thousands of chemicals that are added to our foods, and the dangers, or suspected dangers, of each one. There are several fine textbooks on this subject for those who want to learn more. But be warned: reading them may be hazardous to your mental health, and can destroy any lingering faith or respect you may harbour for regulatory agencies, chemical companies, scientists and food processors.

The list of chemicals in soft drinks is dizzying. Many contain brominated vegetable oils, which have produced large lesions on the kidneys, livers, hearts and spleens of laboratory animals. It would take pages to list all the dangerous chemicals in these innocuous-seeming fizzy drinks. Suffice it to say that many are coal-tar products, which have been known carcinogens for many years.

Soft drinks not only destroy your bones, they also destroy your teeth. If sweet reason won't persuade you and your children to quit drinking them, try these experiments:

- Drop some metal nails into a bottle of cola. In a couple of days they will dissolve.

- Spill some on a concrete surface and watch what happens to a fly that ingests it. And see how clean the surface becomes, too.

- If you're game, spill some on your car and watch what it does to the paint – a car that's destined for the junk yard!

If you and your family persist in drinking soft drinks after these experiments, you need psychiatric help!

It's The Real Thing All Right!

To those who wonder how governments could allow these drinks to be sold if they are so dangerous, I can only say that you must think for yourselves in order to protect yourselves and your families. The food manufacturing industry is huge and powerful and, historically, all governments have been more concerned with protecting industry than consumers.

For example, soft drink companies have, with the help of the government, infiltrated the public school system in the US. Can Australia, and all other 'civilised' countries be far behind? Several school districts in the US have actually signed contracts with *Coca-Cola* that bring in many millions, provided annual sales quotas are met! The result is predictable: school administrators encourage students to drink *Coke*, even in classrooms.

In 1998 the Center for Science in the Public Interest (CSPI) warned that *Coca-Cola* paid the Boys and Girls Clubs of America US$60 million to market its brand exclusively in over 2000 facilities. How do you feel about this? Is it worth taking the time to write letters of protest? Do you feel, as I do, that governments, school districts and these children's clubs are irredeemably sleazy?

Many familiar and loved products wouldn't exist without liberal use of preservatives, particularly canned foods and processed meats, which require potent preservatives to prevent unwanted side effects, such as death. Processed meats are unhealthy on all levels, and best avoided in any case. Some meats are so heavily preserved that the expiry date should read, "You should live so long!"

Setting You Up for Cancer

The oft-repeated excuse used by industry spokesmen and, incredibly, believed by the public and governments, is that because these chemicals are used in such small amounts they are harmless, even though they cause cancer in experimental animals. Some are so poisonous that they would kill humans instantly if eaten in large quantities! The frightening truth is that even tiny amounts of a carcinogen, taken occasionally, are enough to cause cancer in susceptible individuals.

At a meeting of cancer specialists, Dr Hermann Druckery, of Germany, said, "A person absorbing even infinitesimal amounts will still have the cumulative effect and when a certain level is reached and a period of latency has passed, the effect will become evident in the form of a tumour." The chemical you ingest today in that delicious treat you just couldn't resist could be setting you up for cancer ten or twenty years from today. Is it worth it?

Even the director of the US Food and Drug Administration, Toxicological Division, agrees. He says that there is no precise understanding of the ultimate fate of food additives once they are in the body. Years ago it was thought that the body was able to detoxify food additives, and that they were broken down into harmless compounds. It is now known that this does not happen. The processors, chemical manufacturers and governments are playing Russian roulette with our bodies. They can continue doing so *only* if we cooperate.

While it is impossible to establish the cause of most human cancers, statistics tell us that the unprecedented rise in the incidence of cancer closely parallels the huge rise in the incidence of untested chemicals in our food supply. The average person in industrial nations ingests between three and seven kilograms of these additives per year. Prudent people ingest none – so there are lots of people ingesting two or three times that amount. They are courting cancer, and all of the other ills caused by food additives.

Sorry History

There are thousands of man-made chemicals in our food that have never been adequately tested – no one knows their potential to cause birth defects, allergies, genetic damage or cancer. The food processing industry has a sorry history of using chemicals for as long as 75 years before the news leaked out that they caused serious liver damage in experimental animals. Coumarin, dulcin and butter yellow (doesn't it sound appetizing?) are just a few examples.

Many substances which are known to cause cancers in experimental animals are tolerated by governments, in spite of warnings from cancer experts, on the grounds that they are consumed in small amounts and aren't instantly lethal.

Rarely Tested

The processors rarely test additives themselves. They depend upon the manufacturers, and upon 'independent' firms such as Industrial Bio-Test

Laboratories in the US, one of the largest in the world. The executives of this firm were convicted of falsifying the results of over 22,000 tests performed for chemical manufacturers, in spite of the fire that 'accidentally' destroyed all of their records just before the Feds moved in! It's chilling to reflect that the American laboratories are considered the best in the world, and that most other countries rely upon their test results. Honest laboratories have poor track records, too; more often than not, carcinogens are identified only after the product has been tested on an unsuspecting public. Even in laboratories with flawless integrity, cumulative dangers are usually ignored. What may be relatively harmless over a short time could cause cancer over years of ingestion. Interaction has also been ignored in testing – what may be harmless alone could prove deadly when combined with other additives or natural substances. Considering that there can be 30 or more additives in just one kind of food, the permutations are endless!

Poring over labels in the supermarket is an exercise in futility. For example, a pizza maker who uses dough, tomato paste, cheese and vegetables must list them. In many countries he need not list the shocking things that have been done to 'improve' the flour that he used to make the dough, nor the additives in the cheese. If he didn't make the tomato paste, its ingredients may go unlisted. If he uses sausage that someone else has processed, all he must list is 'sausage', and the contents remain the ugly secret of the sausage maker.

Should you or your children be allergic to the sodium nitrate, or any of the many other additives permitted in prepared meat, tough luck. Animal studies show that the young are at much greater risk from additives than mature people. It may be that fully developed organs are better able to resist the onslaught of damaging substances. Whatever the reason, it is well established that all food additives present an unacceptable risk to our children.

When you consider the large amounts of brightly coloured non-foods, sodas, and other highly chemicalised food they consume, it is no wonder we have so high a rate of childhood cancer. Fifty years ago one rarely heard of a young person with cancer, or other degenerative diseases – now it is commonplace.

Into the Mouths of Babes

Even babies are victims of the processors; reading the ingredients of some baby foods, formulas and supplements would make a vulture gag. They read more like chemistry lessons than nourishment. It is known that babies have no taste for salt, yet it is often added, thus starting an early addiction. Even monosodium glutamate (MSG), which has long been known as a dangerous non-food, was used in infant food. After a long fight, consumer groups forced it to be removed in most countries. In the US, executives of prestigious Beech-Nut Corporation were prosecuted because they sold five million jars of artificial colour, sugar and synthetic malic acid, labelled as 100% fruit juice. One was convicted of 429 counts of violating the Food, Drug and Cosmetics Act. Mr Nice Guy. When choosing food for your children, don't trust processors; trust yourself only! If you love your baby, breastfeed for as long as possible, then squash up fresh fruit and vegetables. It's not as quick as opening a can or a bottle, but you will spend less time nursing sick children and protect them from illnesses, surgery, chemotherapy and early graves.

Trap For The Unwary

Probably the most dangerous, and the least necessary, additives are dyes. At least preservatives serve a purpose, dangerous as they are. The only advantage in dyes is to the processor, who is able to mask half-dead, over-processed food so people will buy it, thinking it's fresh and nourishing. Dyes are a trap for the unwary, especially children who are attracted to the bright, shiny colours.

Natural food dyes are rarely used because they are so much more expensive than chemical ones, which are often derived from coal tar, a known carcinogen. *Tartrazine* is just one example among many. It is used to dye food yellow, orange and green, and can be found in sodas, jams, decorations, custard, flavoured milk, and many bakery goods. Approximately 10 percent of the public is intolerant or allergic to it, and no one knows the long-term effect upon people who don't have any immediate, noticeable symptoms. It is an azo dye, and they have all been linked with cancer of the intestinal tract. There are other symptoms, such as skin and respiratory problems. Many consider it a central nervous system poison, as well. It, along with all the other synthetic dyes, should have been banned at inception.

Next time you go to the supermarket, take a look at the mouthwash and plaque cleaners. There they are, lined up in all their synthetic brilliance; hot pink, blazing orange, kelly green, bright blue and scarlet, inviting you to put them in your mouth, swirl them around on your delicate, absorbent membranes, and poison yourself.

Careful people can avoid most food additives, but sulphur is hard to detect. It has been used for years to keep dried fruit from going brown. If the fruit looks plump and the colour is bright, it has sulphur on it. If it looks a bit scruffy and brown, it should be unsulphured. It won't be as soft, but once you become accustomed to unsulphured dried fruit it's lovely, and a bit of a challenge because it's chewy. It's more healthful if you soak it before eating, and that reconstitutes the moisture and makes it soft again. Health food stores usually carry unsulphured dried fruit, but it's wise to ask questions and inspect before buying.

What they call 'sulfiting agents' are a menace which is much harder to detect. Some restaurants use them on salad vegetables to maintain a fresh appearance, and on seafood and fried potatoes. Some people react with diarrhoea, acute asthma attacks, nausea, loss of consciousness and even anaphylactic shock.

Toothless Laws

Deaths have occurred often enough in the United States so that laws have been brought in to protect the public. Unfortunately, they haven't teeth; rather than banning sulfiting agents, restaurants are now merely obliged to post signs stating that they have been used.

Canned foods are chock-full of poisonous chemicals, salt and non-nourishment. Most of the vitamins and minerals are lost through processing, as are all of the precious enzymes, without which the body cannot function efficiently. The cans themselves pose a serious problem because of leaching. This is especially dangerous in canned citrus, berries, or other acidic foods. One hundred and fifty parts per million of tin contamination of the contents was shown in some experiments. Sensitive individuals have been known to become violently ill when exposed to the golden-brown lining which is used to keep the metal from changing the food colour. The seams of the cans are closed with lead, and this leaches into the food, also. Those who store tinned food in the refrigerator are begging for trouble, as contamination increases dramatically each day of storage. In a related incident, a family in Los Angeles, California, brought some pretty pottery back from Mexico. They used one of the jugs to store orange juice in the refrigerator for several days. One of the children died and other family members became deathly ill before it was realised that lead in the pottery had leached into the orange juice. The danger from cans isn't that dramatic, of course. If it were, canned food would be removed from the market and people would be much healthier. But the principle is identical and the dangers are slow and cumulative.

Disgusting things are done by the processors. To facilitate peeling, fruit and vegetable skins may be turned to mush by caustic solutions such as lye. To prevent loss of chlorophyll, magnesium carbonate, or magnesia, is used whether you want a laxative or not. Firming agents, such as monocalcium phosphate, calcium chloride, and citrate may be used in preparation. Since canned food would be an unappetising grey colour without doctoring, soaking in soda or stannous chloride (tin salts) is commonly employed. Most of these distasteful chemicals are not listed on the labels, but you can be sure they are there, just the same. Processors claim they 'dissipate', but processors' track record for veracity and concern for the community leave one unconvinced.

An old saying goes, "The whiter the bread, the sooner you're dead," yet bakers continue producing devitalised, dangerous, deadly white bread, and people go on gobbling it down and giving it to their unsuspecting children. Your mother probably gave it to you, often with peanut butter and jelly, and it was a treat, a part of growing up. Like so many things we grew up with, it's hard to associate it with poison. Yet, poison it is, and it's impossible to build or maintain maximum health while eating the stuff.

Profit Motive

For 30 years flour was bleached with nitrogen trichloride, a central nervous system poison. Now bleaching is done with ammonia, alum, gypsum and chlorine dioxide, all dangerous, in spite of assurances of safety by the food processors. Many scientists deplore this practice, and, in experiments, mice have been shown to suffer stunted growth due to eating flour treated with chlorine dioxide. This makes one wonder why the processors use such harmful chemicals in our foods. Profit is the motive; when using bleaches, it is possible to use very poor quality flours, and the product has a long shelf life. The processors are unconcerned that when they remove the colour from the flour, they also remove the nourishment.

With the exception of the bleaching process, all of the dangers lurking in white flour exist in whole wheat. So, congratulations are not in order for those of you who have been serving your families dark bread, unless you've been grinding your own flour from bio-dynamic grain and baking your own bread, or using a food drier to prepare grain crisps. They maintain all the nourishment as long as the drying temperature is kept below 40° Celsius. If you prefer traditional bread, look at baking day as an opportunity to put some old-fashioned warmth back into family life and get the kids off the street, away from the television and involved in family life.

Of course, at Hippocrates Health Centre we don't advocate the use of any type of cooked bread, however we recognise that not everyone is prepared to stay on an optimum diet, and we prefer those people to eat the least damaging breads. We make dried grain crisps, and they are delicious and healthful for most, but not for gluten-intolerant persons.

Bear in mind, while groaning about the time spent baking, the following facts about commercial flour and baked goods: the original wheat seeds are treated with mercury poison, and in storage bins cyanogen gas is sprayed on them. Later, bakers saturate the dough with mycoban or calcium propionate, which destroys the enzyme that makes it possible for our bodies to assimilate calcium. They use it because it stops mould, unaware or uncaring that anything which retards the growth of a living organism must also be dangerous to people.

There may be as many as 80 ingredients in a loaf of bread, and few of them are listed. Most of them are non-foods, and many are dangerous. There are dyes, preservatives, antioxidants, mould retarders, bread improvers, extenders, emulsifiers, leaveners and conditioners. Some are used instead of eggs, milk and shortenings, because chemicals are cheaper than real food. Others are used to make distribution easier and shelf life longer. These chemical breads remain 'fresh' for a long time, passing the 'squeeze test'. And why not? They're not food anymore, and there's nothing to rot.

By the time everyone has gotten into the act, most bread is unfit for consumption, human or animal. Weevils have more sense than some people – they won't eat white flour. Not only is it chock full of poison, but all the vitamins, minerals and enzymes have been removed in the milling process, and fed to hogs. 'Enriched' flour is a farce. Synthetic coal-tar vitamins are pumped in after the natural nutrients are milled out. Bread made with this kind of flour is the staff of death, and should carry the skull and crossbones.

It is wise to avoid any food that has a numbered ingredient on its label. Those numbers were put on due to consumer pressure – too many people were being poisoned, and even killed, because they didn't know what they were eating – and most of the numbers represent chemicals no sane person would choose to eat or drink. As a tiny example, 'Additive 920' is manufactured from animal hair and chicken feathers. The anonymous 'Bread Improver', which is in so many commercial breads and in many bread maker recipes, is to be avoided, because of the aluminium and other dangerous additives present.

As our appointed 'guardians', governments around the world have failed miserably in their duty of care towards safeguarding our health, by abdicating their role in favour of allowing the chemical companies and food manufacturers to call the shots.

The most important thing to understand when choosing food is that governments will absolutely not protect consumers from the processors. The subject is too complicated for politicians. More sinister, the food processors are too rich and their lobbyists are too powerful and/or generous for politicians to make headway against their dangerous practices, even if they had the motivation, the interest, or the knowledge. They don't, and they probably never will; *as ever, we must protect ourselves!*

As an example of the devil-may-care attitude the Australian government and other governments in 'civilised' countries have adopted, following is a list of a few of the chemicals permitted in our food supply:

Benzyl alcohol; isopropyl alcohol; ethyl alcohol; propylene glycol; glycerin; mannitol; sorbitol; polydextrose; ethyl acetate; glyceryl monoacetate; glycerol diacetate; triacetin; triethyl citrate; edible fats and oils; sugars; sodium chloride; erythritol; modifying agents; natural starches; maltodextrin; gelatin; hydrogenated coconut oil; calcium silicate; potassium caseinate; sodium aluminosilicate; magnesium carbonate; calcium sodium alumino silicate; calcium phosphate; tribasic; calcium hydroxyphosphate.

These chemicals are actually permitted in the food we eat! Do you think your government has any inkling of what damage some, or all of them, may do? Has anyone, anywhere, even considered what interactions these chemicals may have? It is not specifically stated, but I have reason to suspect that some of these chemicals are in *baby food*! Aspartame is permitted in baby food, so why not the above chemicals, many of which are thought to be carcinogens? Do you want to feed these chemicals to your family? I certainly don't, and that is why I never buy any manufactured food. I hope you will follow my example.

6

Oils and Fats

The facts behind all that industry misinformation

Cholesterol is not the enemy. In fact, if you do not provide your body with enough of the right kind of fats, your body will have to manufacture its own cholesterol. And remember, our bodies are a lot smarter than the food industry's hired gun scientists.

What I am about to say regarding oils is not what the food chemists want you to know about, or what the expensive ads postulate. This information flies in the face of the 'conventional wisdom', which may be conventional, but certainly isn't wise: all of the polyunsaturated oils that are now promoted as healthful, are not. In fact, they are dangerous. In order to maintain your health, shun these hyped, manufactured, oxidised, chemicalised products.

The polyunsaturate-pushers don't want you to know the truth. For decades their propaganda has covered up the dangers associated with having low blood cholesterol, and the safety of the old-fashioned fats and oils that have nourished countless generations.

Lost in the shuffle are the hundreds of studies proving that low cholesterol leads to much higher deaths from cancer. These studies have appeared for decades in obscure medical journals and in the books of corporate-neutral scientists. Regrettably, few people are exposed to them. But articles praising the heart 'benefits' of polyunsaturated oils appear everywhere. So, too, do the glossy, full-page advertisements their manufacturers have paid for. Remember, advertisements are the lifeblood of most magazines and newspapers. When the ads are accompanied by favourable articles, it is prudent to look with healthy scepticism upon the products they promote.

A study in Honolulu showed that age-adjusted mortality from cancer was four times higher in the low serum cholesterol group, compared to the high serum cholesterol group. In a Yugoslavian study, as cholesterol levels fell, total mortality rose. In Malmo, Sweden, the lowest serum cholesterol group was associated with the highest death rate, mainly due to cancer and other non-coronary heart disease causes.

Men, are you aware that without the right kind of cholesterol, your body will be unable to manufacture its own testosterone? Apart from the obvious masculinity problems, scientists have identified low testosterone as the cause of 'Irritable Male Syndrome', the grumpy, non-communicative, moody male that makes life miserable for his wife and family.

Shorter Life

Gary Taubes, the author of **The Soft Science of Dietary Fat**, wrote in **Science Magazine**, *2001*, "Men with very low cholesterol levels seemed prone to premature death; the lower the cholesterol the shorter the life… Men with cholesterol levels below 4.1mmol/L tended to die prematurely from cancer, respiratory and digestive diseases and trauma. As for women, the higher the cholesterol the longer they lived.

Dr Robert Jay Rowen agrees. In his newsletter, **Second Opinion**, he writes, "Cholesterol dangers are largely a myth… The majority of heart attacks in this country [*the US*] are incurred by people in the 'normal' range… I see a 67-year-old woman with cholesterol levels over 800 with no signs of vascular disease or hypertension whatsoever!"

Women must have cholesterol. Without this vital nutrient, their bodies will not be able to produce the hormones they need for their reproductive cycle, and to keep them healthy throughout their later years.

Perhaps most telling of all is what leading endocrinologist Dr Raymond Peat wrote in his book, **From PMS to Menopause**: "Unsaturated oils, especially polyunsaturates, weaken the immune system's function in ways that are similar to the damage caused by radiation, hormone imbalance, cancer, aging, or viral infections. The media discuss sexually-transmitted and drug-induced immunodeficiency, but it isn't yet considered polite to discuss vegetable oil-induced immunodeficiency."

The hysterical cholesterol scare campaign gained currency for all the wrong reasons shortly after World War II, and was picked up by the food manufacturers and health professionals who didn't read the research, and blown into a dangerous cult. Sure, some fats are deadly – but they are the *manufactured* fats, such as margarine, homogenised milk, soy oil, corn oil, etc. In short, all of the heavily-promoted oils are dangerous, and the fats and oils reviled by the huge companies – coconut oil, butter and olive oil, are the good fats. But only if they are properly formulated and carefully stored.

For decades, the multinationals who manufacture trans-fats and unsaturated oils manipulated research, in order to promote the sale of their chemicalised, oxidised products, which are unfit for consumption – human or animal! In doing so, they have taken attention away from the real causes of heart disease – sugar, junk food, heavy grain consumption and the wrong kinds of fats. In spite of all the glossy ads and the misinformation campaigns that have led our health practitioners astray, cholesterol, unless it is oxidised, is a valuable nutrient. We need it because it is the precursor of progesterone, oestrogen, DHEA, pregnenolone and other hormones. Our bodies cannot manufacture these invaluable hormones without it.

Can Cause Impotence

According to Dr John Lee, "This decades-long misinformation campaign has been a contributing factor in the meteoric rise in the incidence of heart disease and cancer, and has helped bring billions of dollars in profits to companies selling both cholesterol-lowering drugs and hydrogenated oils." Men who are prescribed these drugs, usually without warning from their physicians, learn the hard way that they can cause impotence. If you are unconvinced, please see *Chapter 14*, *The Perils of Prostate*, to learn what these oils do to the male prostate gland.

For those of you who need any more reasons to embrace a healthful diet, consider this: if you eat and drink yourself into severe heart disease and your physician warns that a bypass is your only option, you run a 42 percent risk of brain damage, neurological complications, and suffering a stroke on the operating table.

Dr Julian Whitaker, of Whitaker Wellness Institute Medical Clinic (*www.drwhitaker.com*), explains why: "There are several explanations for this. Ill effects of anaesthesia may be a factor. Inflammatory chemicals that are released in massive quantities during surgery likely have adverse effects as well. However, the primary culprit appears to be the heart-lung machine... which may introduce air bubbles into the bloodstream that can interfere with blood flow to the brain. Even worse, messing with the aorta loosens embolic matter (small bits of plaque and blood clots), which can break off, travel up the carotid arteries in the neck, lodge in the blood vessels of the brain, and disrupt oxygen delivery."

Be wary of doctors and persuasive glossy advertisements pushing statin (cholesterol-lowering) drugs. They work by blocking an important enzyme the body uses to make cholesterol, but the makers have evidently not considered what other essential work that enzyme may be required to do. Or, perhaps with an eye only on the bottom line, they simply do not care.

Then there are the well-documented side effects: intestinal disease, increased risk of cancer, stroke, suicide and severe Alzheimer's Disease. Bayer had to withdraw its statin drug, *Baycol*, from the US market, when it was found to be responsible for 31 deaths from a muscle-destroying disease. Another, *Cervistatin*, was also taken off the market when it created the same problems. **Public Citizen**, a US consumer watchdog, petitioned the government to force drug companies to warn Americans that they should quit the pills at the first sign of muscle pain or weakness. How about warning them not to take these drugs at all? And, where are the consumer watchdogs in Australia? Recently, one pharmaceutical firm patented the inclusion of Co-Q$_{10}$ in its newest statin. This happened because they finally acknowledged that statin drugs reduce synthesis of this nutrient, which is vital for heart health. This means, of course, that none of the other firms making statins will be able to add Q$_{10}$ to their formulation. Dr Whitaker believes this gives grounds for a huge class-action suit by patients who have been damaged by statins without being warned to take supplemental Q$_{10}$.

Failed to Protect the Heart

Dr Duane Graveline, on American radio show, *The People's Pharmacy*, told of bouts of total amnesia he experienced while taking a statin drug. Pfizer, who make the statin drug, *Lipitor*, deny that there have been any reports of memory loss. But then, they would, wouldn't they? Lipitor brings them in more than US$5 billion per year!

A large Hungarian study, reported in **Dr Peat's Newsletter**, showed that using a drug to lower cholesterol failed to protect the heart, and greatly increased the cancer death rate. "It is now widely recognised that the pattern of blood lipids associated with lower incidence of heart disease – higher blood levels of the High Density Lipids (HDL) and lower levels of the Low Density Lipids (LDL) – is associated with a higher cancer risk. It seems that any intervention – not just excess vegetable oil – which lowers the LDL cholesterol will increase the risk of cancer." Wow! In other words, just the opposite of what the 'experts' say.

The lesson to be learned here is that all of us should consume as perfect a diet as possible, shun drugs, and keep the sickness industry at bay. Don't let them play Russian roulette with your heart and life!

Dr Peat quotes experiments that show even a 'moderate' use of unsaturated oils in the diet accelerates aging. Mice fed soy oil produced offspring with smaller brains and learning difficulties, compared to the offspring of mice given coconut oil. He says, "The brain seems to be especially sensitive to the toxic effects of vegetable oils." Dr Peat also says that if polyunsaturated oils are not eaten, vitamin E needs become low, and he warns that women should shun unsaturated oils during pregnancy, in order to protect their babies.

Mother's milk is rich in cholesterol, and nature didn't put it there because it is bad for infants. It is there to ensure proper development of the nervous system and brain. Whenever women tell me proudly that they have their babies and older children on margarine and low-fat milk I am horrified. These children will never realise their full potential – they are being starved of the kind of fats the brain needs. Denying babies and children the right kinds of fat is child abuse, and any physician or so-called health professional who advises this starvation diet should be ashamed. And, while I'm railing against the health advisors, they have either forgotten or never learned that a major cause of extremely high cholesterol is low thyroid function. Often, just bringing the thyroid up to normal (as discussed in *Chapters 1* and *2*) will bring cholesterol into a normal range.

Rancidity

Flax oil has been heavily promoted for several years as 'essential' for health, and many people force themselves to take a tablespoon each day, even though they don't like the taste. This is misguided, according to Dr Peat, who considers it "…the most carcinogenic of oils"! The British alternative medical newsletter, *What Doctors Don't Tell You,* carried out exhaustive tests on all the brands of flax oil sold in London. They found that most were rancid, which is dangerous because rancidity promotes cancer. Two were not rancid, but the magazine reported that they turned rancid after a few days of refrigeration.

Next time a health professional urges you to consume this oil, ask why it comes in a dark bottle and must be refrigerated immediately. Commonsense dictates that this is because it is highly unstable and readily breaks down into free radicals. If that doesn't scare you, this should: under the influence of unsaturated fats (including flax oil) brain cells swell, and their shape and interactions are altered. For more information on flax, see pages 214 - 215 and 221.

> ### *Radical Facts*
> What are these 'free radicals' we hear so much about? This is Dr Peat's definition: "Free radicals are reactive molecular fragments that occur even in healthy cells, and can damage the cell. When unsaturated oils are exposed to free radicals they can create chain reactions of free radicals that spread the damage in the cell, and contribute to the cell's aging."

As for the so-called, much-touted 'essential fatty acids', consider this quote from Dr Peat's book, *From PMS To Menopause*:

> Essential fatty acids are, according to the textbooks, linoleic acid and linolenic acid, and they are supposed to have the status of 'vitamins,' which must be taken in the diet to make life possible. However, we are able to synthesise our own unsaturated fats when we don't eat the EFA, so they are not 'essential.' The term thus appears to be a misnomer. *(M.E. Hanke, BIOCHEMISTRY, Encycl. Brit. Book of the Year, 1948).*

Intrinsically Toxic

Far from being 'essential', these oils are intrinsically toxic and should be avoided. They inhibit enzymes that are needed for digestion and for the production of thyroid hormones. As Dr Peat writes, these oils "increase the risk of abnormal blood clotting, inflammation, immune deficiency, shock, aging, obesity and cancer... Since the unsaturated oils block protein in the stomach, we can be malnourished even while 'eating well'....

Linoleic acid constricts blood vessels and promotes hypertension... and is specifically associated with serotonin-dependent disorders such as migraine.... Polyunsaturated fats contribute significantly, maybe decisively, to the degenerative changes that occur in aging." Flax oil and all the other unsaturated oils are everywhere – small wonder there is so much serious illness in the 'civilised' world. There's more on flax oil in **Chapter 14, The Perils of Prostate.**

Canola oil should also be shunned, but this is easier said than done, as it is ubiquitous. The only way to keep it out of your diet is by strict avoidance of fast food outlets, by keeping junk food out of your life and by being fussy when choosing manufactured foods. Remember, when you are tempted by a quick snack: **Fast Food = Fast Death!**

Nutritional experts Sally Fallon and Mary Enig, PhD, in a lengthy article in **Wise Traditions**, wrote, "... canola oil is definitely not healthy for the cardiovascular system. Like rapeseed oil, its predecessor, canola oil is associated with fibrotic lesions of the heart. It also causes vitamin E deficiency, undesirable changes in the blood platelets and shortened lifespan in stroke-prone rats... Furthermore, it seems to retard growth, which is why the FDA does not allow the use of canola oil in infant formula." Finally, the FDA did something right!

Margarine, one of the worst offenders, must be avoided. During the many chemical processes used to manufacture this product, hexane and carbon tetrachloride are used as solvents, and traces remain. To achieve a butter-like consistency, hydrogen gas is bubbled over a nickel catalyst, saturating the fat and turning it into an artery-clogger.

These chemical insults create an odoriferous black goop, which must be bleached and deodorised with even more chemicals. Then artificial flavours, dyes and preservatives are added. The result is a plastic, chemical non-food that your body does not know how to deal with or detoxify. You might just as well inject liquid plastic into your veins. Amazingly, many doctors still recommend this stuff for prevention of heart attacks!

Risk of Heart Disease

The New England Journal of Medicine reported that trans-fats (polyunsaturated fats) *increase* the risk of heart disease by damaging arteries. These dangerous fats are in all fast food, fried food and most bakery goods. They are produced when polyunsaturated vegetable fats are artificially hydrogenated. When you see "partially hydrogenated oil" on a label, put it back on the shelf. This is the dreaded trans-fat, and it is a killer. Dr Peat agrees that these oils damage the heart, and adds, "It is now known that polyunsaturated fats interfere with thyroid hormone in just about every conceivable way." Healthy functioning of the thyroid gland is essential for good health. Dr Peat also wrote, "The easily-oxidised short-and medium-chain saturated fatty acids of coconut oil provide a source of energy that protects our tissues against the toxic inhibitory effects of the unsaturated fatty acids and reduces their anti-thyroid effects."

For the sake of your health, ignore the 'experts' who jumped on the bandwagon, and search out the alternative health professionals who know the truth behind one of the most cynical and dangerous publicity campaigns ever mounted. Dr William Campbell Douglass is one, and he has graciously permitted me to reprint the following from his newsletter, *Second Opinion*:

> Coconut oil is the best example of an innocent saturated oil getting the reputation of clogger of arteries because of a misinterpretation of the research. The wrong interpretation was then repeated until it became 'a known fact' that the food manufacturers were killing us by using large amounts of coconut oil. Now there are a lot of things wrong with the food industry, and they do use a lot of unhealthy oils in their foods, but coconut oil isn't one of them. In fact, the seed-oil cartel has managed, by what nefarious method I don't know, to almost eliminate coconut oil from the diet of the American people.
>
> Twenty-five years ago, I was taken in by the seed-oil company propaganda against coconut oil, just like everybody else. It was easy to fool us: coconut oil is a saturated fat; 'saturated fat is bad'. And there's the economic factor; that's the one that really counts. Coconut oil is relatively expensive. Soy bean, peanut and corn oils are not. But these cheap oils that are used in processed foods today are very unstable. They can become rancid in just a few hours, even in the refrigerator. So the answer to that problem, you may have already guessed, is the addition of a lot of preservatives.
>
> Coconut oil, for reasons not completely understood, does not become rancid, even though it contains a small amount of unsaturated oils. Coconut oil has been left at room temperature for a year without developing any rancidity. The five percent of unsaturated oils in coconut oil should turn rancid, but they don't. It is theorised that the saturated oil in coconut oil has an antioxidative effect and thus prevents the oxidation of the unsaturates present in the oil.
>
> Unsaturated oils cause cancer; the research is there to confirm it, but few people have seen it. **The 'essential' fatty acid, linoleic acid, when fed to experimental animals, gives them heart disease.** But if you give the animals saturated fat, in the form of animal fat or coconut oil, they will be protected from the harmful effects of the 'essential' unsaturated linoleic acid. This is clearly understood in the organ transplant field. Emulsions of unsaturated oils are used specifically for their immuno-suppressive effects. Is that what you want on your salad – oils, such as canola and soy bean, that suppress your immune system? Or would you prefer an oil, like coconut oil, that protects you against the ravages of immune suppression?
>
> Fifty years ago, farmers attempted to fatten their livestock by using coconut oil, which was a lot cheaper than grains. They reasoned that fat (any fat) would make the animals fat, a simple and self-evident postulate. But they were wrong. What they got instead was lean and perky, rather than fat and indolent. Granted, the cows were hungry all the time, and ate a lot, but they didn't get fat.
>
> So, back to the drawing board. They next tried drugs that would suppress the function of the thyroid. It worked; the animals got fat on less food. But the compounds were found to be carcinogenic and it was feared that the meat would in turn give cancer to

the consumers. So they decided to try various cheap beans, such as soy, and cheap vegetables, such as corn.

Both soy beans and corn worked. And here is the point of all this animal husbandry: the soy beans and corn suppressed the thyroid gland, just like the drugs, and the animals got fat without consuming a lot of food. So do you wonder why it's hard to lose weight on these oil-based vegetarian diets? You don't lose weight if your thyroid gland is suppressed, you gain it. What the farmers already knew was later 'proven' with animal studies. The animals fed unsaturated vegetable oils, such as soy and corn, were fat; the animals fed coconut oils were lean. The total amount of fat eaten was not the controlling factor. The higher the ratio of unsaturated oil to coconut oil, the fatter the animal, no matter what the quantity of oil ingested.

And there are other reasons not to use the unsaturated oils. The seed oils block proteolytic enzymes, which is probably why they block the production of thyroid hormone. But they also block digestive enzymes and affect the clotting mechanism.

Even worse is the effect of the unsaturated oils on the brain. Soy oils are incorporated directly into the brain, making the brain structurally abnormal. Children fed exclusively on unsaturated oils are not going to develop normally unless they get the protective effect of coconut oil.

As expected, the drug companies have fractionated coconut oil to obtain patentable products, such as butyric acid, because it's well known that coconut oil contains many important nutrients. But you don't need purified products; you just need coconut oil. The natural coconut oil acts as an antihistamine, an anti-diabetic, an anti-cancer agent, and an anti-infective.

The *Journal of the American Medical Association* agrees with Dr Douglass: "Coconut oil may be one of the most useful oils to prevent heart disease because of its antiviral and antimicrobial characteristics (*JAMA 1967 202:1119-1123*; *American Journal of Clinical Nutrition 1981 34:1552*).

"In Framingham, Massachusetts, the more saturated fat one ate, the more cholesterol one ate, the more calories one ate, the lower people's serum cholesterol... we found that the people who ate the most saturated fat weighed the least and were the most physically active." (William Castelli, director of *The Framingham Study*).

"The diet-heart hypothesis had been repeatedly shown to be wrong, and yet, for complicated reasons of pride, profit and prejudice, the hypothesis continues to be exploited by scientists, fundraising enterprises, food companies and even governmental agencies. The public is being deceived by the greatest health scam of the century." (George Mann, MD, renowned researcher).

"An analysis of cholesterol values in 1,700 patients with atherosclerotic disease revealed no definite correlation between serum cholesterol levels and the nature and extent of atherosclerotic disease." (Michael DeBakey, MD, famous heart surgeon).

The pioneering *Townsend Letter for Doctors and Patients* states: "Coconut oil is particularly useful as it has an essential saturated fat, lauric acid.

Trans-fat is the fat that should be absolutely avoided at all times. Read labels. Any time you see partially hydrogenised fat - that means trans-fat. Avoid it... Organic, unrefined coconut oil is safe. However, most other coconut oil products are hydrogenated. Coconut oil has been subjected to a smear campaign by commercial vegetable oil producers, but the research studies cited have used *hydrogenated* coconut oil, which has skewed the results."

Skin Care

Dr Peat has this advice for women; he suggests avoiding skin creams containing polyunsaturated botanical oils because they promote aging of the skin by intensifying the effects of the sun's ultraviolet rays. He recommends coconut oil as the best for skin care, and so do I. It's the only cleanser or moisturiser I use, and I always give it to my massage therapist, because I don't want any dangerous oils absorbed through my skin.

The Health Centre's interest in coconut oil started years ago when we read the following story in **Health and Healing Wisdom**, the journal of the Price-Pottenger Nutrition Foundation:

More On Rancidity

Regarding the rancidity in most oils, Dr Peat said, in one of his informative *Newsletters*, "The fact that saturated fats are dominant in tropical plants and in warm-blooded animals relates to the stability of these oils at high temperatures. Coconut oil which had been stored at room temperature for a year was found to have no measurable rancidity. Since growing coconuts often experience temperatures around 100 degrees Fahrenheit, ordinary room temperature isn't an oxidative challenge. Fish oil or safflower oil, though, can't be stored long at room temperature, and at 98 degrees F the spontaneous oxidation is very fast."

"When an AIDS sufferer found that his viral load had reached almost 700,000, he decided that the best use of his money and remaining time on Earth was a relaxing vacation. He chucked all the vitamins and drugs he was using – including *Naltrexone* – packed his bags and headed for an Indian village in Surinam. There he dined on fresh coconut meat every day. Within two days his peripheral neuropathy was gone and within two weeks, he was 'running through the jungle'. Back home, and continuing to consume at least one-half of a coconut per day, his lab tests showed that the viral load had dropped to just over 300,000. Within another month the viral load had dropped to non-detectable levels and he had gained 32 pounds."

This little paragraph came like a bolt from the blue. Knowing the integrity of this non-profit foundation I decided to research coconut, starting by turning myself into a guinea pig – not for the first time! Within minutes, I was on the way to our local supermarket. Unfortunately, green, soft flesh coconuts are hard to find in cities so dried nuts are the next best thing.

A coconut novice, I didn't have the sense to ask the produce man to saw the coconuts in half and empty the liquid into a jar. (Some will cooperate, some won't, I later discovered). Fired with enthusiasm, I rushed home, not giving a second thought to the task ahead – how to open two incredibly hard spheres.

After trial and error I discovered the way to proceed, and the following are my recommendations, but first, when choosing your coconuts, shake them to make sure there is plenty of liquid inside. If not, they are old and probably spoiled. Be sure to keep your sales slip because sometimes even those with liquid are found to be spoiled, and the market will return your money.

Preparation

If your produce man is uncooperative, you will have to fend for yourself, this way:

Take the nuts outside, along with a hammer, screwdriver and a jar. Prop the coconut between your knees, place the screwdriver on one of the eyes, and hammer it into the eye, until it slips in easily. Then do the same with the other two eyes, being careful not to spill the liquid. Up-end the nut and pour the liquid into the jar. Taste it. If it's sweet, you have a good nut. If it smells or tastes sour or offensive, you have an old nut. If it's good, drink the liquid while it's fresh. If you have eyestrain or cataracts, put some of the water in a glass dropper bottle and use the healing water as eye drops. After removing the water, cover the nut with an old towel or a plastic bag and hit it, hard, with the hammer until it breaks into pieces.

Then you will have to remove the meat from the husk, which is easier said than done. But persevere, it will come out. Don't be concerned by the thin, brown coating on the outside of the meat. There is nothing wrong with it. And, please, don't attempt to chew the meat – you run the risk of cracking a tooth that way.

Once you have the meat separated from the husk, the best approach is to shred it. I use a *Champion Juicer*, with the 'blank' on. This shreds beautifully. If you use a different shredder, make sure it doesn't heat up, and don't under any circumstances use aluminium; it is toxic and will contaminate the coconut. I then put my coconut in a food drier, although it isn't necessary. Undried, it will keep well in the fridge. It tastes better, and is slightly crunchy, dried, and appears to keep better. But remember, if you opt for drying, be sure the drier doesn't have aluminium trays, and keep it at a low temperature so the nutrients aren't destroyed, 40° Celsius (104° Fahrenheit) or under. Most Indian stores sell a great and inexpensive coconut scraper that gets the meat out simply, if you first saw the coconut in half. For those of you who do not have this equipment, or the time to go through this exercise, there is another way – buy pure, unadulterated coconut oil. More about that below.

At the health centre we stick to the Hippocrates Programme, which has been incredibly successful since it was established by Ann Wigmore in 1960. We do not experiment on anyone. This does not deter *me* from meddling, however, in my private life, and I started recommending the coconut I had prepared to acquaintances with symptoms of viruses. Without exception, their symptoms vanished. Because of this, I keep a supply of dried coconut in the freezer, and use pure coconut oil daily. Both taste delicious, and who knows when I might overwork, get run down, and encounter an opportunistic virus? Or a microbe, or a cancer cell or a protozoa? Those meanies are everywhere, more than ever with jet travel commonplace, and it's wise not to issue any invitations to the dirty, rotten scoundrels.

Lauric Acid

Every illness is different, as is every case. Fortunately, experimentation is not dangerous, and you will have to figure out for yourself how much you need, and how often. Proceed slowly, bearing in mind that coconut flesh is rich, and too much can be hard on susceptible digestive systems, and the liver. I prefer the oil to dried coconut as it is easier and perfect for cooking.

After proving to my satisfaction the benefits of coconut, I wanted to know – *why*? So, I rang the Price-Pottenger Foundation and talked to their dedicated, helpful editor, Pat Connolly. She suggested that I read a back issue of their journal, which contained an article by Mary Enig, PhD, an expert of international renown in the field of lipid chemistry. Dr Enig, who has impeccable credentials, is able to practice pure science, as her research is not 'bought and paid for' by the food conglomerates.

Dr Enig has done an enormous amount of research on coconut oil. She has found the oil to be not only antiviral, but anti-microbial, anti-protozoal and anti-carcinogenic. This is extraordinary information, and Dr Enig quotes other research studies made by many other prestigious scientists. She cited studies which found the lauric acid in pure coconut has adverse effects on various micro-organisms, such as bacteria, intestinal yeast overgrowth, fungi and enveloped viruses. She states that it was found that lauric acid *causes the disintegration of the virus envelope!*

Important Nutrient

"Some of the viruses inactivated by the lipids in lauric acid are measles virus, herpes simplex, vesicular stomatitis virus, visna virus and cytomegalovirus," she says. There are also several studies described in this article which found that dietary coconut oil, as widely used in island communities, does not cause high cholesterol levels. Breast milk contains lauric acid for the protection of babies, indicating that nature considers this an important nutrient.

It is nothing short of criminal that the medical profession has ignored the healing properties of coconuts. According to Mary Enig, immune-compromised people should ingest about 25gm of lauric acid per day. She based this figure on comparative levels found in human breast milk. If using oil only, this would amount to four tablespoons per day for an adult. It can be used in soups, as salad dressings, and for sautéing food and in drinks.

Coconut milk, if you can find a pure one, is another option, as four ounces contain about 11gm of lauric acid. Fresh, shredded coconut contains about 6gm per ½ cup. Although I don't approve of it myself, since I don't know what 'they' have done to it, another possibility is desiccated coconut. It, too, contains about 6gm of lauric acid per ½ cup. But please remember: **no** hydrogenated coconut oil, and **no** 'lite' oil!

These large amounts are recommended by Dr Enig only for those with severe immune system problems. Smaller amounts are adequate for others.

Those of you who remain phobic about cholesterol, even after the evidence I've compiled, must now be trying to decide which is worse – eating an oil which is not recommended by the multinational food industry and by ill-informed health professionals, or the virus or bacteria you are trying to banish.

When you consider what commercial food processors do to coconuts before they reach the stores, it's small wonder that proprietary coconut oils, grated coconut and other end products are toxic. They burn the coconut, dry it at extremely high temperatures, store it in dirty sacks, then bleach and deodorise it, because the manufacturing processes make it look and smell disgusting. And, in the case of oil, after all the above insults, they homogenise and hydrogenate it. They call it *RBD Oil* (Refined, Bleached, Deodorised) and it's a disaster – everything decent has been killed.

For years, we were unable to find a good coconut oil. They all smelled of chemicals, and now I know why. Finally, after months of phone calls to several countries, I was able to locate a superb oil, and the Hippocrates Health Centre is importing it. It is made by native South Pacific communities, using very old and safe methods. Nothing is done which can hurt the oil, and the presses are washed only with hot water, never the benzene or other poisons most oil processors use. These poisons, of course, end up in small amounts in most of the conventionally-processed oils. Manufacturers stress the minute amounts, ignoring the cumulative effects of years of poisons our bodies are expected to detoxify.

Dr Peat has this to say about coconut oil: "This oil contains immunity-boosting lauric acid, also found in mother's milk. For these reasons, its regular use offers protection against disease and premature aging." Dr Peat recommends taking about an ounce each day, as salad dressing. Many people have reported to me that they take much more than this and claim that it has helped them greatly.

Dr John R Lee concurs with this, and also with Dr Douglass, that "An added bonus is that by increasing the metabolic rate via the thyroid, coconut oil, in spite of being a fat, has been known to bring about an amazing loss of excess weight. Farmers, in fact, who thought it would be an inexpensive way to fatten their animals, found it had just the opposite effect!"

Addressing the irrational fears most people have regarding this oil and heart attacks, Dr Lee also states, "Equatorial people, whose main source of fat is unrefined coconut oil, tend to be very free of heart disease."

The Good Oil on Oils

So, what oils and fats can you eat and maintain your health? The Hippocrates Health Centre does not use any oils, because they have no place in a healing centre, where the students need to detoxify. Avocado is used at the centre, and is an ideal vegetable fat, containing no cholesterol, for those who are *still* afraid of this much-maligned substance. It is delicious cut up in salads, and we have many recipes for sauces made with avocado and other ingredients to make a tasty salad dressing.

Once Hippocrates graduates go home, however, they want to know if they can use any oils and fats in a 'transition' diet and still stay well. To these people we recommend the following:

Olive Oil

Buy only green olive oil, or extra virgin for salads, and make sure it is in a dark bottle, to avoid the oxidation that occurs when oil is exposed to light. Be sure to refrigerate after opening. Please do not cook with olive oil, as heating oxidizes it and creates free radicals, which we all need to avoid.

Butter

This fat, recommended by all the oil experts I trust, contains the valuable A and D vitamins, which are vital for the proper absorption of calcium, and efficient functioning of the thyroid gland. The fatty acids in butter are valuable to the immune system, and the lipids in butter protect gastrointestinal health. These fatty acids are burned for quick energy, rather than stored as fat. According to the American health journal, *Health Freedom News*, "The notion that butter causes weight gain is a sad misconception." But this does not confer open slather – moderation is essential. Tragically, 'they' have ruined this nourishing food by taking the cattle out of grassy pastures where, in the 'good old days', they were free to absorb the life-giving nutrients nature provided. They are now fed the cheapest, most unhealthy grains, dosed with drugs, and treated inhumanely. If you can locate a dairy that allows their cows to live according to the laws of nature, their butter will be high in life-giving omega-3 fats and will nourish your family.

New Zealand's butter and meat are said to be from grass-fed livestock. The Americans, in some States, are fortunate to have certified dairies, as well as organically raised meat. In Australia some health stores carry meat and butter from properly raised animals. Please let us know if you are able to find any. Always purchase the unsalted variety, and do not use it for frying.

Because of my well-founded mistrust of the food manufacturers, my recommendation is for people to churn their own butter. Ideally, find a dairyman willing to sell you pure, uncontaminated milk. The big problem for most of us is finding time for such things!

Coconut Oil

For all the reasons already mentioned, and from a great deal of experience, I am convinced that this is the most healthful oil available. Nature has wisely provided the coconut with protection against tropical heat, so its oil does not turn rancid or oxidise in hot weather. Nor does it create free radicals when heated. Because of this, coconut oil is the only oil I consider safe to use in cooking.

Storage is also not a problem. Although I do not recommend it, I have stored it un-refrigerated for four years without noticing a rancid smell or flavour.

Dr Peat urges people to eat at least one ounce (30ml) per day in order to maintain health. I believe much more is safe and extremely beneficial. Do not allow yourself to be taken in by the seed oil propagandists who claim it contributes to high cholesterol. On the contrary, Pacific Islanders, who rely on this oil, have amazing heart health. Those who have reported results to me of using it in large quantity assure me that their cholesterol has dropped! I eat two to four tablespoons per day and my cholesterol is lower than it has ever been, yet not so low that it will compromise my health. Yes, it turns hard when exposed to cold, but the moment it is heated in warm water, or placed in the sun for a while, it liquefies, and when it is in the body it is in its liquid state. Do not purchase commercial coconut products because of the processing which can turn it deadly.

> For additional sound information on oils I recommend Dr Peat's books and newsletters, and the work of Mary Enig, PhD, and her co-writer, Sally Fallon, all of which you will find listed in *Resources*.

(Also see polyunsaturated fats in Chapter 12.)

7

Bone Health 1
Demineralisation
... and why most popular osteoporosis treatments are not only ineffective but damaging, too

There is a clearly defined profile of the osteoporosis victim. The main genetic factors are: ancestors from Northern Europe, Britain, China or Japan, family members with the disease, long, slender bones, thin, fair skin, and female sex. The latter is the most influential factor.

This dreadful affliction is eight times more likely to strike women than men. This has proved to be most unfortunate for women, because if it were a 50/50 illness, male-dominated science would presumably have tried harder to learn the causes. To appreciate the truth of this, one has only to observe the way women's physical problems have been neglected through the ages. Men split the atom, built weapons of unimaginable destruction, and spent billions on ego trips through space. Yet, we are still waiting for an effective female contraceptive that doesn't have potentially dangerous side effects.

> **Early Warning Signs of Osteoporosis**
> - **Height Loss**
> - **Unexpected Fractures**
> - **Brittle Fingernails**
> - **Insomnia & Restless Legs**
> - **Leg Cramps at Night**
> - **Periodontal Disease**
> - **Joint Pain**
> - **Unexpected Loss of Teeth**
> - **Transparent Skin**
> - **Back Pain**
> - **Excess Plaque on Teeth**
> - **Heart Palpitations**

There are many examples of this bias, such as the great emphasis that has been placed on preventing heart disease, which has traditionally affected more men than women. Nowadays, there is hardly a doctor who doesn't hand out diet sheets to susceptible persons. Yet, should a female patient enquire about preventing osteoporosis, dairy, calcium tablets and HRT are pushed, with only the rare doctor mentioning the many natural things which can be done to prevent and reverse bone loss.

The unpalatable truth is that we women are on our own in the cold hard world, and it is not a nice feeling. I remember how I felt when I understood that I was a prime genetic candidate for osteoporosis. It was a chilling moment, and it was obvious that I was not going to get help from the medical/pharmaceutical establishment. I had to help myself. We all do.

But first, what is this disease, so much in the news, and the scourge of our middle and old age? The name gives an apt description: *osteo* means bone and *porosis* means porous. Put them together and they spell deep trouble for women, and for men too, if they live into old age, and persist in habits which promote the disease.

A common misconception is that our bones are formed in childhood, grow until we mature, and then do not change. It's natural to get that impression from observing a skeleton. But this is not the case. Our bones are alive! This is why they can develop osteoporosis. Our skeletons are composed of dynamic tissue that is constantly breaking down and regenerating. If our health habits are contrary to what nature demands, there will be more breaking down of our bone cells, and insufficient regeneration to keep our skeletons strong enough to support us. The bones become so porous that the spaces between mineral deposits enlarge and the bones look honeycombed.

When this occurs, a cough or a slight movement may be enough to fracture a bone. The resultant fall may lead to prolonged hospitalisation, and the immobility may lead to pneumonia and death. Many sufferers are never able to walk again.

> ## *Osteoporosis Risk Factors*
> - Early menopause (natural or through surgery)
> - Irregular or absent menstrual periods
> - Never having children
> - Liver disease, coeliac disease, kidney disease
> - Family history of osteoporosis
> - Premature grey hair (half grey by age forty)
> - Thyroid problems
> - Wrong food and beverage choices
> - Exposure to tobacco smoke
> - Caucasian or Asian heritage (those living on Western food)
> - Lack of exercise
> - Thin build, small bone structure short stature
> - Fair skin, blonde or red hair; freckles
> - Lack of sunlight
> - Females more susceptible than males
> - Environmental toxins and heavy metal absorption
> - Sodium fluoride exposure
> - Certain medications

Until adulthood this breaking down (which is called resorption) and regeneration remain equalised. But, starting around age 30, women and men begin to lose approximately one percent of bone per year. Post-menopause, women's loss goes up to approximately five percent per year. Frightening! Men, who have high levels of sex hormones into old age, do not have this hormone-related bone loss. Further, their bones are heavier, initially, and this gives them additional protection. They are not immune, however, because more and more men are now succumbing, due to distorted eating and drinking habits and sedentary lives.

Take Control of Your Health and Escape the Sickness Industry

Because this terrible disease is rampant, it is thought by many people to be unavoidable, a natural outcome of the ageing process. It is not. It is a degenerative condition, and can be avoided and even reversed. So take heart.

As mentioned earlier, genetics plays a large role in your predisposition to osteoporosis. But please do not allow yourself to become complacent if you have no family members with the disease, or are swarthy, short, chubby and have heavy bones. Just remember that the majority of women, and men, in the Western world are constantly in the process of assuring that their bones will crumble, due to ignorance or indifference to the dangers of poor health habits. Don't be one of them. There are lots of things you can do, starting right now, no matter what your age, to ensure a sturdy and productive middle and old age. First, we will start with a vitally important list of no-nos, beginning with one of the worst offenders: sugar – *White Death*.

✗ *Sugar*

Sugar leaches the body of precious minerals and vitamins because of the heavy demands its detoxification and elimination make on the entire system. To protect the blood, so much calcium is leached from the teeth and bones that osteoporosis and decay, and weakening of the entire body, results.

Avoidance of this dangerous substance requires constant vigilance. Often, people are unaware they are eating sugar, because it can be listed as fructose, glucose, levulose, maltose, dextrose, galactose, maltodextrine, corn syrup and maple syrup. Even some vitamins and medicines contain sugar in these disguised forms. It takes effort to banish sugar from your life, but do it for the sake of your bones, if nothing else. See **Chapter 25**, *The Banned List*, for more reasons to avoid sugar.

✗ *Artificial Sweeteners*

Please don't decide to substitute artificial sweeteners like aspartame for sugar. They are even deadlier, and it is impossible to maintain health while ingesting them in any form. It is imperative to read labels carefully because they are in most 'diet' products, chewing gum, and even in medicines, especially those for children. For more information on these deadly products, by far the worst in manufactured foods, see **Chapter 4**, *Excitoxins*.

✗ *Thyroid Medication*

It has been known for decades that synthetic thyroid medications stimulate osteoclast activity, accelerating bone resorption. Only natural, porcine thyroid hormones are safe for your bones. See **Chapter 1,** *That "Mystery Illness",* and **Chapter 10,** *Hormonal Havoc*, for more on this.

X Caffeine

You know that caffeine occurs in coffee, tea, cola and chocolate. Heavy consumption of this chemical doubles your need for calcium because, as the body strains to eliminate what it perceives as poison, it flushes calcium from your body, via the kidneys. It also allows more calcium to be secreted into the gastrointestinal tract. Because of this, three cups of coffee per day increases your osteoporosis risk by 82 percent!

Caffeine is often hidden. For example, according to an article by Jill Margo in **The Australian**, *February 2000*, a 25-year-old West Australian woman died following a massive dose of caffeine. She had not, however, been drinking coffee, but a fashionable drink called *Race 2005 Energy Blast*. This drink, like some other sports drinks, contains guarana, which is high in caffeine. Had she known the drink contained caffeine she would not have drunk it, because she knew caffeine was dangerous for her health. But caffeine was not listed as an ingredient. This woman, according to the inquest into her death, paid with her life due to this omission. The Commonwealth Department of Health concurred, ruling that caffeine was considered likely to have contributed to her death.

Please do not decide to switch to decaffeinated drinks! Dangerous chemicals are used to remove the caffeine, and government regulations permit traces of it to remain. The US National Cancer Institute has warned that these chemicals cause liver cancer in mice.

When asked to comment on this warning, a General Foods spokesman said, "It is most regrettable that consumers have to have their confidence undermined by this kind of information." He didn't even try to deny that his company used cancer-causing chemicals; he was just upset that the public found out about it.

X Soft Drinks

Everything said about the dangers of caffeine also applies to soft drinks, since they contain caffeine in abundant quantities. The caffeine in cola drinks is even more harmful because it is more concentrated, and not wrapped up with tannic acids as in coffee and tea.

The phosphoric acid in soft drinks combines with calcium in the body and causes it to be excreted in the urine, leading to demineralization of the bones. Phosphoric acid also leads to kidney and bladder stones, and stones which get caught in the urethra. Not a pleasant experience!

There are approximately five teaspoons of sugar in every 250ml bottle of non-diet soft drinks. The sugar is necessary because the phosphoric acid makes the acidity of soft drinks approximately that of vinegar, and it would be undrinkable without lots of sugar and flavourings. Persist in drinking this rubbish and your bones will crumble.

X Chocolate

There are four bone enemies in that tempting chocolate treat; sugar and caffeine, lecithin to make it smooth and oxalic acid, which is notorious for combining with calcium and magnesium and rendering them useless, and *theobromine*, an alkaloid related to caffeine which has been shown to cause genetic damage. Next time you get a chocolate attack, don't give in to it – turn to carob, which is delicious and actually beneficial, and it contains lots of calcium.

X Grains

High grain consumption is bad for bones. Gluten intolerance leads to osteoporosis because it causes malabsorption of a wide variety of nutrients that are vital for bone health. This extreme condition, properly called coeliac disease, usually goes undiagnosed, because it doesn't cause gastrointestinal symptoms. There is a non-invasive test for gluten-intolerance that is conclusive, and if you find you have latent coeliac disease you will have to give up all gluten-containing grains (wheat, rye, barley, spelt and oats). Please don't whinge – you will be much healthier in every way, as cooked grains are the enemy of almost all people. Please read *Chapter 16*, *Against the Grain*, for more on the dangers of grains.

X Alcohol

Because our bones constantly break down and renew themselves throughout our lives it is essential to avoid any substance that retards new bone formation. Alcohol does this in several ways; it decreases intestinal absorption of calcium, it damages the liver, thus stopping the metabolic process that supplies your body with vitamin D, which is vitally necessary for calcium utilisation. Alcoholics are known to have ten times the risk of contracting osteoporosis! If you drink alcoholic beverages, cut down to practically nothing or quit altogether. Your bones and the rest of your body will thank you in many ways you can't even imagine.

X Tobacco Smoke

Smokers, and even those exposed to second-hand smoke, have up to 30 percent less bone mineral content than non-smokers. Cadmium, one of the many poisons in tobacco smoke, interferes with new bone formation. Oestrogen levels and vitamin C are decreased by tobacco smoke. This is serious – we need the natural oestrogen, and vitamin C is essential for calcium absorption. Smoking accelerates bone demineralization by decreasing intestinal absorption of calcium. So, if you smoke, please stop. You will be much healthier and your family will benefit enormously. If your friends smoke, lay down ground rules, and if they persist in exposing you to thousands of cancer-causing, bone-destroying chemicals, dump them. Remember, second-hand smoke diminishes the blood supply to the bones and cuts off vital nutrients. There's a lot more on many other awful effects of tobacco smoke in **Chapter 22**, *Smoke Gets in Your Eyes*.

✗ Salt (Sodium Chloride)

Excess table salt causes the loss of large amounts of calcium in the urine, and when calcium is excreted that way, blood levels of calcium drop. This then causes the parathyroid hormone to be released, which has to break down bone in an effort to restore the level of calcium in the blood. An intake of 200mg of salt a day does not apparently affect calcium excretion, but at 2000mg a day there is a noticeable increase of calcium in the urine. This may negate the high calcium in bony, tinned fish, such as sardines. If you eat them, look for the brands that are packed in water and little or no salt. They can be doctored with herbal seasonings and pure, triple virgin olive oil (from a dark bottle, please) to make them quite delicious.

Never use bleached, chemicalised white table salt. If the sodium chloride doesn't get you, the dangerous additives will. Celtic salt is still the way to go, and make sure it is free from chlorine bleach and contains the valuable sea minerals. Alternatively, use the large salt crystals from the Himalayas that have just become available (see **Resources**). Do not go salt-free, as that will lead to adrenal exhaustion.

✗ Dairy Products

For decades we have been bombarded with ads telling us we must drink lots of milk and eat yogurt and cheese in order to get our calcium. The ads don't mention that the calcium in dairy products is altered by pasteurisation and homogenisation and is turned into a hard mineral. When this denatured form of calcium gets into the bloodstream, it cannot be used to build bones, so it gets deposited along the insides of the blood vessels. These deposits can lead to arteriosclerosis or, when it gets deposited in the joints, it can lead to arthritis.

And, of course, dairy products can create mucous, which leads to colds and flu and asthma, which can lead to steroid over-use, which leads to bone demineralization. It's a vicious circle, and the only winners are doctors, hospitals and the drug companies. We are the losers. Some cheeses have the added disadvantage of having aluminium added by manufacturers, for reasons which remain obscure to me, and which should be illegal.

Powdered milk, which is highly advertised and recommended as a non-fat source of calcium, is especially hazardous. In order to thicken the consistency of powdered milk, oxidised cholesterol is added, and this creates a build-up of plaque in the arteries. Avoid this non-food.

Remember that billions of people throughout the third world never drink milk once weaned, and have little osteoporosis, while milk-guzzlers in Western countries are afflicted in ever-increasing numbers. It would not be an exaggeration to state that osteoporosis is in epidemic proportions now in industrialised nations. If you can't give up your milk, stick to goat or sheep yogurt, and be sure it hasn't been denatured.

Failing availability, if you must use milk products, remember that calves fed only pasteurised milk do not survive beyond six weeks. If the milk is also homogenised, they live only two to four weeks. Further, an expert on pasteurisation said that the process destroys 34 enzymes in milk, making it indigestible. I suggest that the 'authorities' who are making it so difficult for us to obtain old-fashioned milk, butter, cheese and cream, should give some thought to why there is such a rash of lactose intolerance, which is no doubt simply an intolerance to the dreadful things done to what used to be a pure food.

X Calcium

This brings us to the contentious and contradictory subject of calcium supplements. For decades there has been a great deal of propaganda about our supposed need for large amounts of calcium, in the form of dairy products and supplements of very doubtful safety and benefit. Because of this, people have been brainwashed to think they must take calcium tablets containing between 800 and 1200mg per day. Contrary to industry's relentless advertising campaigns, the truth is that when large amounts of calcium are administered, the body turns off its production of vitamin D hormone, stopping the bone remodelling process. This results in an unhealthy skeleton.

Excess calcium can be redistributed in the body, and can lead to bone spurs, tendonitis, tennis elbow, arthritis, bursitis, arteriosclerosis, glaucoma and kidney stones. Merely quitting calcium supplementation can bring about a 'miracle' cure of pains of long standing. Susceptible people sometimes feel pains in various parts of the body shortly after ingesting calcium pills. I am one of them – even a tiny amount gives me joint pain in just one day.

Dr John Lee, in his *Newsletter*, says, "The majority of calcium available is almost un-absorbable, so people get very little out of it. What's not used and converted into bone material will end up being excreted through the kidneys. I find it common that women who are put on high calcium supplements develop kidney stones after a year or two." In his newsletter, ***Second Opinion***, Dr William Campbell Douglass warns that calcium phosphate reduces iron absorption by 62 percent, causing life-threatening anaemia in elderly women. He writes, "Don't take calcium supplements unless you have a disease of the parathyroid gland that requires it – which is highly unlikely. You get plenty of calcium from your diet." I agree completely.

This is what the ***Journal of the American Medical Association*** said about calcium: *(284-11-:1425-29)* "Researchers obtained calcium supplements derived from a variety of sources and produced and distributed by a variety of manufacturers and analysed them for lead content. In this study, sea bed 'oyster shell' calcium supplements varied in lead content, from undetectable to high levels. 'Refined' (calcium carbonate) supplements also varied considerably in lead content, and name brands offered no protection from lead – some brand products tested had much higher lead content than did generic brands. The researchers also noted that consumers 'cannot assume that a given brand is uniformly safe, because some products may have high and others low lead levels.' Even individual formulations within a given brand may vary in lead levels over time, because of batch-to-batch inconsistency in lead levels of materials used in manufacture."

One of my closest friends, film actress Allison Hayes, died because of a calcium supplement, which contained large amounts of lead and the pesticides dieldrin and aldrin. She sued the company and won, but she didn't live to enjoy the money.

A serious aspect of calcium overload is that it can imbalance stores of other minerals in the body – minerals which are more critical than calcium for building bone. Further, calcium tablets can suppress the thyroid gland, and glandular health is essential for the maintenance of strong bones, and for overall health.

There are several different forms of calcium available. Some health professionals prefer calcium citrate because it appears to be better assimilated. Studies have concluded, however, that this calcium significantly increases absorption of aluminium from dietary sources.

It seems clear that mega-dosing on inorganic forms of calcium can be dangerous and doesn't appear to work. One example, of many, is a British Institute of Radiology study, in which women of all ages were tested for calcium levels. It was found that none had low calcium levels, whether they supplemented with calcium or did not, and whether they were osteoporotic or not. What they did find, in the osteoporosis sufferers, was low levels of the other, more important, nutrients – magnesium, zinc, manganese and vitamins C and D. Another study, reported in the *American Journal of Public Health*, found that hip fractures tended to be more common in women consuming higher calcium supplementation.

There have been so many studies proving that calcium supplementation is ill-advised, that it is difficult to know whom to quote. For example, in his *Second Opinion Newsletter*, Dr Robert Jay Rowen tells of a study at Penn State University which started following women at age 12. They found no significant effect on the bone density of these women through to age 20, whether their intake of calcium was at the low end of 480mg or at a high end of nearly 2000mg. Lead researcher Thomas Lloyd suggested that young girls' bones "do not benefit from more than 500mg calcium daily." He also quoted a study at Harvard University showing that "women who drank the most dairy products suffered the most fractures."

Bill Sardi, in a well-researched article in the *Townsend Letter for Doctors and Patients*, *January 2003*, quotes from many studies. One, from the *International Journal of Cardiology*, *33:19, 1991*, says, "The countries with the highest calcium consumption (from dairy) have the highest mortality rates in the world (Scandinavian countries, USA and New Zealand), while the countries with the lowest calcium consumption (Japan, Portugal) have the lowest mortality rates." And, from the *Journal of Clinical Endocrinal Metabolism, 81:2149, 1996*, "Among men less than 50 years of age, high blood calcium levels are associated with a 30-200% increase in mortality from cardiovascular disease." The Japanese have the longest disease-free lifespan and only consume around 400mg per day.

In case you have been popping calcium supplements, these, according to *Nutrition Reviews 55:1, 1997*, are some of the symptoms of overdose: "Anxiety, muscle cramping, migraine, heart flutter, eyelid twitch, leg cramps and constipation. Calcium is a smooth muscle constrictor."

Most health advisors recommend calcium to women who want to maintain bone density. But just remember, that "… as bone mineral density increases, so does the risk for breast tumours", according to the *Journal of the American Medical Association, 276:1404, 1996*.

✗ Coral Calcium

There has been huge hype over coral calcium recently. Please don't be duped – this product contains several minerals and vitamins that are questionable, and high levels of aluminium. According to *Hypertension Research, March 2002*, "Another myth is that calcium protects against diabetes. Actually diabetes has been defined as a disease of excessive calcium influx into cells. There is a relatively high rate of diabetes among the people of Okinawa who are purported to consume large amounts of coral calcium."

Bear in mind that a large proportion of the people on earth live in the equatorial zone, where cow's milk is not used and calcium pills are unheard of. Yet, these people have strong bones – certainly stronger than ours in the industrialised world. The calcium our bodies need and can utilise is the kind of calcium these people get. You'll find more on foods that provide a natural source of calcium in the next chapter - *How To Build Healthy Bones*.

✗ Bone Meal/Dolomite

If, after all the above evidence, you still want to take calcium, please at least avoid supplements made of bone meal – ground bones of animals – they are life-threatening. They can be heavily contaminated with lead, as well as with *Dieldrin* and *Aldrin* – two deadly pesticides. Because animal bones act as a metabolic sink, by the time the animals are slaughtered, the poisons they have ingested through fodder spraying and from the lead contamination in the air, have settled in their bones. So, if you take calcium supplements, check carefully to make sure there is no bone meal in them. Unfortunately, it isn't always on the label, so it's rather like playing Russian roulette to take them. Dolomite is also dangerous, as it often contains aluminium, arsenic, cadmium and lead.

✗ Sodium Fluoride and Aluminium

The chemical pushers maintain that fluoridated water strengthens bones, and they back up this cynical misinformation with X-rays of bones, before and after exposure to fluoridated water. And sure enough, the bones do appear to be thicker, but the truth is that they have been made softer by the fluoride, and fracture much more easily. Four studies reported in the *Journal of the American Medical Association* showed strong links between hip fractures and fluoride. The *New England Journal of Medicine* reported that people given fluoride to cure their osteoporosis actually wound up with an increased fracture rate.

Many other respected organisations concur. In highly-fluoridated New Zealand, hip fractures have tripled since fluoridation was forced on the people by the government. And, of course, osteoporosis is epidemic in Australia, most of which is fluoridated.

One of the reasons for this increase is that fluorides destroy enzymes that are vital in bone formation. So, shun fluoride in your water and toothpaste, antiperspirants and baking powder. And don't forget that the aluminium in cookware is also dangerous, as the aluminium leaches out and is bad for your general health, as well as your bones. For more on fluoridation see *Chapter 19*, *Water Woes*, and please support the Australian Fluoridation News (see page 331 in *Resources*).

✗ Soy

Don't be fooled by advertisements and ignorant health professionals who say that soy products prevent osteoporosis. They *all* leach calcium out of bones! And that includes lecithin, which is *everywhere*. Please watch labels carefully, because soy flour and soy oils are in many products and most breads. A full exposé of the dangers of soy is in *Chapter 9, Soy - The Abominable Bean*.

✗ Imbalance of Omega-3 and –6 Fats

One of the reasons that osteoporosis has become a modern day calamity is the way our food supply has been altered. Junk food and drink and junk oils have contributed mightily to the western world's epidemic of crumbling bones. The highly-advertised polyunsaturated oils are in most processed foods and bakery goods. This means that, unless you stay away from all manufactured food, your body will be overwhelmed by the worst kinds of fats and oils.

Further, your A and D will be compromised, and no matter what supplements you take, or how good your diet is, the result may be osteoporosis. This subject is vastly complicated. I would need a PhD in Lipid Chemistry to explain the complex actions of oils on the human body. And I would need a full-length book to do it, and you would be bored speechless. The best advice I can offer is that you study ***Chapter Six***, *Oils and Fats*, and live according to the suggestions made there.

Depending upon your age, it's likely your parents, grandparents or great-grandparents did not have to think about which foods were safe. It probably never occurred to them. They ate a natural, traditional diet that maintained their bones for life. Artificial fertilisers and pesticides were not used. Most cooked with lard, which was second only to cod liver oil as a source of vitamin D. Today most lard is hydrogenated, altering any vitamins it may contain.

Processed oils did not exist and natural hand pressed oils from seeds, grains and legumes, such as sesame and sunflower, were uncommon. Polyunsaturated oils were used in small amounts and were fresh pressed just before using. They were never processed and never stored.

In the 'good old days', people ate meat from animals that grazed on grass and hay, which is natural to ruminants. Meat from these animals was safe and contained healthful fats. Then agribusiness took over and, in order to promote rapid growth and high profits, they started penning the animals, injecting them with antibiotics, growth hormones and who knows what else? New drugs come along all the time, and the consumer is always the last to learn what industry is up to. The poor animals are stuck in pens, and forced to eat the worst kind of grains. These grains have turned what used to be a wholesome food into a dangerous one that overloads your body with drugs and bad fats. If you are a meat eater, and if you are unable to find or afford grass-fed raised meat, don't eat any. And, tell your butcher the reason. Eventually, if enough people protest, this dreadful practice will be stopped.

And here is the worst news – fish is no longer a wholesome food. It is contaminated with mercury. Did you know that there is an 'allowable' amount of mercury in our fish? When I checked with the government, I discovered they permit a scary percentage of mercury in imported fish. I don't know if they check local fish at all. Mercury is the second most toxic element on Earth, next to radiation, and there shouldn't be *any* permitted in our food!

Don't kid yourself that farmed fish is safe. In order to maximise profits, farmed fish are fed junk grains. What used to be an excellent source of Omega-3 oils, is now causing Omega-6 overload in our bodies. Remember what salmon tasted like when it was caught in icy cold, unpolluted waters? Things have changed – salmon are now treated like livestock, fed pellets that turn their flesh pink, and inoculated to ward off diseases. Often, pens are so close together, and the fish so crowded, that currents cannot flush the water out, and faeces accumulate. Because the fish are living an unnatural life, there are frequent outbreaks of parasites and diseases, which leads to antibiotics in the feed. The last thing we need is *more* antibiotics in our bodies!

Farmed fish are fed canola oil, soy meal and corn gluten meal, as well as bait fish that have picked up pollutants, such as polychlorinated biphenyls (PCB), flame retardants and dioxin. These chemicals are neurotoxins. According to **Dr Joseph Mercola's Newsletter**, *Aqua Bounty Farms* have sought permission to produce an Atlantic salmon implanted with a special gene that could cause a 10-fold increase in growth. So, watch out! Halibut, sea bass and tuna are also being farmed. It looks as if it won't be long before we won't be able to get wild fish unless we catch it ourselves. And, what about poultry and eggs? Same deal. When chickens were permitted to scratch at grass and herbs and eat bugs, their flesh was a source of Omega-3 fats, and their eggs had dark orange yolks and a strong taste. Now, penned up in the most inhumane way, and fed the worst grains and drugs, they are no longer fit for consumption. Their eggs are pale and tasteless, and their flesh and eggs now contain the Omega-6 fats we are trying to avoid. Poultry meat grown this way, and their eggs, are bad for our bones, and it serves us right for treating a fellow creature so cruelly!

What does all this mean for your bones? It means that, if you eat meat or chicken, unless it is produced naturally, you will suffer from Omega-6 overload, and the best diet and supplementation will not be able to overcome the damage. These foods have gone multinational, and have been destroyed!

Vegetables and fruit have also been degraded by agribusiness. Try to grow as much as possible yourself, and if you can afford organic, that's the way to go. Wheatgrass juice is chock-full of important nutrients. It is not hard to grow, and the juicers (see **Resources**) are not expensive.

✗ Mercury Fillings

Excellent general health, which includes dental care, is essential in order to avoid osteoporosis, as well as all other health problems. It is impossible to achieve true health in the face of constant, low-level mercury poisoning. This is what occurs in those who have mercury-amalgam fillings, as discussed in **Chapter 17**, *Dental Health*.

✗ Drugs

There are so many reasons to shun drugs that **Chapter 20,** *Legal Drugs*, is devoted to the subject. Here, however, we'll look at those that have an adverse effect on our bones, starting with those pharmaceutical money-spinners, antacids – which are also discussed in more detail in **Chapter 3**, *Stomach Acid*.

When I first learned that some people take antacids to get calcium, I was astounded. First, the calcium in antacids is in a poorly-absorbed form. Second, they contain sugar, dyes, preservatives and aluminium. The H_2 blockers, such as *Tagamet*, *Zantac* and *Pepcid*, suppress the secretion of stomach acid, which is vital for digestion and calcium absorption. Tagamet actually causes breast enlargement in men because it interferes with estrogen metabolism and excretion in the liver.

In 1998 the professional journal, ***Bone, *22(6) 695-698*, reported the case of a pharmacist who self-treated her ulcer and stomach symptoms with antacids for eight years. Her intake was only slightly above the maximum recommended dose, yet over that period it produced an estimated intake of 18 kilograms of aluminium hydroxide and 15 kilograms of magnesium hydroxide. She developed muscle weakness, back and limb pain, loose stools and stress fractures. Subsequent examination showed that the aluminium had been substantially absorbed into her bones, resulting in the typical long-term accumulation symptoms of toxicity, phosphate depletion and osteomalacia.

If you believe the advertisements you will think that heartburn is caused by too much stomach acid. This is an advertising executive's fantasy; usually heartburn is caused by *too little* stomach acid. Used regularly, antacids disturb your acid/alkaline balance, which is so important for maintaining strong bones. To keep your bones strong, never take them. Eat properly, and you won't have to.

Digoxin, isoniazid, methotrexate, phenobarbital, medrol, aspirin, dilantin, tetracyclines, epilepsy drugs, laxatives and blood thinners all play a part in damaging bones. If in doubt, just remember that anything you do which is not bone-friendly, whether in drugs, diet or exercise, is likely to be bad for your bones, because they will only be as strong and healthy as you are.

The use of diuretics leads to an increased risk of bone fractures, because they create a serious loss of calcium. People taking pharmacologic strength cortisone drugs over a long period will definitely develop osteoporosis. These drugs dissolve bones by causing calcium to be withdrawn from them and lost in the urine. The result of prolonged use is spontaneous bone fractures. The only good news is that the loss of minerals stops when the pharmacologic strength cortisone is discontinued and a good nutritional program is followed.

Every time I hear of asthmatics being given pharmacologic strength cortisone I get the urge to kill. The doctors who so cavalierly prescribe these dangerous drugs to people, without saying a word about controlling their health problems with diet, amaze me. It is well documented that asthma and arthritis are easy to help with diet. Sometimes, merely taking a child off milk and cheese will clear symptoms. There is no excuse to use drugs unless natural methods have been investigated first. And then, only in a life-threatening attack on a temporary basis.

Contraceptive drugs are also dangerous for bones. The *Norplant* contraceptive contains a synthetic form of progesterone that can make women miserable, probably due to the way it interferes with the monthly cycle. Some doctors report that their patients say Norplant makes them feel as if a black cloud has settled over them, according to Burton Goldberg, in his informative series of books, ***Women's Health***. This product is associated with an increased risk of blood clots and cardiovascular disease, like all synthetic progesterones. Some of the symptoms women complain of are irregular bleeding, water retention, weight gain and depression. Possibly worst of all, Norplant is known to interfere with thyroid function, which is vitally important for our health.

The pharmaceutical companies offer a variety of drugs to treat osteoporosis. They all have unpleasant side effects and doubtful effectiveness. Some are:

DIDRONEL / ETIDRONATE / DIDROCAL:

These drugs slow bone loss by sticking to the bone surface and making the osteoclasts less effective. This allows osteoblasts to build up more bone, leading to retention of old bone and an apparent modest increase in bone mass. The accumulated old bone is, however, poor quality and results in increased hip fractures by the third or fourth year of use.

Long-term toxicity is unknown, and the side effects include nausea, Paget's disease, increased risk of bone cancer, blood dyscrasias, fracture risk, leg cramps, diarrhoea and headaches. Further, it is hard to use and expensive.

FOSAMAX / ALENDRONATE:

The instructions for this drug warn patients to stand upright for thirty minutes after taking, to keep it from burning the oesophagus. It is supposed to prevent old bone being taken away by osteoclasts, but it hardly seems worth it, as side-effects include gastrointestinal disturbances, muscular and bone pain, headaches, nausea, vomiting, oesophagitis, ulcers, liver damage, renal failure, hypocalcemia and eye problems, from blurring of vision to painful swelling and even blindness if untreated. And it doesn't even *work*!

Dr John Lee told women for years not to take Fosamax. Unfortunately, however, he was in the minority due to the aggressive marketing which encouraged doctors to prescribe this drug. According to Dr Lee, the advertising is misleading and research indicates that Fosamax does not reduce the risk of hip fractures, and increases the risk of wrist fractures. If it burns the oesophagus it can cause permanent damage as well as chronic gastrointestinal problems. Many women have told me that they had to discontinue Fosamax due to extreme burning when they swallowed it. Small wonder, considering that it is used to kill osteoclast cells with poisons that are the same class of abrasive chemicals used to scrub mildew off tiles! .

FORTEO:

A new one to watch out for. According to Dr Jonathan Wright in *Nutrition and Healing*, "None of the presently sold patent medicines for osteoporosis actually stimulate new bone growth. They all 'work' by slowing the destruction of bone, called 'inhibiting bone resorption'. At any rate, there are some distinct and serious risks involved with Forteo. After singing its praises, the media also reported that 'FDA officials said the drug, given by injection daily, will carry a special warning because in laboratory tests it caused cancerous bone tumours in rats.' Of course, the 'consolation' is that the cancerous tumors hadn't yet been seen in the 2000 people injected with the drug in clinical trials."

If your doctor suggests this daily injection, I advise that, instead, you follow the instructions in this book and save yourself from becoming the first non-rat to develop a cancerous bone tumour from Forteo.

CIBALCIN / CALCITONIN:

Side effects include flushing, GI disturbances, site reaction, and urinary frequency. Results are patchy, with a brief period of new bone formation after the first injection, followed by progressive loss. When the drug is discontinued benefits are lost quickly.

CLODRONATE/BONEFOS:

The side effects with this drug are elevated parathyroid hormone, renal dysfunction, GI upsets and asymptomatic hypocalcaemia. Again, hardly worth the risk.

IPRIFLAVONE:

According to Dr Joseph Mercola, this is yet another highly-touted 'bone building' supplement, but it doesn't build bone. It is reputed to be natural, but it is not, and studies have proved that it doesn't work, and may suppress immune function.

To most people, it seems easier to take a drug, rather than learn to avoid illnesses by living according to nature's laws. It isn't. Ultimately, it is much harder, due to debilitating illnesses and a shortened life. Just remember when considering popping drugs, that it wasn't long ago when mercury and laudanum were considered cure-alls. Now, of course, they are known to be poisons, as are so many drugs used in the past – even drugs prescribed enthusiastically in the recent past. That drug you took today, will probably be banned next year.

And what does all this have to do with your bones? Consider the words of Dr Raymond Peat, who wrote, "Practically any kind of poisoning causes cells to take up calcium from the blood." In this instance, he was referring to drugs, whether legal or illegal.

The following is reproduced with permission from *Dr Peat's Newsletter:*

"No topic can be understood in isolation. People frequently ask me what they should do about their diagnosed *osteoporosis/osteopenia*, and when they mention 'computer controlled' and 'dual photon X-ray' bone density tests, my attention tends to jump past their bones, their diet, and their hormones, to the way they must perceive themselves and their place in the world. Are they aware that this is an X-ray that's powerful enough to differentiate very opaque bones from less opaque bones? The soft tissues aren't being studied, so they are allowed to be 'overexposed' until they appear black on the film. If a thick area like the thigh or hip is to be measured, are they aware that the X-ray dose received at the surface where the radiation enters might be 20 times more intense than the radiation that reaches the film, and that the 90 or 95 percent of the missing energy has been absorbed by the person's cells? If I limited my response to answering the question they thought they had asked me, I would feel that I had joined a conspiracy against them. My answer has to assume that they are really asking about their health, rather than about a particular medical diagnosis.

"Neurologists are famous for making exquisitely erudite diagnoses of problems that they can't do anything to remedy. The owners of expensive dual photon X-ray absorptiometer diagnostic machines are in a very different position. *The remedies for osteoporosis are things that everyone should be doing, anyway, so diagnosis makes no difference in what the physician should recommend to the patient.*

"Most often, estrogen is prescribed for osteoporosis, and if the doctors didn't have their bone density tests, they would probably prescribe estrogen anyway, 'to protect the heart', or 'to prevent Alzheimer's disease'. Since I have already written about estrogen and those problems, there's no need to say more about it here, except that **estrogen is the cause of a variety of tissue atrophies, including the suppression of bone formation**.

"General Electric, a major advocate of X-ray screening for osteoporosis and breast cancer, has advertised that 91 percent of breast cancers could be cured if everyone used their technology. Breast cancer has not decreased despite the massive application of the technology, though the US government and others (using crudely deceptive statistics) claim that the War on Cancer is being won. Similarly, during the last decades when the 'high technology' X-ray machines have been more widely used, the age-specific incidence of osteoporosis has increased tremendously.

"I think there are several reasons for avoiding X-ray tests of bone density, besides the simple one that everyone should eat a bone-protective diet, regardless of the present density of their bones.

"Even seemingly identical X-ray machines, or the same machine at a different time, can give very different estimates of bone density. Radiologists evaluating the same images often reach very different conclusions. *Changes in the tissue, water and fat content can make large differences in apparent bone density, and estrogen, which affects those, could appear to cause improved bone density, when it is merely causing a generalised inflammatory condition, with edema.* A machine that is accurate when measuring an aluminum model, won't necessarily give meaningful results when the composition of the tissue, including the bone marrow, has changed. Calcification of soft tissues can create the impression of increased bone density. Studies of large groups of people show such small losses of bone density (around 1 percent) especially in the neck of the femur (which is important in hip fractures) that the common technical errors of measurement in an individual seem very large.

"**Ultrasound devices can do an extremely good job of evaluating both bone density and strength, rather than just density. Ultrasound stimulates bone repair. X-rays accelerate the rate of bone loss. X-rays do their harm at any dose; there is no threshold at which the harm begins.**"

The Latest on Fosamax

Use it at your peril: the US Food and Drug Administration has issued a strong warning that Fosamax can cause osteonecrosis (ONJ) of the jaw (also known as Dead Jaw) which is even worse than it sounds. ONJ is a painful and irreversible decay of the jaw, which can make dental restorations impossible. Fosamax is a bisphosphonate drug, as are Zeneta, Aredis and Actonel. Persons damaged by taking any of these drugs for osteoporosis, cancer or multiple myeloma can file for compensation from anywhere in the world.

Email: info@jeffbogertlaw.com phone USA: 1-800-421-4505.

As you will have learned from this chapter, your skeleton is under constant attack, even from so-called 'bone-building aids', and it is little wonder that osteoporosis has lately become rampant in our modern society. In the following chapter we look at some of the positive things you can do to restore and maintain strong, healthy bones.

Frightening headlines about the dangers of drugs cause problems for doctors, who then must spend valuable time answering the questions of concerned patients.

- Editor of JAMA
The Journal of the American Medical Association

"A depressing number of scientists are greedy, unethical, selfish, egocentric, intolerant, racist, narrow-minded – all the way to evil. Scientists cheat, plagiarise work on poison gasses or for tobacco companies, advise and support tyrants and dictators."

Leon Ledermen, Physicist

New York Times, 24 July, 1999

AMEN!

Elaine Hollingsworth
Gold Coast, Queensland, Australia

8

Bone Health 2
How To Build Healthy Bones
… with a lot of help from vitamins A, D, K and sunlight

If you do not provide your body with sufficient vitamin D, you might as well kiss your bones goodbye. If you live in a part of the world where UV-B rays are plentiful all year round (and there are precious few), and if you get adequate sun throughout the year, without sunscreen, your skin will synthesise your vitamin D from sunlight.

Caryl Nowson, of Canberra's Deakin University School of Health, speaking about the value of vitamin D in preventing osteoporosis, said, "Nursing home patients and veiled women are among high-risk groups... The main source for Australians is exposure to sunlight." And this, of course, means without sunscreen (see *Remedies*).

In Australia, if you live north of Coff's Harbour, the sun will provide you with sufficient vitamin D for maintaining and building your bones all year long. That is, provided you do full body sunning (as much as modesty permits, and don't neglect your tummy) for 10 to 15 minutes on each side three to four times a week, between 10am and 3pm. Yes, that's right – just the opposite from government recommendations. You will not be able to soak up beneficial rays on overcast or polluted days, and you will need to avoid the scorching summer sun. Do not allow your skin to burn, or even tan. If it does, you are getting too much sun for your skin type.

For overseas readers, the rule of thumb is this: check your atlas and find yourself in relation to the latitude lines. If you are living between 30° and the Equator, your year-round sun will be superb. If not, you will have to supplement carefully. Many health professionals think that the more D, the better, when the truth is that willy-nilly supplementation is dangerous. Nature, in her infinite wisdom, knows when to stop; if you are getting your vitamin D from the sun, synthesis in your skin provides its own brakes against D toxicity. But, if you are obliged to depend upon supplementation for this crucial vitamin, you must test, treat and test again.

This is where my research on osteoporosis gets good. It has been my great good fortune (and yours, too, if you are concerned about your bones) to discover one of the world's foremost experts on this subject, Krispin Sullivan, an American clinical nutritionist, lecturer and teacher. According to Krispin, with whom I have had many long conversations, vitamin D storage is genetically variable and deficiency is commonplace, even in warm climates. She told me that only two out of 220 of her patients' tests show D in optimal ranges. Her research was done with Northern Californians, so their D would be lower than people in, say, Queensland, Australia, or Florida.

Krispin's book, *Naked At Noon, The Importance Of Sunlight and Vitamin D*, is now available (see **Resources**). Prior to its publication, I read some of her voluminous research papers, which she kindly mailed to me, and I believe this book will be definitive on osteoporosis.

If you are unable to get sufficient sun exposure all year, or if your skin does not synthesise vitamin D well, due to advanced age or genetics, you will need to take special care to eat foods that contain vitamin D several times each week, or take supplements. This becomes a bit tricky, because before vitamin D supplementation is started, you need to be sure that your calcium intake is equal to, or greater than, 1000mg per day (from supplements and food combined). You have already learned about inorganic calcium, so derive your calcium from the recommended raw vegetables, nuts, sardines, etc., and from Maca, which is a fine source. The reason for this reliance on calcium intake is due to the way low calcium can mask as low vitamin D. If you are uncomfortable with this, bear in mind that my female friends and I all place great emphasis on raw vegetables and Maca, and no supplements, and all of us test high in calcium.

The definitive vitamin D test is called *25-Hydroxyvitamin D* or *25(OH)D*. This, according to Krispin, is vital. Some physicians are not familiar with this test, so it may be your job to gently educate. Then, you must be certain that the lab you take the prescription to understands which test it is. **The test you do not want is called** *1,25 dihydroxy*.

Once your 25(OH)D result is in, get a copy for yourself, or at least write down your level for your records. This test should be available in all countries, but the technicalities differ.

In Australia, and in many other countries, the levels are measured in *nmol/l*. In this instance, according to Krispin, the desirable range is no lower than 75nmol/l, and no higher than 150nmol/l. She says that the optimal is still being determined, and is probably 100-150nmol/l. With a level below 75nmol/l, you would be wise to take steps to improve your levels of vitamin D, whether by sunlight or food/supplements. If your level is below 75nmol/l, there is a likelihood of bone loss. Holick, a longtime vitamin D researcher, however, is suggesting the new value for deficiency be set at 50nmol/l. Levels below 25nmol/l indicate clinical deficiency and possible *osteomalacia* (adult rickets).

"*In the US*, and in some other countries," says Krispin, "the levels are known as *ng/ml*. A range between 40 and 60ng/ml is optimal, perhaps dropping into the 30-40ng/ml range in winter months. Below 30ng/ml there is a significant chance bone loss will occur. Levels above 60ng/ml are excessive, unnecessary, and in people very sensitive to vitamin D, have the potential to cause bone loss or otherwise contribute to disturbed calcium metabolism. 25(OH)D levels below 10ng/ml are considered a clinical deficiency and are associated with osteomalacia. 28ng/ml is just below the the lowest acceptable range and only a small adjustment from current supplements, food or sun is needed." Krispin can assist people in the US whose doctors won't prescribe the test.

A friend of mine, who lives on the Gold Coast in Australia and should get enough sun, evidently doesn't, or is unable to absorb D effectively, due to her advanced age. She was tested, and this is the result:

REFERENCE RANGE - 70nmol/l   35-150

The 70nmol/l refers to her vitamin D level, and 35-150 is the range the lab checks for. When I rang Krispin with this result she said that my friend's level is just below the lowest acceptable range, requiring the small adjustment from current supplements, food and sun mentioned above. Krispin said my friend should not get more than 400iu (international units) of D daily and testing should occur every six months for the next three years to make sure the additional D is enough and not too much. That means no more vitamin D than 400iu per day from *all* sources – *sun, food and supplements* – without physician guidance. This is not easy to figure out, but well worth the effort, and frequent testing will monitor progress.

Egg yolks are the second most potent source of vitamin D. If you raise chickens, see to it that they get plenty of sun. Those who live in areas where sun exposure is not possible year round can compensate by feeding the chickens cod liver oil as two percent of their ration. This gives a five-fold increase in vitamin D in the yolks, and I have discovered that the chickens love it!

We all know about cod liver oil. Many of us were given it as children, some have given it to their own children, and it has the reputation of a benign, effective product. Well, it is, and it isn't. Under certain circumstances it can be your answer to osteoporosis. But there is a downside: most fish are contaminated with mercury and cod liver oil can go rancid easily. I prefer other sources (See chapter end) so it has to be approached carefully.

The Downside of Vitamin D

The action of vitamin D, whether it is from cod liver oil, sunlight, food or supplements, is not the same as the action of a conventional vitamin, because it is actually a pro-hormone, and has to be treated accordingly. **There are no symptoms of chronic marginal overdose, which can be serious and irreversible**. Too much or too little vitamin D will cause calcium to be diverted from your bones into your soft tissues, where you do not want it. Acute overdose causes death rapidly! This is the reason sunlight is such a good source. Nature knows how to apply the brakes, but Man doesn't, and the latest craze of vitamin D injections – *"One shot a year, to get all the D you need!"* – can cause irreversible damage to soft tissues and premature aging of arteries. D injections send the vitamin/hormone levels way above normal, then way below, in a dangerous yo-yo.

After testing, if your physician approves, and recommends a dosage of vitamin D, it will be necessary for you to be tested again in six months for your follow-up *25 hydroxyvitamin D* level. This way, you and your physician will be able to make sure that the cod liver oil or other supplements are having the desired effect, and will not cause an overdose. But do not take any vitamin D at all if you suffer from *Sarcoidosis*, or any other disease associated with D toxicity. Taking vitamin D when it is not needed is dangerous!

What's The Upside?

Cod liver oil is considered by many health professionals to be the finest, most-assimilable form of preformed vitamins A and D, which are crucial for prevention and reversal of osteoporosis. It contains 21% saturated fatty acids and 57% monounsaturated fatty acids, which provide stability, and has the great advantage of being easy, because a small amount each day will provide all the A, D and Omega-3 oils you need for the day. These important nutrients are hard to come by because, as the **Merck Manual** clearly states, these vitamins in an assimilable form are found only in animal products, such as cold water fish and liver, and in egg yolks, cream and butter, but *only from animals allowed to graze on grass*. Many people don't do well on dairy foods and even if they do, many cannot find products from grass-fed animals. And, as shown elsewhere in this book, our fish are hopelessly poisoned by mercury.

Vitamin A

You already understand why vitamin D is so important, but vitamin A is equally necessary for your health, and not just for preventing osteoporosis. Deficiency can lead to serious thyroid malfunction, eye diseases, night blindness, birth defects, cardiovascular diseases, skin problems and immune system dysfunction. This has been known for years, but rarely used by establishment medicine to help people.

As an example, in 1997 *The South African Medical Journal* reported on a study of vitamin A as a therapy for excessive bleeding. They wrote that Johannesburg General Hospital had documented a 92 percent cure rate, over a ten-year period. This is encouraging news for women who are being bullied into having hysterectomies for excessive bleeding, when vitamin A therapy, combined with a good diet, can normalise the flow quickly. This knowledge is especially valuable for women with low thyroid function, because they are not able to convert the beta-carotene in food and most vitamin pills into real vitamin A. These women are at extreme risk of unnecessary reproductive organ surgery.

I can only recommend cod liver oil because we have an accurate test that can monitor what it is doing to your body. If you are not prepared to take this test (which Medicare pays for in Australia), please do not use it at all: get your vitamin A from egg yolks, liver, cream and butter. This is my preferred method, as I am able to get these nutrients from properly-grown animals.

Downside Of Vitamin A

Experts have widely differing opinions about vitamin A toxicity. Studies have shown A to be toxic in large doses, but synthetic A, in the form of the toxic *retinol* (which can cause birth defects) was used in the studies, so this skewed the results. To further complicate this subject, many fabricated foods and most vitamin products contain this unnatural form of vitamin A. This means that, if you eat manufactured food and take vitamins, you could possibly get an overdose, if you then add cod liver oil, which contains lots of vitamin A. My recommendation – never eat 'fortified' food. Toxic vitamins are used and it's impossible to measure intake.

Krispin told me that too much vitamin A can cause a deficiency of vitamin D. Because A accumulates very slowly, people can do well on it for two years, then the same dose can move into excessive. This is complicated, and health professionals who understand these interactions are rare and extremely valuable. You may have to become your own expert.

Beta-carotene is not vitamin A. It is only a precursor of vitamin A, and hard for people with liver problems, under-active thyroid glands and nutrient deficiencies to convert into 'the real thing'. Have you ever noticed the way some people who drink lots of carrot juice have yellow complexions? This is because their livers are unable to convert the beta-carotene in the carrots into vitamin A. Misguided health professionals sometimes advise this practice for those with weak eyes and poor night vision. This is not good advice, as it would take a carload of carrots to affect the eyes, and the carotene would probably not be converted anyway. Those who have problems metabolising vitamin A may be helped by taking zinc.

How To Protect Yourself

Your physician will know about toxicity and can order the right kind of tests. As Krispin says, "Cod liver oil can be toxic to anyone with liver problems, anyone on prescription medications, aspirin, or other NSAIDs, or those who consume alcohol or take multi-vitamins containing vitamin A, or beta-carotene." Never combine cod liver oil or vitamin A from supplements with oral or topical medications for acne or other skin disorders treated with retinoid acid derivatives. Krispin counsels that the **maximum** dose is one tablespoon per day, except in very unusual circumstances, with the above considerations. Your physician will know that you must not take any cod liver oil if you are diabetic (it can raise blood sugar), or if you are on *Warfarin* (cod liver oil is a natural anti-coagulant).

Good Oil

The only good cod liver oils are bottled in Norway immediately after the fish are caught. Krispin says that *Carlson Laboratories* (see **Resources**) makes a fine Norwegian oil, and they use only cod fish caught during the winter and early spring because the liver oil content is highest at that time of year. The oil is separated from the liver tissues without the use of chemicals. To ensure maximum freshness, the air inside the glass bottles is replaced with nitrogen before bottling. It even tastes all right, which is more than I can say about the cod liver oil I choked down as a child.

Dr Joseph Mercola is a cod liver oil enthusiast, too. He says that Carlson's oil is put through a molecular distillation process that cleans out mercury, if any, and that this oil is also tested routinely to ensure freedom from detectable levels of cadmium, lead, PCBs and 28 other contaminants, including mercury. Carlson's Cod Liver Oil contains 2000-2500iu of vitamin A and 400-500iu of vitamin D in each teaspoonful. One teaspoonful should be adequate for most people. In extreme cases, those with very low vitamin D levels, who live where they cannot get enough sun, should take no more than one tablespoon, making sure to test regularly. If you choose this method, be sure to combine cod liver oil with butter from grass-fed cows to aid assimilation.

If you cannot, or do not wish to take cod liver oil, eating three ounces of liver twice a week will give you the A and D your bones need. Due to the well-founded concern people have about poisons in animals, liver has suffered bad press in recent years. According to Krispin, this is undeserved, because ingested poisons do not accumulate in liver, they merely pass through as the liver processes them. She counsels looking carefully at the liver before buying it – if it looks firm and deep red, it is from a healthy animal. If it is mushy and pale, the poor animal has had a hard life and it isn't fit to eat.

For those people who have problems digesting liver, Dr Peat has this suggestion: "Liver doesn't have as much fat as other meats. The digestive system works best with roughly equal amounts of fat, sugar and protein present at the same time, so it helps to have fruit or fruit juice and some kind of fat along with the liver." It can be simmered in pasture-raised butter, as long as the heat is extremely low and there is no bubbling to cause oxidation, or it can be cooked at a higher temperature in pure coconut oil. Be aware that all livers contain purines, which can cause gout.

Krispin Sullivan's monumental research is not just about vitamins D and A, but concerns all aspects of bone health. I cannot, in just these few pages, do justice to her work. I can only cover a few of the main points. Many health professionals read my book, and I sincerely hope that all of them will send for hers. It is cutting edge. Her information is so new that it will take up to seven years for it to disperse, just in the US. Imagine how long it will take to trickle down in Australia! So, doctors, be the first on your block – take advantage of Krispin's research, and do your bit to stem the terrible epidemic of osteoporosis in Western countries. (And, while you're at it, lobby the government to stop poisoning our water supply with osteoporosis-causing sodium fluoride).

Vitamin K

Vitamin K is essential for calcification of bones. People who have suffered from osteoporotic fractures are often found to have a deficiency of vitamin K. Those who have had their gall bladder removed, or who have difficulty digesting fats, are unable to absorb and utilise vitamin K. Aspirin destroys this vitamin, and this explains why people who take it habitually bruise so easily. Antibiotics inhibit vitamin K production, so that's one more reason to avoid them. The elderly frequently have large black and blue patches just beneath the skin, and this should be a clue to their doctors that they need supplemental vitamin K. But it rarely is, as few health professionals know how to treat this deficiency.

There are conditions and symptoms that can indicate a shortage of vitamin K in the body, many related to excess bleeding. Excessive menstrual flow and clotting, bloody vomit and stools, nose bleeding, eye haemorrhages and even the occurrence of mini-strokes and hardening of the arteries can be caused or aggravated by lack of vitamin K. And remember, if you are unable to digest fats, you will need to address that problem before you will be able to assimilate vitamin K.

Spinach, Brussels sprouts, endive, cabbage, broccoli and lettuce all contain vitamin K, but if you depend upon food for this vitamin, be aware that high intakes are necessary in order to get sufficient. Wheatgrass and chlorophyll contain adequate amounts, but be careful to avoid all polyunsaturated oils, as they stop K absorption dead.

Krispin says that fermented foods, especially if the ferment is lactic acid, contain vitamin K. Unfortunately, however, it is close to impossible to get sufficient K from food, unless you are on a traditional diet. By that, I mean a time-tested native diet that includes all necessary nutrients, taken from natural sources – animal and vegetable. Dr Weston A Price investigated diets such as these in his ground-breaking *Nutrition and Physical Degeneration*, a book Hippocrates Health Centre highly recommends to all those interested in the study of nutrition. It is available from *Wise Traditions* (see *Resources*).

In her research, Krispin found that the minimum active dose of vitamin K is 1 milligram per day, preferably taken as 500 micrograms, twice daily. She said that any vitamin K, with the exception of K_3, is acceptable, and that this amount reverses calcium loss in urine. But remember, vitamin K must be taken with a meal that has some fat in it (refer to *Chapter 6*, *Oils and Fats*), for proper absorption. And, before you start hyperventilating about fat, remember that your calcium levels will *not* go up on a low fat diet, and that skim milk is a disaster.

In vitamin K deficiency, osteocalcin cannot direct calcium into our bones, where we need it. This means that, even if your D values are acceptable, your calcium will end up in your arteries, soft tissues, kidneys and urine, if your level of K is low. When supplementing with vitamin K, there is an important caveat: **people on anti-coagulants must not use vitamin K without physician approval and guidance**. If you are unable to find a source of K where you live, check *Resources* for a supplier.

In addition to maintaining a good vitamin intake and balance, there are other things you can do to ensure healthy bones.

Progesterone Builds Bones Too

Please review what I have written about Dr Peat's *Pro-Gest* oil. It is essential for your bones, as well as for your overall health.

Maca

See *In Other Words…* for details about this amazing cruciferous root vegetable from Peru, where it is used for bone building as well as for all its other health benefits.

Hydrochloric Acid

You can take the best supplements and eat the best food until the cows (grass-fed, of course) come home, but if you do not have an acid environment in your stomach you will not assimilate the nutrients vital for bone health (see *Chapter 3*, *Stomach Acid* for more details).

Protein

A great deal of twaddle has been written about how protein damages bones – almost as much twaddle as has been written about the importance of taking bucket loads of calcium. As Dr Robert Jay Rowan reports in his ***Newsletter***, "Bone density, largely mineral related, contributes only 70 percent to bone strength. The bone matrix, which is made up of protein, determines the remaining 30 percent of bone strength. Thus, some relatively low-density bones with excellent protein matrix may be quite resistant to fracture, while high-density bones with poor protein quality may break!"

This fits right in with an experience I had with two strict vegan women I knew who lived on fruit. I couldn't even persuade them to eat nuts, and it wasn't from want of nagging. They were both in their early thirties, and it was disturbing to watch them destroy themselves. Over a period of several years, their hair became lifeless and fell out by the handful, they lost lots of teeth, and their bones fractured spontaneously. Even in the face of such compelling evidence, they would not accept that their lack of protein and minerals had caused their problems. Both stopped menstruating, and pointed to this as 'proof' of health, when it is proof of the opposite – their bodies were not strong enough to bear and raise children, so nature curtailed their ability to become pregnant. They belonged to a group of committed vegans – all sweet people, but a sickly bunch!

There have been many studies proving the need for concentrated proteins for bone health, too numerous to detail here. One, from Dr Herta Spencer, of the Veterans Administration Hospital in Hines, Illinois, is instructive. She found that studies concluding that calcium was lost due to high protein diets were flawed because, as is so often the case, the protein used came from isolated, fractionated amino acids from milk and eggs. These are unnatural substances. In her studies, she found that when the protein used is from meat, there is no increase in excreted calcium, or any change in serum calcium, even long-term. The ***American Journal Of Clinical Nutrition***, *April 2002;75:609-610,773-779*, reported that "Bone mineral density may be improved by increasing protein intake in many older men and women, as long as they meet the recommended intakes of calcium and vitamin D... You need both calcium and protein for bone, and if your diet has plenty of both, then your bones are likely to be in better condition than if you are short on one or both of these nutrients... This study and other recently published research go a long way toward refuting concerns that animal protein is bad for bones."

Just make sure that the animal protein is raised properly and the calcium is from food, not toxic supplements.

Magnesium

About half of the magnesium in the body is found in the bones. They act as a reservoir for the mineral, and when the diet is deficient in magnesium the body will draw calcium from the bones. All of the research I have reviewed concludes that adequate magnesium intake is more important than calcium intake. Most Western people are deficient in this mineral due to our dreadful farming methods.

A deficiency of magnesium impairs utilisation of calcium for bone building, and results in calcium being deposited in soft tissue, rather than in bone, where it belongs. Calcium levels rise, even without supplementation, when magnesium is supplied. As an illustration, this experiment was described in *Metabolic Aspects of Health*: A calcium-rich diet was given to chickens, with the result that they laid thin, weak-shelled eggs. The chickens which were given no calcium, but a diet of magnesium, silica, and various other minerals, laid eggs with calcium-rich shells. This proved that the animal kingdom is capable of transforming magnesium and other minerals into calcium, and explains why a vegetable-rich diet builds strong teeth and bones.

As well as being essential for the development of healthy bone, magnesium can help reduce cramps and muscle tremors, insomnia, migraine headaches and stress, and is essential for the prevention of heart disease. Chocolate craving is a sign of magnesium deficiency, and often fades when sufficient magnesium is given. Dosage is individual, and the advice of a well-qualified professional is advised. For example, if you are sedentary, your needs are smaller than for those who use lots of energy exercising. Further, some magnesiums act as bowel cleansers and will create diarrhoea if used in excess. Professionals often recommend taking magnesium to bowel tolerance – which means learn your individual dose and do not exceed it.

Grains were originally high in magnesium, but the scandalous refining processes used to extend shelf life and our mineral-deficient soils, has left us with a legacy of magnesium deficiency in all industrialised societies (see *Chapter 16, Against the Grain*). This crucial mineral occurs in greens, and sprouted grains, nuts, beans, dried fruits and vegetables and is especially high in wheatgrass juice. Supplementation, especially for menopausal women who are not on perfect diets, is necessary to maintain bone integrity. Magnesium chloride is the best, according to biochemist Walter Last, as it is easily assimilated. Never use the excitotoxin, magnesium aspartate.

Boron

The mineral boron is essential for bone metabolism, including efficient use of calcium and magnesium, and proper functioning of the endocrine glands. As well, boron is required for bone maintenance, and normal blood levels of oestrogen and testosterone. Within eight days of supplementing boron it was found that women lost 40 percent less calcium and 33 percent less magnesium through their urine!

Women getting boron supplementation had blood levels of estradiol 17B, the most active form of oestrogen, doubled to levels found in women on oestrogen replacement therapy. Further, levels of testosterone almost doubled with boron supplementation. It is important to emphasise that these are natural hormones, made by the body, not dangerous hormones made by the drug manufacturers.

About 35 years ago, Rex E Newnham, of Perth, Australia, developed arthritis. A botanist, he knew that boron was necessary for calcium metabolism in plants, so he began taking boron twice daily. In three weeks, all his swelling, pain and stiffness had disappeared.

Because of this experience he returned to school and took degrees in osteopathy and naturopathy and earned a PhD in nutrition. Eventually, he was selling 10,000 bottles of boron tablets per month, curing thousands of people with arthritis.

Then the drug companies, who earn billions each year on cortisone (which, as mentioned earlier, when taken in pharmacological doses dissolves bone) and pain killers for arthritis, used their immense influence to change the law so that boron became illegal. Dr Newnham was heavily fined, put out of business and moved to England, where he has continued helping people.

Exacerbating the problem of osteoporosis, Australia is the most highly fluoridated country in the world. Fluoride remains in the bones and leads to skeletal fluorosis, which mimics arthritis. Boron antagonises fluoride by the formation of complex ions, which is probably the reason it helps with arthritis symptoms.

Put simply, boron helps control bone formation and repair by removing other elements, such as fluoride, from circulation, and by stimulating natural processes. Obviously, it would be better to take to the streets and riot to force authorities to stop poisoning our water (see **Chapter 19**, *Water Woes*). But, until that unlikely day, boron is a necessary element, both for prevention of osteoporosis and for general health.

Boron is richest in vegetables and fruits, especially grapes, apples, dates, peaches and raisins, and nuts such as almonds and hazelnuts. But not in Australia, because of our notoriously depleted soil, where we get little or no boron from food.

Boron capsules are easily available in the USA, Canada, England, New Zealand and many other countries. But not in Australia, thanks to our government. They do permit tiny amounts of it in a few supplements that contain other ingredients, which we do not recommend. It is legal for Australians to have it mailed here for personal use only. Please buy plain boron only, with no other minerals added (see **Resources**).

Since writing earlier editions of this book, Dr Newnham and I have been in touch. He is a fine man who is dedicated to helping people. He told me that for those who do not wish to buy boron capsules, it is safe and effective to use simple borax powder. He recommends taking 6mg of borax daily, well below toxicity levels. He said that people can simply wet a finger, put it in the borax powder and lick it off, twice a day. Cheap as chips and, according to Dr Newnham and several other physicians and naturopaths I've spoken to, safe. Dr Newnham says, "The toxicity of borax powder is about the same as for sodium chloride, namely 40-60 grams is a lethal dose." (Please confirm this with your own physician). I use Borax myself, rather than importing Boron.

According to Dr Newnham's research, boron/borax is a must for those afflicted by osteoporosis, arthritis, allergies and even SLE (*systemic lupus erythematosus*). He says that 9mg per day caused great improvement in a patient in only three weeks, with complete recovery later. Please do not take a high dose without a physician's clearance. It is still not known how many other conditions can be caused by boron-deficient soil, which is common all over the developed world, due to poor farming methods. I believe everyone should take this trace mineral as an insurance policy.

Silica/Silicon

Silica is crucial in keeping bones strong because, without silica, the deposition of mineral salts, especially calcium, cannot take place. The silicon in silica acts similarly to vitamin D in the hastening of bone formation. It produces new bone tissue in the bone matrix.

Silicon alone can regenerate the structure of the body, including the skeleton and skeletal appendages, collagen (the glue that holds us together), nails, skin, hair, cartilage, tendons and ligaments. Studies in the US and Europe point to silicon as an essential factor in dealing with bone loss. The older we become, the more our silicon is depleted, so we need to supplement. Fortunately, the Australian government has not banned silica. At least not yet.

We recommend *Flora Sil Vegie Caps*. They are on sale in Australia, or through the manufacturer (see **Resources**).

Manganese

Manganese is required for the repair of bones and connective tissue, as well as for normal growth and development. Studies have shown that it helps to maintain bone density in post-menopausal women. Diets high in refined carbohydrates do not supply adequate manganese. Further, manganese is poorly absorbed, so supplementation is advised, especially for those at risk of osteoporosis.

Fruits and vegetables contain some manganese, but unless it is organically grown, Australian produce is unlikely to contain enough for bone health. Other sources are hazelnuts and pecans, seaweed, avocadoes, oats, whole wheat and buckwheat. But not, of course, refined grains. The phytates in grains, unless they are soaked and sprouted, interfere with manganese absorption. The way grains are prepared at the Hippocrates Health Centre is bone-friendly.

The optimum daily intake of manganese is thought to be 15 to 30mg, and manganese gluconate is gentler to the digestive tract.

Zinc

Zinc phosphate plays a critical role in the development of collagen, which, as Professor Stryer, of Stanford University in the US, wrote in his book, **Biochemistry,** "is required for the deposition of calcium phosphate to form bone." Bone contains 40 percent of the total body collagen, so you can see how important it is to the strength of our bones. As it is degraded during the aging process, it is replaced, but only if the body has the proper nutrients. Put simply, low zinc creates poor collagen, which leads to demineralised bones. Since collagen is the glue that holds the body together, this is an important mineral to take for bone health.

Do not overdose on zinc, because a high intake can reduce calcium absorption if your calcium intake is low. As with all supplementation, it is wise to consult an expert. The Hippocrates Centre always recommends looking to nutritional sources, if possible, rather than to manufactured supplements. Zinc is found in pumpkin seed kernels, nuts, sprouted wheat, egg yolk and wheatgrass juice.

Copper

Crucial for bone development, copper is also important for the maturation of collagen. Supplementation is problematical because many people drink water from copper pipes, and it is important to keep your copper/zinc ratio correct. According to Dr Raymond Peat, no synthetic copper supplement has been proven to be safe. Hit and miss mineral supplementation is not advisable, particularly in this case. The best way to ensure that all your mineral uptake is sufficient and natural is by embracing the Hippocrates Health Centre diet. Failing that, it is advisable to take a mineral supplement or, preferably, grow wheatgrass and juice it.

Calcium

The calcium we need, the calcium our bodies can assimilate and utilise for bone health, is the calcium from the soil of our earth. This is the calcium used for aeons by native peoples to build perfect bones. The broad leaf vegetables contain this superior calcium. They also contain vitamins and minerals and other energy-rich compounds that haven't even been identified yet.

Manufacturers, with their puny efforts at formulating an effective calcium supplement, can never hope to approach nature's perfect answer to our calcium needs. A large and varied selection of raw vegetables, sprouts and wheatgrass juice is a perfect bone friendly diet.

Sesame seeds are reputed to be one of the richest sources of calcium, but this is not correct. The outside of the seed contains most of the calcium, but it has to be removed, and the inside contains only 110mg of calcium to 100gr. Raw kale, watercress, spinach, parsley and Swiss chard are excellent sources (please do not cook these vegetables as cooking brings out the oxalic acid). Most vegetables have smaller, but still useful, amounts of calcium.

Pumpkin seeds, sunflower seeds, Brazil nuts, walnuts, pecans and hazelnuts are good sources, as are almonds. Dried figs contain significant amounts as do dried apricots. Other calcium-containing foods are okra, turnips, parsnips, red kidney beans, chick peas, lentils, barley, brown rice and egg yolk. Sardines, of course, contain lots of calcium, but be careful to buy only those packed in spring water because canners use unhealthy oils. Also, buy low-salt ones. Carob powder contains lots of calcium, and is delicious when put in desserts. But avoid confectioneries that contain carob, because they always contain other ingredients, such as lecithin, sugar, etc, which are dangerous for your bones. Make your own carob treats from unsweetened carob powder – it's naturally sweet.

If you have room and time for an organic garden, you can grow your own calcium. Even if you only have a tiny space, go to your local herb growers and tell them you want herbs that have a large calcium content. I did, and came home with three different dark green, heavy-leafed herbs that are delicious in salads. One, called South American Crinkle Lettuce, is particularly crunchy and nice. But don't neglect the humble dandelion, a perennial herb that has a long and distinguished history as a food and medicine in many countries. It has been considered a panacea for centuries, as it contains more vitamins and minerals than most vegetables. Plant it in your garden (if it isn't already thriving) or in a pot, and eat four leaves each day in salad for an easily-assimilated calcium/potassium/mineral supplement. It tastes all right and the price is right.

Niacin (Nicotinic Acid)

The late Dr John Whitman Ray, a scientist whose work we respect, said that there is no use taking any nutrients at all, unless you also take niacin. The reason is that the vasodilation, which causes a flushing reaction, carries the nutrients out to the cellular level. You will need to find your own dose, starting very slowly. If it does not cause your skin to turn red and burn slightly, you are not taking enough (but please refer first to important information on Page 342). This nutrient has the added benefit of protecting us from radiation. But be sure the bottle says *'Nicotinic Acid'* not just *'Niacin'* or *'Niacinimide'*. Take in the morning before eating, just once per day. Cut the tablets and gradually increase the size until you find the dose that creates a flush.

Vitamin B₆ (Pyridoxine)

Vitamin B6 is a facilitator in the production of progesterone and promotes collagen repair. People with osteoporosis are often low in this vitamin. If supplementation is needed, a complete B complex should be taken because the B vitamins work in synergy. But be aware that some people suffer from insomnia from B-12 supplementation.

Vitamin C

Most people are aware of the importance of vitamin C to our health, and know that our bodies do not have the capacity to manufacture it. Further, since we cannot store vitamin C, as we can other vitamins, it is necessary to replenish our supply daily. But this is not possible on a diet of stored, canned, packaged, processed foods. This means that most people in industrialized nations are deprived of the vitamin C-rich food many primitive societies have in abundance. Even those of us on good diets can be deficient in vitamin C due to our poor soil quality. This has serious ramifications for our tendency to osteoporosis, because vitamin C is essential to the synthesis and repair of bones. As well, it facilitates the absorption of various essential minerals, especially magnesium, which is so important in bone maintenance. The diet advocated by Hippocrates Health Centre is rich in fresh, organic fruit and vegetables, so those enjoying this diet need not be concerned with supplementing vitamin C. Those people not so disciplined would be well-advised to take a supplement of vitamin C.

For years we were unable to recommend any vitamin C supplements because all those we have known about have been poorly formulated, using the cheapest chemicals. Many sensitive people get serious bladder and kidney irritations from them, and even kidney stones. Gastric distress can also be caused by improperly-formulated vitamin C. The late Dr John Whitman Ray preached for years against manufactured vitamin C, as have many other scientists (Dr Ray blamed C for the high incidence of bowel cancer).

The Australian (20 March 2000) printed a report on the danger of vitamin C: "New research by the University of Southern California has shown vitamin C supplements might do more harm than good by clogging the arteries. During the recent study, the artery walls of 583 people – aged 40-60 – with no symptoms of cardiovascular illness who took a typical 500mg dose of vitamin C per day thickened at more than twice the rate of those who took none." The article did not mention what kind of vitamin C was used. We assume synthetic.

Fifty years ago, 'everyone' said vitamin C was a panacea. Not having learned my lesson about what 'everyone' said, I took some, and was rewarded by a dreadful bout of cystitis. This painful bladder infection, which often afflicts women, can easily become chronic. Nothing daunted, I tried different supplements over the years, which people assured me were different, and all caused the dreaded cystitis. During the many years since then I must have cured at least fifty women of chronic cystitis by simply telling them to quit taking vitamin C.

Because Dr Ray believed that vitamin C is essential for health, and because so many of his patients were not on good diets, he conducted extensive research on various vitamin C products, and concluded that all killed the vitally important gut flora we need to sustain health. Then, he discovered a product from the Andes, had it tested, found that it did no harm, in fact is beneficial, and was finally able to recommend this vitamin C to his patients (see **Resources**).

I first heard about this vitamin C from one of Dr Ray's instructors, but was afraid of cystitis and not game to try. Bless her, she gave me some of the granules, encouraged me, and I screwed up the courage to try a tiny amount. No problem. Each day I took a tiny bit more, until I had worked up to a normal dose without any repercussions. I then told friends who also had not been able to tolerate any kind of vitamin C, and not one encountered problems.

Exercise

Your bones will become sluggish and stop building bone mass if you do not stimulate them by weight-bearing exercise. It is necessary, however, to do the right kind of exercise; a ladylike stroll will not build bone, nor will swimming, which is a great cardiovascular workout, but not much help to your bones. Exercise improves blood circulation to the bones, and this is vital, due to bones' limited blood vessel network. Isometric exercises, properly designed to pull on bones and stimulate growth, can be excellent, as can judicious use of light weights (as detailed in **Remedies**). Dr Robert J Rowen, in his **Second Opinion Newsletter**, puts it very well when he says that even on the best diet program, "… without the subtle electrical stimulation of the bone formers through exercise, the osteoblasts would have no stimulation to pick up the available calcium… My recommendation is to rely far more on exercise for maintaining bones than calcium."

Housework, gardening and walking in the shopping mall don't count! A brisk walk four or five times each week will go a long way toward strengthening your bones. If you have been sedentary, start by walking ten minutes, adding ten minutes each day until you have worked up to at least 30 minutes, preferably 40. Please, no moseying!

When you're just not in the mood, remember what happens to the bones of immobilised people, astronauts and any bones in a cast – they begin losing calcium in two days. You'll find more on the many other benefits of exercise in **Remedies**.

If you have plans for the future that do not include osteoporosis, nagging illnesses, dangerous medicines, hospitals and untimely death, eat a large proportion of your food raw, as nature intended.

Cooking kills the enzymes in food that are absolutely essential for life. Food enzymes become catalysts in the body – substances that help maintain the tissues and general body functions and digest food. After maturity there is a gradual decrease in the enzyme content of our bodies. Death occurs when it becomes so low that metabolism cannot proceed.

When we eat cooked foods, the pancreas must create the enzymes necessary to digest it. This puts a strain on the body, depletes our enzyme supply, and causes the pancreas to enlarge. Raw food is bursting with these life-giving enzymes, and protects us from illnesses, as well as prolonging our productive years and our lives.

Billions of our cells die daily and must be rebuilt in order to maintain health. Food is one of the fuels used to replace these cells, and cooked and/or junk food will build junk cells, which lead to the cemetery.

Before grumbling about the time it takes to prepare a healthful salad, rather than popping a TV dinner into the oven, please reflect upon all the time stolen by illnesses. How much time do you throw away each year incapacitated by colds, flu, headaches, indigestion, allergies, hangovers, PMT, menstrual cramps and just feeling icky? How much time do you spend nursing children, spouses and other family members when they're ill? How many time-consuming trips are you obliged to make to doctors, specialists, laboratories and hospitals? None, repeat none, of this is necessary (excepting accidents, of course) for those who eschew junk and embrace raw fruit and vegetables. Reflect, also, upon the extra years, possibly decades, of life that you and your family will gain through healthful habits. Looking at it from this perspective, preparing fresh, wholesome food saves time.

The medical magazine *Nature, 22 September 2000*, reported on a study that was carried out in Switzerland, at the University of Bern, by Roman Muhlbauer and Feng Li. They head the Department of Clinical Research on Bone Biology. Following are some details from their research paper:

"Calcium consumed in dairy products has only a small effect on the risk of hip fractures, and soy has not been shown to be effective in humans. Here we show that a variety of salads, herbs and cooked vegetables that are common in the human diet can alter bone metabolism in rats.

"The consumption by rats of onion, for example, increases their bone mass: in male rats fed 1g dry onion per rat per day for 4 weeks, bone mineral content increased by 17.7%; mean cortical thickness increased by 14.8%; and the mineral density of trabecular bone increased by 13.5% relative to controls.

"Vegetables eaten by humans can significantly inhibit bone resorption in the rat. A mixture of 500mg each of onion and Italian parsley, and a mixture of lettuce, tomato, cucumber, arrugula (rocket), onion, garlic, wild garlic, common parsley, Italian parsley and dill (100mg of each daily) significantly inhibited bone resorption, indicating that the effect was additive. There was no inhibition by soybeans at the same dose, or by foodstuffs of animal origin, and even milk powder had no significant effect, despite its 1.29% calcium content. The mean 20% inhibition by 1g onion per day is slightly higher than the effect of calcitonin at doses (per kg body weight) used to treat postmenopausal osteoporosis... Onion therefore inhibits resorption not only in male rats, but also in females in which bone resorption is stimulated by oestrogen withdrawal.

"Our results indicate that several common vegetables in the human diet alter bone metabolism in the rat. If this also happens in humans, then including an appropriate amount of these vegetables in the daily diet could be an effective and inexpensive way to decrease the incidence of osteoporosis."

The *American Journal of Epidemiology (vol 146, 1997)* reported, "It's a well established fact that consumption of fruits and vegetables is associated with lowered risk of lung cancer, skin cancer, colon cancer and others." A study conducted in the United Kingdom found that people who consumed fresh fruit and vegetables daily had one third fewer strokes, one quarter fewer heart deaths and one fifth the deaths from all causes. We could add that as a source of vital minerals and vitamins they also contribute mightily to the health and strength of your bones.

There are hundreds of studies proving the value of eating much, if not all, food raw. One study, which is apt for those concerned with osteoporosis prevention, involved two groups of rats. One group, fed on raw vegetables, had significantly less bone loss than the other group, which ate soybeans and milk powder, among other foods, and had a great deal of bone loss.

Many Hippocrates Health Centre graduates, after losing weight and greatly improving their health during their attendance, have told me that they intend to continue eating the Hippocrates way. Not all do, of course, but they have learned enough to shun harmful foods and beverages, and how to grow wheatgrass and make the delicious dishes served at the centre. When they leave, we counsel them to at least always eat salad before cooked food, in order to activate their enzyme systems. The Hippocrates diet has all of the nutrients necessary to build and maintain buoyant health and strong bones. The sprouted grains and the wheatgrass juice are filled with vitamins and minerals. Those who cannot or will not stay on a perfect diet need to take other measures, as detailed in this chapter, to protect their health, and the integrity of their bones.

Enzymes

One last thought about supplementation: enzymes, which are referred to many times in this book, are so important that their depletion leads speedily to a breakdown of health and premature death. Without this "spark of life", there is no point in taking mineral supplements, as they will go unabsorbed. Further, enzymes are essential before food can be broken down and enter the blood without causing allergies. In perfect health, the stomach, the pancreas and the small intestine produce the digestive enzymes we all need. But cooked food, and the wrong kinds of food, destroy our enzymes and impair absorption and digestion, and accelerate aging.

Even those on perfect diets need to take food enzymes, because they help eliminate toxic wastes and correct long-standing enzyme deficiencies. The food enzymes Hippocrates Health Centre imports are formulated to the specifications of famed enzyme expert, Edward Howell. They are plant-based and contain no fillers (such as rice bran or rice powder) and no preservatives, and are encapsulated in vegie-caps.

Dr John Whitman Ray used these enzymes extensively in his practice, experimenting with them and testing them laboriously, using his renowned expertise as an iridologist. He explained to me that because they are a food, rather than a laboratory-engineered product, they have a natural vibration, which enhances all of the body's functions. They are now available through Hippocrates Health Centre (see **Resources**).

Mary's Story

Some time ago, 58-year-old Mary came to me with an all-too-familiar sad tale. She had just been to her doctor to get the news about her bone scan, and was told that she had the bones of an 80-year-old. Mary wasn't surprised, because she was suffering incapacitating pain and walked with great difficulty. Her doctor told her to take HRT, Fosamax, lots of calcium, and sent her on her way.

Instead, she came to ask my advice and (after a strict lecture about diet) I recommended the 'Big Five' of osteoporosis – Dr Peat's progesterone, magnesium, boron, hydrochloric acid and Maca. This was the most she could manage on her budget. Six months later Mary had another bone scan and when her doctor compared it to the original, she was convinced the lab had sent the wrong one. "This can't be right," the doctor said, "no one improves like this."

The doctor re-checked and once she realised that it was, indeed, the right scan and that Mary's bones were infinitely better, she said, "You must have done what I told you to do." "No," said Mary, "I went to Elaine Hollingsworth and did what *she* told me to do." This did not go down well, and the doctor said, "Oh, yes, I've heard about *her!*"

Three things are instructive about this true story: (1) Osteoporosis can be reversed, even using only diet and the 'Big Five'; (2) Mary's pain had gone and her bone scan had improved out of sight; (3) Yet her doctor, a fellow woman who could reasonably be expected to care about her patients, did not care enough to ask her how she did it.

More on Vitamin D

For those of you who live in areas where it is not possible to get sun all year (see the first page of this chapter for specifics) a dedicated vitamin D lamp has recently come on the market. It has few damaging UVA rays, has peak UVB outputs in the range that optimally triggers vitamin D production in the skin, and makes large amounts quickly. It is called Sperti KBD C/UV Lamp, and can be located on the internet.

For cutting edge information on vitamin D, I highly recommend that you key in Vitamin D Council and subscribe to their free newsletters.

> If your head is swimming with all the pros and cons of supplementing, and the sometimes difficult-to-implement rules about food, and you think it's all just too much trouble, please bear in mind that there are few things in life more difficult than dragging around with a crumbling spine, or a broken hip that lands you in a nursing home, prematurely and permanently. But, when designing your own osteoporosis treatment, do not guess; it is essential to *Test, Treat And Test Again* when using Krispin's vitamins D and A therapy.

> "I have always told my patients that they should avoid hospitals as they would avoid war. Do your utmost to stay out of them and, if you find yourself in one, do everything possible to get out as soon as you can. Understandably, modern medicine is so fearful that you'll discover its role in spreading disease that medical texts caution doctors not to allow the phrase hospital-acquired infections to pass their lips."
>
> *Robert Mendelsohn, MD*
> *Author of MALE PRACTICE*

9

Soy – the Abominable Bean

A terrible tale of corporate greed,
bad science, regulatory misconduct...
and how we've all been conned!

To see, read and hear about it in most mainstream and 'alternative living' media you'd think that the ubiquitous soy bean and its derivatives are the most versatile, natural, heart-friendly, health-improving, fat-preventing, growth-promoting and generally loveable foods ever grown on our good earth. A simple, easily-cultivated bean which has been part of our diet since the dawn of civilization, promising health and vitality to the lactose-intolerant, the new-born, the aged, the menopausal, the frail, the athletic, the health-conscious and just about everyone else as well.

It's inexpensive, available everywhere, on its own or as a vital ingredient in thousands of other food products, such as our daily bread, cakes, confectionery, baby formula, milk and meat substitutes, breakfast cereal, sauces, snackfoods, pasta; it forms the basis of non-stick cooking sprays. It is widely used in stockfeeds and is in most petfoods. Doctors, farmers, nutritionists, athletes, respected companies whose household names have become part of our culture, government authorities – all make a point of telling us how safe and health-giving this wonder-food is for us. It's so good and harmless, they tell us, that it's often not even listed as an ingredient in many processed foods. And even when it is we don't mind; everyone knows it's safe. Our health watchdogs happily accept the assurances given by companies who produce and process it that it is 'GRAS' – Generally Regarded As Safe – so it must be.

Around the world, hundreds of millions of acres are devoted to its cultivation, providing a secure cash crop for millions of farmers who cheerfully pay a levy to the developers of their genetically-modified strains to help Monsanto Chemical Company and other huge companies spread the gospel that *'Soy is Good For You'*.

Too bad that for decades these same developers and corporations have known of and deliberately suppressed the evidence that prolonged ingestion of soy causes cancer and countless other life-threatening illnesses, destroys bone, creates havoc with the hormonal systems of humans and animals alike, represses the sex drive and, even if eliminated from our diets overnight, is so entrenched in the food chain and the bodies of everyone who has ever ingested it, that its adverse effects would still plague the health of generations yet unborn.

The truth behind the blatantly commercial integration of the *Abominable Bean* into the Western diet is a disturbing tale of fraud, corporate irresponsibility, greed, bad science, public and media manipulation, corruption, intimidation, political opportunism, suppression, legal manoeuvring, regulatory inaction and governmental incompetence which makes the tobacco companies look like Good Guys.

Find that hard to believe? Maybe after you've been acquainted with some of the evidence for these assertions you'll share my outrage over the fact that not only is yet another proven life-endangering product allowed to be cultivated, manufactured and sold in the first place, but that in this case its producers and pushers have so successfully created their own mythology around it that government regulators and so-called health watchdogs have evidently buckled under and given them virtual *carte blanche* to continue to misinform, confuse and poison not only those who are suckered into consuming their noxious products, but also everyone who is unknowingly obliged to partake of this toxic time bomb through its placement in all manner of basic foodstuffs and in the feed of animals and poultry destined for human consumption. Passive smoking is one thing; forced feeding quite another.

Since my interest in the promotion of safe natural alternatives to many of the manufactured elements of Western diets and medical treatment has become widely known, I now receive a daily influx of desperate pleas for help or accounts of terrible personal tragedies directly connected to the use of soy.

Physiological Havoc

And, yes, I do hear from a few people who tell me I've got it all wrong and send me reprints of magazine articles quoting 'solid scientific evidence' which 'proves' how wonderful and safe soy is for everyone, or assure me that "Sanitarium wouldn't sell it if it wasn't OK." It doesn't seem to have occurred to them, or maybe they don't care, that almost all this 'evidence' and the 'research' on which it is based has been published, and usually funded by, the very same corporations who are producing and selling the stuff. Or that they are perpetuating the 'everybody knows' urban myths so helpfully placed in appealing editorial features liberally scattered through the pages of mainstream media and, regrettably, repeated in many health-oriented and alternative lifestyle public-cations that should know better!

So, if you're one of those who feels bound to harangue me with the 'well-known fact' that Asian people have thrived on soy for centuries, hold on to your pen for a while and be prepared to learn just how wrong that particular 'Furphy' is. It's one of the most widely-believed 'scientific facts' touted by the proponents of soy – and one of the best examples of how successful they've been in brainwashing the public.

Far more distressing, and never mentioned in the producers' "solid scientific evidence" are the tales I hear, almost daily, from parents whose baby daughters have commenced menstruation, developed pubic hair, underarm odour and breasts from as young as four and five years of age. Or whose teenage sons are too embarrassed to shower with their mates because they have grown breasts of female proportions or because their genitalia haven't developed.

For example, following my appearance on the Australian Channel 7's **Sunrise** breakfast program in August 2002, our office was flooded with phone calls and e-mails backing my warnings on the dangers of soy. The most upsetting were from mothers whose children suffer from the usual soy symptoms, and by far the worst was the testimony of a shocked mother who described her son's tragic childhood. She had drunk copious amounts of soy milk during pregnancy – unknowingly poisoning her son with a female hormone. Then, because the oestrogen had damaged her reproductive system, she was unable to breastfeed and her baby received more oestrogen (the equivalent of five birth control pills each day) from the soy baby formula her doctor told her to use. Her son's genitalia did not develop, but his breasts did and he refused to go to school until he had had a double mastectomy. Unaware of the cause of their health problems, the family continued drinking soy milk and now, at 21, her son needs another double mastectomy, but they can't afford it.

The soy pushers, who know *exactly* what their products do, have ruined his life as well as those of millions of other unfortunates – but I bet they don't lose a wink of sleep over it!

True, such disasters do not befall *every* child who is fed soy. But neither are they rare, isolated or anecdotal instances. They are the documented, widespread, frequent and in many cases predictable results of hormonal imbalance caused by the assimilation of high levels of oestrogen. And where did the oestrogen come from? From the baby formula and soy drinks fed to these unfortunate offspring by their caring parents – often on professional medical advice. Presumably the same source of 'professional' advice that apparently sees no contradiction in recommending that the identical ingredient prescribed to menopausal women to manipulate their hormonal levels can be safely fed to men and newborn babies!

If you want to persuade your health professional, point him or her to this website: http://vm.cfsan.fda.gov/~djw/pltx.cgi?QUERY=SOY

In simple terms, though obviously not simple enough for some in the medical profession, feeding an infant soy formula is the equivalent of giving it five birth control pills a day.

The Swiss Health Service put it this way: "100gr of soy protein has the oestrogenic equivalent of one contraceptive pill", and there are numerous other studies published since the early 1960s which confirm this undeniable fact. Many enlightened scientists and medical professionals argue that the continued use of soy in baby formula is a form of genocide, since these effects have been known and published within the scientific community for decades. **The finely tuned endocrine system depends upon hormones in concentrations as tiny as one trillionth of a gram to influence the womb environment, and the money-hungry soy propagandists urge women to destroy this delicate environment with oestrogen-laden soy!**

"I didn't know..."

Frequently, as in the case cited above, drinking soy milk during pregnancy can cause a failure to produce breast milk, which then leads to feeding the baby soy formula. It's tragic that so many of the most distressing cases of soy damage that I have heard personally are those of women who have had precisely that experience. Often these women cannot restrain their tears when describing the dreadful health problems their children suffer. They keep repeating to me, "I didn't know, I just didn't know; the doctor told me to drink it for my bones and to feed baby the soy formula."

As you will see shortly, one of the major culprits when it comes to why soy is so dangerous is the fact that the bean contains high levels of aluminium absorbed from the soil in which it is grown. In 1997 no less an authority than the American Academy of Pediatrics' Committee on Nutrition reported, "Aluminium in breast milk is 4 to 65 ng/mL. Soy-based formulas contain 600 to 1300 ng/mL."

Similarly, a recent study at the University of California-Irvine led by Francis Crinella, professor of Pediatrics, pointed to the increased risk of significant behavioural problems such as ADHD being triggered by high concentrations of manganese in soy formula. According to Crinella, "Soy milk formula contains about 80 times the levels of manganese found in breast milk, posing the risk that infants could receive too much manganese in the first weeks of life."

Apart from the ravaging of delicate hormonal systems, serious gastrointestinal disturbances suffered by babies on soy formula are now commonplace.

Money Spinner

The multinational Nestlé corporation, which owns the Carnation brand, is a major soy advertiser; you may remember them as the company which brought infant formula to third world countries, discouraging breast feeding and killing, according to the World Health Organisation, 1.5 million babies each year. Well, they're still at it, shamelessly flogging their soy milk formulas such as *Alsoy* in spite of all the evidence that it is deadly. Little wonder, really, when one considers the size of the market for infant formula. The Washington Times' investigative magazine, **Insight on the News** *(June 26 2001)*, quoted an independent expert's estimate that soy-based formulas account for about $750 million of the annual $3 billion sales revenue for all formulas.

Surely risks such as those mentioned above should have been sufficient for the use of this killer bean to be outlawed years ago, at least in baby formula? And even if the regulators are not prepared to act, despite all the well-known and easily accessible compelling evidence, how can it be that physicians are still prescribing soy formula – and do you wonder that my website is called *doctorsaredangerous.com*? Only the UK government, so far, has begun to take seriously the warnings of independent scientists and is considering a ban on the sale of soy-based infant formulas.

Unfortunately, outrageous and preventable as are these crimes against infants, they are only the tip of the iceberg. The bad seed within the Killer Bean has no regard for the age or gender of its victims.

I am not a scientist, nor will I subject you to a long technical dissertation, but a basic understanding of the physiology of the soy plant and its subsequent processing is helpful in understanding why the bean is far from being the 'white knight' its producers and proponents would have us believe.

Aluminium is one of the most prevalent minerals in soil, but it doesn't affect most crops. The soy plant, however, has an affinity for aluminium, which it extracts from the soil and concentrates in the beans. This contamination is exacerbated when the beans are dumped in aluminium holding tanks and subjected to an acid wash during processing. Inevitably, traces of aluminium from both sources are absorbed into the body through the consumption of soy.

Seen a Soy Cow Lately?

Soy milk contains 100 times more aluminium than untreated cow's milk. And, while on the subject of so-called soy milk, have you ever seen a soy cow? You cannot milk a soy bean; in order to obtain that pure-looking, inviting stream of white liquid pictured so appealingly in the ads, many processes are needed. It is necessary to grind the beans at high temperature, and then extract the remaining oils with dangerous solvents, some of which remain in the meal. Then the meal is mixed with an alkaline solution and sugars, in a separation process designed to remove fibre. Then it is precipitated and separated, using an acid wash. At each stage of processing a tiny amount of poison remains within the soy. Government regulators say it's so small an amount that it doesn't count. I wonder who told them that? And why don't they take notice of the scientists who say it *does* count, due to its accumulation in the body over long periods of soy ingestion? Are you really happy to accept the manufacturer's assurance that it's safe to eat a tiny amount of poison each day, perhaps several times a day, until you have a serious health problem?

During my research for this book I came across twelve chemicals that are added after these processes, most of them unpronounceable, and the majority known to be dangerous, if not deadly. I won't bore you with the names but, trust me, you wouldn't want them anywhere near you, much less in your body.

It's also worth mentioning here that a by-product of soy processing is a form of *lecithin*. Unlike the naturally occurring variety found in free-range eggs, nuts, seeds and avocados, this by-product is always rancid, and is extracted from the sludge left after the oil is removed from the beans. It contains high levels of solvents and pesticides. And guess what? Rather than consign it to the toxic waste dump where it belongs, the manufacturers have instead created another hugely-profitable market for it as a 'healthy' food additive. Among its delightful qualities is the ability to induce severe joint pains (often mistaken for arthritis), and serious gout. (During many years as a natural health advocate, I have counselled countless people who thought they had incurable arthritis. Their doctors prescribed strong drugs, without discussing improvement through diet. All reported cessation of symptoms after quitting soy, and/or lecithin; but it requires time, and lots of water).

But back to the bean. Putting in additional poisons is bad enough, but the killer bean hardly needs them to accomplish its deadly purpose. It is already riddled with potential carcinogens and lots of other plant chemicals guaranteed to wreak havoc within the human body. Yet in the face of overwhelming evidence of catastrophic effects resulting from their prolonged ingestion by humans and animals, the soy pushers continue to assert the exact opposite – that all these things are not only harmless *but are actually good for you!*

The fact is that the soy bean contains numerous *phytoestrogens* – a descriptive name for plant chemicals having *oestrogenic (oestrus-inducing)* effects. They occur in nature to help regulate animal breeding cycles and, in synthetic form, are used in farming for the same purpose. The ubiquitous birth control pill is, of course, the human synthetic version. At high dosage or over long periods phytoestrogens become anti-oestrogenic. Much higher doses are used in chemotherapy to kill cancer cells.

The class of chemical compounds called phytoestrogens contains dozens of sub-classes, such as *coumestans, isoflavones, lignans* and *sterols*, each of which contains further sub-classes. Soy contains many isoflavones, including the sub-classes *genistein, coumestrol* and *daidzein*.

Scientists have known for years that isoflavones in soy products can depress thyroid function, causing autoimmune thyroid disease and even cancer of the thyroid. As far back as the 1950s phytoestrogens were being linked to increased cases of cancer, infertility, leukaemia and endocrine disruption.

Charlotte Gerson, of the Gerson Cancer Clinic in the USA, has published detailed research *(Gerson Clinic: Cancer Research, June 1, 2001 - 61 (11): 4325-8)* proving that the phytoestrogen genistein is more carcinogenic than DES (*diethylstilbestrol*), a synthetic oestrogen drug that was given to millions of pregnant women primarily from 1938-1971. Few would be unaware of the death and misery that particular drug inflicted on countless women and their daughters.

Forbidden Food

Ms Gerson also wrote the following in the *Gerson Healing Newsletter*: "Soybeans contain *hemagglutinin*, a clot-promoting substance that causes red blood cells to clump together. These clustered blood cells are unable to properly absorb oxygen for distribution to the body's tissues, which can damage the heart." In his classic book, *A Cancer Therapy – Results of 50 Cases*, Charlotte's late father, Max Gerson, MD, put soy and soy products on the forbidden list of foods for Gerson Therapy patients.

No less an authority than the US Department of Energy Health Risk Laboratory has published research showing that isoflavones in soy act in the same way as the outlawed insecticide *DDT* to cause breast cancer cells to multiply. In 1988 a Taiwan University team led by Dr Theodore Kay remarked that for more than half a century soy has been known to cause thyroid enlargement, especially in women and children.

Dr Mike Fitzpatrick, a respected toxicologist who is at the forefront of the New Zealand campaign against soy, wrote a paper in 1998 citing much of the published work on the dangers of soy isoflavones, which he submitted to the US Food and Drug Administration (FDA). This paper was also published in the *Price-Pottenger Nutrition Foundation Journal* under the title *Isoflavones: Panacea or Poison?*, and subsequently as *Soy Formulas and the Effect on the Thyroid* in *The New Zealand Medical Journal (February 2000)*. It is long, detailed, and frightening.

Here are just some of the things he has to say: "The toxicity of isoflavones to animals first raised the awareness of the scientific community to the fact that soy isoflavones are endocrine disruptors... There have been profound negative endocrine effects in all animal species studied to date."

In plainspeak, this means that your glandular system can be damaged by soy, and if your glands don't function properly, your health will suffer drastically. There is more: "Soy isoflavones increase the risk of breast cancer... Soy isoflavone disrupts the menstrual cycle during, and for up to three months after, administration... Dietary concentration of genistein may stimulate breast cells to enter the cell cycle... Concern was expressed that women fed soy protein isolate have an increased incidence of epithelial hyperplasia."

Neither Safe Nor Natural

With these and numerous other credible studies warning women of the adverse effects of prolonged consumption of soy, how, in all conscience, can Australian household brands like *Herron, Novogen* and those self-proclaimed icons of good health, *Blackmores* and *Sanitarium*, continue to promote the use of soy and isoflavones extracted from soy as 'tonics' for middle-aged women in menopause? Or health professionals endorse claims that soy is a safe, natural alternative to HRT. What they are pushing is neither safe, nor natural and they should be ashamed for suggesting that it is either.

Phytic acid is another jolly little part of the abominable bean's makeup – and also totally destroys the credibility of the manufacturers' claims that soy products are a good source of calcium and help prevent osteoporosis. Because soy contains more phytic acid than any other grain or pulse, and because phytic acid impairs absorption of all minerals, especially calcium, soy actually strips your body of calcium. The enzyme inhibitors in soybeans block *trypsin* and other enzymes essential for good health. This can produce serious gastric distress, reduced protein digestion, and chronic deficiencies in essential amino acids.

All the foregoing assertions, and more, are well-documented, and have been available for many years, with new evidence becoming available almost every day. Detailed references for all the papers and extracts on which I have drawn for this chapter are too numerous to be included here, but many of them can be found in a special section on my website, which contains the equivalent of 16 A4 pages of references (almost the length of this chapter) to scientific studies attesting to the dangers of soy, covering a 50-year period to date.

For reasons I will explain shortly, most of this 'subversive' material has not achieved wide circulation, being the work of corporate-neutral or independent scientists, who are not in the pay of the multinationals, and who are as voices in the wilderness. Their papers often appear only in esoteric professional journals, or 'alternative' publications, such as the Australian *Nexus Magazine* which also publishes editions in New Zealand, the UK and US, who have been courageous in pursuing a 'publish and be damned' policy by enabling publication of arguments against the lies of the big corporations.

> *Attention Animal Lovers*:
> Be vigilant when buying pet food. Most contain soy, because it is dirt cheap. It will shorten your animal's lives and make them miserable while they are here!

Nevertheless, through the efforts and dedication of many enlightened, qualified, courageous, independent and highly-respected scientists, researchers and medical practitioners, it has been possible to unearth volumes of credible research and evidence which demonstrates clearly the criminality of the actions of companies, spearheaded by the mighty Monsanto Corporation, whose genetically-modified cultivar is the prime source of all this misery.

Bringing the covert actions of the soy industry into the public arena has been an undertaking of truly David and Goliath proportions. The public relations machine extolling the virtues of soy has been global and relentless. It has to be – there are at least 100 million acres of soy under cultivation in the United States alone, much of it genetically engineered.

In Australia it is estimated that about 50,000 acres are being cultivated. Displaying the kind of ingenious duplicity which even Machiavelli would surely applaud, and conscious of the public unease regarding genetically modified foods and the trend towards organically-grown produce, Monsanto Corporation has 45 million acres of genetically modified soybeans growing in the United States. American law permits these crops to be mixed with a small amount of organic soybeans, and the resultant combination may then be labelled organic! And you still think the government wouldn't let them lie to you?

Radio activity

Although getting the anti-soy message across is unbelievably difficult, there have been a few occasions when I have been given air time on Australian radio and television to bring this particular piece of corporate skullduggery to public attention – notably on Alan Jones' 2GB Sydney Breakfast Programme, Yvonne Adele's evening programme on 3AK Melbourne and Channel Seven's national breakfast show, 'Sunrise'.

In all cases, the audience response was phenomenal – and without exception, supportive of my claims. The broadcasts also elicited many more instances of health problems directly attributable to the abominable bean.

And I was able to gain some satisfaction from seeing that one major Australian soy-pusher was so concerned that its customers might suspect the truth that it was forced to take expensive full-page ads in national newspapers to 'reassure' listeners and viewers that its products were blameless.

With these levels of production at stake a market must be found, increased and maintained. To this end, American soy bean farmers contribute approximately US$80 million per year to finance what is one of the most effective propaganda campaigns ever known to the Western world. The resultant high-powered publicity blitz ensures that 'news' stories about soy's benefits are everywhere, reinforced by multi-million dollar advertising campaigns.

Thumb through any popular women's magazine, read the newspapers, watch the television commercials and count, for example, those for soy drinks alone. Soy producers, processors and manufacturers spend billions of dollars advertising the 'goodness' of their products. The economics of the mass media ensure that such expenditure guarantees the regular placement of news and feature items extolling the claimed health benefits of soy. The same economics also guarantee that the chances are minimal of any extensive publicity being given to reports of tragic cases such as those mentioned earlier, and the dire warnings of hundreds of corporate-neutral scientific and academic researchers. What media mogul is going to risk offending the Goose that lays these particular Golden Eggs by appearing to question the worth of the product or the truth of the ads?

Sure, occasionally, a report of adverse scientific findings or medical evidence may be too newsworthy to be ignored and will find its way into the inside pages. No problem; in the interests of balanced reporting, the manufacturer will receive their Right of Reply and has an army of in-house or retained 'independent' experts ready with a rebuttal. Even if the rebuttal is unsubstantiated, or based on limited or inaccurate research, it will be published and we're all expected to drink up our soy milk and go back to sleep.

Believe me, this industry has secured the services of some of the best scientific prostitutes money can buy. And if that doesn't work, the usual 'Plan B' is simply to attempt to discredit the whistleblower. But it's not only the media who bear responsibility for helping the soy industry carry out this mass-manipulation and brainwashing. Most of our health professionals appear so busy, or so unconcerned, that even if they were prepared to question what you're told in the glossy handouts the suppliers give them to hand to you if you ask for information, they probably wouldn't consider it worthwhile. People who wouldn't believe anything else Monsanto Chemical says swallow, hook line and sinker, their self-serving lies about soy.

Consider the words of Dr Raymond Peat, the noted endocrine physiologist at the University of Oregon who was one of the first to blow the whistle on the dangers of HRT, years before it finally made headlines:

> "There is a distinct herd instinct among people who 'work in science' which makes it easy to believe whatever sounds plausible, if a lot of other people are saying it is true. Sometimes powerful economic interests help people to change their beliefs. For example, two of the biggest industries in the world, the estrogen industry and the soy bean industry, spend vast amounts of money helping people to believe certain plausible-sounding things that help them sell their products."

We could add to that the tendency for people to believe what they want to believe. Especially when it's comforting, reassuring and comes from 'someone who knows'.

Which brings me to my well-intentioned but badly misled critics mentioned earlier. Those who are so offended that I should dare to question the masses of 'independent scientific research' extolling the virtues of their favourite health-giving food. Or that I should choose to dismiss the 'well known fact' that people in Japan practically live on soy and don't suffer from any of the problems I go on about.

The Asian Myth

Many of the subjects I debate with students during my lectures at Hippocrates Health Centre and at public speaking engagements are controversial. There are always some who disagree, but they accept these findings when presented with evidence. The soy controversy, however, is another matter, and some simply can't accept what I say. Their arguments always centre on their perception that 'everyone' says soy is good; they've read glowing press releases on soy; listened to what health professionals have told them; and surely there's no question about the 'fact' that Asian women do so well on soy food and have few problems with menopause or osteoporosis.

These arguments are so fallacious and so dependant on what the world's most effective commercial publicity machine would have us believe that it's hard to know where to begin. But here goes.

To begin with, soy does *not* comprise a major part of the Japanese, or any other Asian diet. And it is likely that very little of the domestically produced soy is grown from the genetically modified cultivar which dominates the Western market. In any case, except in poverty and during times of famine, Asians consume soy in tiny amounts – 7 to 8 grams per day – and most of this has been fermented for from 3 to 5 years to remove the toxins. The fermentation process also reduces the growth depressants in all soy products, but does not remove them entirely. The Japanese eat a small amount of tofu and miso as part of a mineral-rich broth, followed by meat or fish, which offsets some of the dangers.

Dr Raymond Peat and others have shown that tofu (a soy derivative) consumption is associated with dementia. In a major US study, eight thousand Japanese-American men from Hawaii were assessed for mid-life tofu consumption and its relation to brain function and structural changes in later life. Researchers performed radiologic brain neuro-imaging, extensive cognitive function studies, and post mortem follow-ups. Among the subjects of the study, an increased level of tofu consumption was found to be associated with indications of brain atrophy and cognitive impairment in later life. They even found, at autopsy, swelling of the brain cavities and a decrease in brain weight among heavy tofu eaters. This study was reported in *The Journal Of The American College Of Nutrition*, *April 2000,* and reprinted in Dr William Campbell Douglass' *Second Opinion Newsletter*.

Whilst on the subject of soy consumption in Asian countries, one real and bitter truth that does not appear in the producers' handouts is that an abnormally high incidence of cretinism in parts of China where soy is widely consumed because the people are too poor to get other forms of protein, has been linked to brain damage caused by the iodine-depleting effect of soy-based goitrogens on the thyroid. New Zealand toxicologist Dr Mike Fitzpatrick says, "An epidemiological study in China has shown that high soy intake is not protective against breast cancer. There have been several similar studies, which have refuted the theory that soy helps prevent breast cancer."

Furthermore, Asians, unlike Westerners, do not guzzle soy protein isolate as a milk substitute. Milk is not a part of their culture.

Bad Science

So how do these 'myths' originate? In recent years, several studies have been published regarding the soybean's effect on human health. Thanks to the power of the well-oiled PR machine, the most widely-published results are those of the studies *underwritten by various factions of the soy industry*. Not surprisingly, they are always presented as being overwhelmingly in favour of soy, even when this is not the conclusion of their own researchers! The primary claims about soy's health benefits are based purely on bad science or 'skewed' interpretation.

Although arguments for cancer patients to use soy focus on statistics showing low rates of breast, colon and prostate cancer among Asian people, there are obvious facts being utterly ignored. While soy-funded studies boast that Asian women suffer far fewer cases of breast cancer than do American women, they neglect to point out that these Asian women eat a diet that is dramatically different from that of their Western counterparts. The standard Asian diet consists of more natural products, greater amounts of vegetables and more fish. Their diets are also lower in chemicals and toxins, as they eat far fewer processed foods. It is likely these studies are influenced by the fact that cancer rates rise among Asian people who move to the US and adopt American diets. Ignoring the remarkable diet and lifestyle changes, to assume only that reduced levels of soy in these American-Asian diets is a primary factor in greater cancer rates, is bad science.

As for the osteoporosis/menopause protection myth, it is absurd to infer that soy protects Asian women. Their habits and diets, as mentioned above, containing little junk food, are totally different from those of Westerners. Further, they rarely smoke or drink alcohol, and have not replaced vitamin D-containing butter with the damaging soy oil margarine so popular with misguided Westerners.

Need more evidence of the soy producers' dominance of what you can read about their product? A widely circulated article, **Scientists Suggest More Soy in Diet**, by Jane E. Allen, *Associated Press'* science writer, cites numerous speakers in the course of a symposium discussing the probable advantages of soy under the topic, **Health Impact of Soy Protein**. Their deliberations are still widely quoted as proof of soy's beneficial effects. Less well publicised is the article's comment that the US$50,000 symposium "…was underwritten by Protein Technologies International of St.Louis," *a DuPont subsidiary that makes soy protein!* What price impartiality?

Allergenic

Other popular arguments in support of soy state that fermented soy products like tempeh or natto contain high levels of vitamin B_{12}. However, these supportive arguments fail to mention that soy's B_{12} is an inactive B_{12} analog, not utilised as a vitamin in the human body. Some researchers speculate this analog may actually serve to block the body's B_{12} absorption. It has also been found that allergic reactions to soybeans are far more common than to all other legumes. Even the American Academy of Pediatrics admits that early exposure to soy through commercial infant formulas may be a leading cause of soy allergies among older children and adults.

And while on 'Furphys', one persistent critic tells me that he "knows for sure" that allowing the bean to sprout removes all the toxins. He remains unconvinced by the scientific evidence that shows that sprouting allows genistein to metamorphose into coumestrol, which happens to be 30 times more oestrogenically potent!

A while back, as information regarding the dangers of soy started leaking out, the public relations machine went into overdrive, churning out stories about how the 'baddies' known to be in soy are removed during processing. This is a complete untruth, which has been refuted by many studies, yet is fervently espoused by the soy adherents. As described earlier, processing actually *adds* more deadly ingredients to an already potent toxic cocktail.

There are many more 'truths' that the pro-soy lobby will trot out as the answer to just about any health concern, and if you still believe the claim that taking soy will improve hormonal health in men and women, consider this. Eating soy with that intention is not only dangerous, it is futile, as reported in **Nexus Magazine**: "Celibate monks living in monasteries and leading a vegetarian lifestyle find soy foods quite helpful because they dampen libido."

In developed countries such as the USA, Canada, Australia and New Zealand, governments have established statutory bodies with the power to ensure the safety of proprietary food and drugs made available to the public. Sadly, as far as the marketing of soy is concerned, the FDA in the US and the Australia-New Zealand Food Authority, ANZFA (now renamed Food Standards Australia New Zealand – FSANZA), have both displayed a willingness to put the commercial interests of manufacturers ahead of those of the consumers, even to the extent of falsifying data or withholding commercially unpalatable information.

In our own region, one recent extraordinary and blatant case of deliberate government deception has come to light – and been totally ignored by the media. It concerns, once again, the use of soy in baby formula, and should be considered carefully by anyone who is still under the impression that "they wouldn't be allowed to sell it if it wasn't safe."

Hiding the Truth

In March 1999, ANZFA prepared a document with the catchy title, *An Assessment of The Potential Risks to Infants Associated with Exposure to Soy-Based Infant Formulas*.

In Section 3.1, *Hazard Identification*, some potential hazards are listed:

3.1.2 Stimulation of oestrogen-sensitive tissue; Infertility; Sexual differentiation; Sexual maturation.
3.1.3 Neonatal brain development.
3.1.4 Thyroid alterations: Immune responses.
5.1.1 Dietary exposures: An exposure to hormone levels 240 times higher than breast milk.
6.0 Risk Assessment: "It is clear that phytoestrogens pose a potential hazard to the consumer of soy foods".

The signatories to this document included the Chief Toxicologist, Dr Luba Tomaska, together with Dr Fiona Cumming (ANZFA), Dr P Tuohy of the New Zealand Ministry of Health, and five academic experts in food safety from both Australia and New Zealand. Among the authoritative references examined by this committee was a 1999 assessment from a US Federal government laboratory, *Anti-thyroid Isoflavins From Soybean: Isolation, Characterisation and Mechanism of Action*, which examines 50 years of medical reports of thyroid harm and describes how it occurs.

The committee's final report was clear and unambiguous in its conclusions that the inclusion of soy in infant formula was potentially hazardous.

Yet, in May 2002, this same body, ANZFA, prepared a document for the signatures of all the Health Ministers of the Australian States and Territories and for the Australian and New Zealand Federal Health Ministers, setting standards for infant formulas which contained no hint or mention of the hazards detailed in their own expert committee's Risk Assessment document.

Following ANZFA's recommendations, all these health ministers, presumably unaware of the hazards that someone in ANZFA considered not worth bringing to their attention, signed the document. The result is that the agreed Standard for the composition of infant formula sold in Australia and New Zealand, now approves the inclusion of ingredients which its own expert committee (as well as many other authorities) have labelled severely detrimental to health.

Such approval flies in the face of Australian food safety and practice laws and puts our children at risk of permanent endocrine disruption and infertility.

Barefaced Lies

But it gets worse! Australian politicians, spurred by worried constituents who were questioning the inclusion of soy in baby formula, asked ANZFA for more information. The Authority's standard response was unbelievable – and a barefaced lie:

> *"...there is no evidence that exposure of healthy infants to soy-based infant formulas over 30 years has been associated with any demonstrated harm."*

Isn't it good to know that we have such honest and ethical watchdogs to safeguard our children's health? And why is this body prepared to continue to totally disregard not only its own qualified advisers, but also those of a high-powered UK government committee, whose report is noted on the final page of this chapter?

The Americans fare no better in trusting their government-appointed watchdogs. Their Food and Drug Administration has control over what claims are permitted to be made for food and drug products. They employ scientists and researchers to investigate and validate the claims made by manufacturers for their products and ingredients.

But, when it suits, the agency apparently has no compunction in ignoring, and pillorying, its own experts in order to please a manufacturer. As in the case of two FDA scientists, Daniel M Sheehan, PhD, director of the FDA's Estrogen Base Program in the Division of Genetic and Reproductive Toxicology, and Daniel R Doerge, PhD, a member of the Division of Bio-chemical Toxicology. In 1998, they protested the FDA's handling of a cardiovascular health claim by the giant DuPont soy manufacturing subsidiary, Protein Technologies International (PTI).

After examining the claims and making their own tests, Sheehan and Doerge sent a   letter to the FDA management vigorously opposing the claim, which centred largely on claimed beneficial effects of isoflavones in relation to lowering cholesterol levels. Both specialists in oestrogen research, they suggested instead that a warning might be more appropriate.

The FDA's response was to make the unprecedented move of rewriting PTI's petition, substituting all reference to isoflavones with the words 'soy protein' – a move in flagrant contradiction of FDA's own regulations, which then resulted in the health claim being allowed. They also banned Sheehan and Doerge from making public comment on the issue.

In a more passive action, the FDA has now become so acquiescent when it comes to helping the soy peddlers they have even allowed them to 'self regulate'. A manufacturer or processor is, with little, if any, supporting evidence, allowed to declare their product '*GRAS*' – Generally Regarded As Safe – a nomenclature which basically says, "This is OK and won't harm you because nobody has complained about it." Only in America? Don't you believe it!

Many of those who have dared to speak and act against the industry and its political protectors have suffered both physically and financially as a direct result. The story of a New Zealand couple, Valerie and Richard James, who devote their lives to exposing the evils of this trade, is worthy of honourable mention. Much of the suppressed research and evidence has been brought to worldwide attention through their single-mindedness and courage, and they have been a great source of inspiration, advice and information to me and to many others in our efforts to spread the word.

The James' Experience

I first became aware of the James' work from an article in **Nexus Magazine**. Breeders of tropical birds, the couple had been alerted to the genetic effects of soy when they switched to bird feed which was based on soy protein – with disastrous results: "…deformed, stunted and stillborn babies and premature deaths among females, with the result that the total population in the aviaries went into steady decline." They then realised that many of the symptoms suffered by their birds were similar to the symptoms suffered by their children, who had been fed soy formula. Understandably, they were deeply disturbed by what soy had done to their children and their birds, and enlisted the aid of toxicologist Mike Fitzpatrick, PhD, whose work is detailed elsewhere in this book. Together they formed an alliance to investigate and expose what big business and government preferred to hide.

While preparing the sixth edition of this book, I rang Valerie and Richard in Whangarei, New Zealand, to introduce myself and ask a favour. I needed a paragraph on the reaction of the soy industry and the New Zealand Government to their nine-year crusade against feeding babies soy formula. As Richard said, "It's impossible to compress years of fear and a constant feeling of menace into a paragraph." So they sent me, instead, a huge envelope stuffed full of the most horrifying information, which instilled in me a feeling of menace which remains with me to this day.

Even I, with my knowledge of cosy industry/government connections, was shocked by what I read. The James' enclosed a copy of the painstakingly-researched scientific proof they had presented to the government. This document is so damning that I was astonished they had been unable to persuade the government to even consider the problem. They enclosed hair-raising details of industry/government threats, lies from officials who were and are protecting the soy industry, and details of careers that were destroyed, grants withdrawn, and research papers censored or not published.

The pressure on one of the scientists with whom they worked was so great that his assistant suffered a nervous breakdown and had to flee the country. Yet the New Zealand government was and still is prepared to go to any lengths to protect the soy industry and their multi-billions in annual profits. Even their Federal Health Minister was firmly aligned behind the baby killers!

Threats and Lawsuits

As they have become recognised as serious threats to the continued dominance of the pro-soy lobbyists, the James' have faced all manner of threats, personal vilification and legal actions. Their own government actually allowed a soy producer to use government-funded Legal Aid to sue them for telling the truth about their product! They, of course, had to fund their own crippling legal defence. Despite this, and with increasing public support, they are preparing to lead a class action against Monsanto and others on behalf of thousands whose lives have been affected by the Killer Bean.

Visit Dr Fitzpatrick's website, *www.soyonlineservice.co.nz* , and you will be able to see not only the mountain of credible evidence he and the James's have assembled against the actions of the multinationals, but also get a sense of some of the lengths to which their detractors will go in their attempts to discredit them. This courageous couple are being pilloried for trying to save millions of babies from the crippling effects of soy formula! They should be thanked, instead of being sued and threatened. It's not only depressing: it's outrageous.

It would seem that there is no way decent people can win against the multinationals when these corporations are backed by governments.

Truth Will Out

But maybe there is hope yet. Slowly, and despite the power of the vested interests and the complacency and *laissez-faire* attitude of governments, the truth is beginning to emerge. The UK government is considering restricting the sale of soy-based infant formula, and the US Congress is now taking seriously a plethora of complaints and legal actions being instituted against Monsanto on behalf of millions of Americans whose lives have been ruined through the corporate greed of this legalised drug pusher. This is largely due to the efforts of the Weston A Price Foundation, a Washington public interest charitable organisation, which has conducted an unrelenting political lobbying campaign in Congressional Committees.

In other countries, notably Australia and New Zealand, as well as the USA, class actions are being prepared which will finally make public the human toll and the extent of cover-up, falsification, manip-ulation, harassment, threats and other illegal activities undertaken

> ### *Attention Men!*
> The Soy propagandists neglect to mention that their product contains a potent female hormone – phytoestrogen – that will adversely affect your fertility and your sex drive. If you fall victim to their billion dollar ad campaigns, YOUR TESTOSTERONE LEVELS WILL DROP, AND YOU MAY DEVELOP BREASTS And your son, if fed soy while in the womb, and then fed soy formula, will be in danger of having a penis no larger than its size in infancy, and may also develop breasts!

by powerful multi-nationals in order to maintain the multi-billion-dollar profits generated by this innocuous-looking, genetically modified and deadly poisonous bean.

Numerous former advocates of the inclusion of soy in our diet have been prepared to re-examine the evidence and are now publicly admitting they were misled by false claims, incomplete and fraudulent research. Which, paradoxically, seems to have hardened the resolve of less enlightened proponents to bury their heads even deeper in the sand and continue to ignore reality.

The words of one former soy user and prescriber are well worth considering. Here are some extracts from a letter sent by US hospital dietician Joyce Gross, MA, RD, LD/N, to her own patients and friends, which she has kindly allowed me to publish (you can read the full text on my website):

> "Some of you may remember that last year I was touting soy along with the rest of the medical profession regarding its beneficial effects. I was consuming soy for its phytoestrogen effect to alleviate menopausal symptoms. I was duped like so many other non-suspecting consumers.

> "I have developed Hashimoto's Disease or acute Hashimoto's Thyroiditis which is an acute autoimmune disease that affects the thyroid gland. (In basic terms this means that my thyroid is attacking itself and I can no longer produce thyroid hormone). My initial symptoms included things like severe joint pain especially in my hands, "trigger" finger(s), carpal tunnel syndrome, excessive weight gain (I gained about 25 lbs. in 3-4 weeks …"

After describing how her self-diagnosis and research established the cause and condition that physicians she consulted had at first failed to recognise, Joyce advised her friends:

> "… I have since found out that Hashi's can take 8 years to diagnose (we don't build up the antibodies overnight to it)…

> "The soybean industry is a multi-billion dollar industry in this country so they are trying to keep this quiet, even though there have been doctors in the FDA who have written position papers regarding the dangers of soy.

"With so many new products coming out containing soy, and the continued 'touting' of it as a major benefit, more and more women are going to become hypothyroid. I am currently working as a nutrition expert in treating depression, bi-polar disorder and substance abuse problems. I can't tell you how many of the women who are admitted for depression are also hypothyroid to the point now that the medical doctor automatically first checks their TSH before the psychiatrists even start prescribing their meds. If I hadn't been so adamant about taking over my own health issues last August, I could have very easily wound up being a patient in my own hospital."

Would that other influential health professionals had her courage and honesty.

Buyer Beware

In conclusion, I'd like to share with you a true story indicating the extent to which members of the soy lobby will go in order to mislead the consumer about the claimed benefits of their products. In Australia and New Zealand, the *Sanitarium Health Food Company* (a commercial, tax-free offshoot of the Seventh Day Adventist Church) makes a wide range of products containing soy – all of which are claimed by Sanitarium to provide health benefits.

In 1998, the New Zealand Commerce Commission launched a prosecution against Sanitarium for publishing over 150 misleading advertisements for its *So Good* soy milk, in which various unsubstantiated health-related claims were made. The NZCC action was settled out of court after Sanitarium signed a consent decree and entered a Deed of Trust promising not to repeat the claims.

Then, in 1999, Sanitarium formed and financed the official-sounding *International Soy Advisory Board*, which sent Sue Radd and others to New Zealand in May that year to promote Sanitarium's products. (Ms Radd is an Australian nutritionist whose media articles, books and public appearances invariably promote the 'goodness' of soy.)

In a cooking program on TV NZ's **Good Morning** show, Ms Radd, appearing as a 'nutritionist guest expert', spoke glowingly of the claimed benefits of soy consumption. Cartons of *So Good* were prominently in view of the camera.

The following are direct quotes from the published decision of the NZ Broadcasting Standards Authority in response to complaints about the program:

"The benefits of soy consumption were said to include a lower incidence of heart disease, improved reproductive health, reduction in the incidence of osteoporosis, and alleviation of the symptoms of menopause… The material discloses that the Nutritionist was closely aligned to Sanitarium, makers of 'So Good'…If an expert is aligned to product promotion, that ought to be made clear… By failing to disclose this relationship in a programme where she spoke positively of 'So Good', apparently as an 'independent' nutritionist, the Authority concludes that the broadcast, through this omission, breached the requirement of Standard in Sec G.1 to be truthful and accurate on points of fact.

"Where making claims about the health benefits of ingredients which are themselves a matter of controversy, then the Authority considers that the broadcast should at least acknowledge the existence of that controversy... those claimed benefits are a matter of contention and there is controversy... the Authority notes that no effort was made on the programme to point out that there is significant disagreement among the experts about the claimed health benefits of soy. As these criticisms were not raised or discussed, the Authority concludes that the programme lacked impartiality and balance, and that the Standard (G 6) was breached."

On 23 August 2002, both Sue Radd and I appeared on the Australian Channel 7 programme *Sunrise*, where she was again credited as a spokesperson for the *International Soy Advisory Board*. My attempts to clarify her credentials and cite the above case were gagged by the presenters and the 'independent' Ms Radd strongly denied she had any formal links to Sanitarium.

There's more. Sanitarium admits that it is the 'convenor' of the *Australasian Nutrition Advisory Council*, another supposedly independent public advisory body on nutrition. And, from Sanitarium's own website: "In 1987...Sanitarium established the *Nutrition Education Service* in order to provide the community with reliable, easy-to-understand nutrition information." So much for all that 'independent' research and advice (and let's not forget that many of their 'health' products are also laced with artificial sweeteners).

Shun Soy Protein Isolate! (SPI)

The stuff is poisonous! If you doubt that it is possible for the "authorities" to allow such a substance to be mixed in almost every processed food, read THE WHOLE SOY STORY. This impeccably-researched book explodes every lie told by the soy growers/pushers, and if we could just persuade our legislators to read it and act in our best interests for a change, all soy would be outlawed. Kaayla T. Daniel, PhD, CCN, is to be congratulated for the monumental work she has done, and for the way she takes readers by the hand and leads them to the truth. This is science writing at its best and it's entertaining too.

Dr. Daniel explains that SPI contains "...some 38 petroleum compounds including, but not limited to: butyl, methyl and ethyl esters of fatty acids; phenols, diphenyls and phenyl esters; abietic acid derivatives, diehydroabietinal, hexanal and 2-butyl-2-octenal aldehydes; dehydroabietic acid methyl ester; dehydroabietene and abietatriene."

Dr. Daniel exposes the way SPI increases the requirements for vitamins E, K, D and B12, and details the way carcinogenic nitrosamines and lysinoalanines are created during processing. Not surprisingly, severe mineral deficiencies appear in test animals fed SPI. (And, presumably, in people as well.) Yet, if you buy processed food, you will not be able to avoid SPI and it will not necessarily appear on the label. This deadly "food" belongs in the toxic waste dump, but the multi-nationals are disposing of it in **YOU, YOUR FAMILY AND IN BABY FORMULAS**. I call this genocide.

For those who ask if organic soy is safe, I say, "Would you eat organic arsenic?"

10

Hormonal Havoc

A close look at the symptoms, treatment and prevention of various hormone-related conditions:

Endometriosis	*Menstrual Irregularities*
Endometrial Cancer	*Vaginitis*
Fibroid Tumours	*Ovarian Cysts*
Uterine Cancer	*Urinary Tract Infection*
Fibromyalgia	*Incontinence*

Men, please do not skip the next three chapters because, even though they are more specific to women than to men, there is much of importance for men's health in them as well. Further, I hope that male readers will find that understanding the problems perhaps suffered by their partners may inspire kindness and a willingness to assist in preventing and overcoming these distressing conditions.

Endometriosis

According to the American Endometriosis Association, this painful, chronic disease affects 5.5 million women and girls in the USA and Canada, and millions more worldwide, and is frequently associated with infertility. It often occurs when tissue like that which lines the uterus (tissue called the endometrium) is found outside the uterus – usually in the abdomen on the ovaries, fallopian tubes, and ligaments that support the uterus; the area between the vagina and rectum; the outer surface of the uterus; and the lining of the pelvic cavity. Other sites for these endometrial growths may include the bladder, bowel, vagina, cervix, vulva, and in abdominal surgical scars. Less commonly, they are found in the lung, arm, thigh, and other locations.

This misplaced tissue develops into growths or lesions that respond to the menstrual cycle in the same way that the tissue of the uterine lining does: each month the tissue builds up, breaks down, and sheds. Menstrual blood flows from the uterus and out of the body through the vagina, but the blood and tissue shed from endometrial growths has no way of leaving the body. This results in internal bleeding, breakdown of the blood and tissue from the lesions, and inflammation – and can cause pain, infertility, scar tissue formation, adhesions, and bowel problems.

David Smallbone, MD, from Buxton, England, has been in medical practice for more than 30 years. For the past 25 years he has successfully and almost exclusively used nutrition, herbs and homeopathy, combined with diet and lifestyle changes, to treat his patients. He has been using natural progesterone for nearly a decade, and is well-versed in the finer points of using nutritional supplements to reverse illness and create health. Interviewed in ***Dr John Lee's Newsletter***, Dr Smallbone said this about endometriosis:

> "I'd say that three-quarters of the women with endometriosis that I put on natural progesterone are 20 percent improved over six months. The more prolonged and widespread the problem is, the slower the response.

> "I think that endometriosis is caused by an incorrect stimulus of blast cells, which are pre-differentiated cells that can be stimulated to turn into any type of cell, given the right circumstances. It's a combination then of estrogen – and specifically estradiol – over-stimulation and failure to control the cell itself. It's similar to the process that produces some cancer cells. I believe one of the factors in this is a failure to produce enough progesterone early in life. These would be women who have a lot of non-ovulatory cycles, girls who have early onset of menstruation but then have a lot of non-ovulatory cycles, and girls whose menstruation seems to start and stop a lot. It's in the earlier half of life that you get the first symptoms of it.

> "This is one reason why good nutrition is so important for teenagers. Those blast cells will be much better equipped to resist stimulation by estrogen if they are well-nourished. I also believe that birth control pills have an over-stimulating effect and should be avoided.

> "As always, by far the most effective approach to this debilitating illness is prevention."

So, eat your fruit and vegetables, with emphasis on raw; keep your immune system strong; and your digestion thorough.

Endometrial Cancer

Cancer of the womb is due to unopposed oestrogen and/or oestrogen dominance, conditions that are explained in the *Menopause* chapter of this book. As is the case with so many female illnesses, this can be prevented by diet and progesterone. Even the synthetics, progestogen and progestin, may help prevent this cancer, but they are most certainly not recommended, as they have serious side effects. The natural progesterone is the only healthful option.

We strongly recommend that any woman faced with a decision about endometrial complications read Dr John Lee's book, ***What Your Doctor May Not***

Tell You About Menopause. He has a most educational chapter on this subject, in which he states that any doctor recommending a hysterectomy for this problem is self-serving. "In pretending to act as protector of his/her patient, he/she manages to convert a side effect of a drug he/she administered (estrogen) into a lucrative surgical operation."

Fibroid Tumours

Dr Lee states that fibroid tumours, like breast fibrocysts, are a product of oestrogen dominance. Oestrogen stimulates their growth and lack of oestrogen causes them to atrophy. When natural progesterone is supplied, fibroids no longer grow and can be kept from growing until after menopause, at which time they gradually atrophy.

Dean Ornish, MD, in *Obstetrics and Gynecology, September, 1999,* states, "Fibroids are linked to hormones, such as oestrogen, and while they might not cause any problems they can contribute to conditions such as anaemia, pelvic pain and infertility... A diet rich in green vegetables appears to be particularly effective in preventing uterine fibroids, one of the most common reasons for hysterectomies."

Brenda Beeley, in her book, *Menopause And Osteoporosis*, recommends the following remedy: "Castor oil packs used 3–5 times per week over a period of 3–6 months help shrink fibroids. To make a castor oil pack, wet 2–4 layers of 12-inch-square cotton or wool flannel with castor oil. Place the wet (but not dripping) flannel on the abdomen. Cover it with a piece of plastic, then place a hot water bottle or heating pad on top of the plastic. Wrap a towel around the entire pack to hold in heat and leave it in place for one hour. Limiting one's intake of estrogen, which is found in birth control pills, estrogen replacement therapy, and dairy and meat products (from cows fattened with hormones) also helps shrink fibroids". Sounds like a pain, but certainly preferable to surgery!

Burton Goldberg, in his *Alternative Medicine Guide to Women's Health Series*, states, "As in endometriosis and breast lumps, the conventional medical treatment for fibroids is to cut them out, even though **almost all cases of fibroids are benign** (fewer than 0.5% of fibroids become cancerous). However, it may be difficult to remove just the fibroid, so the physician may want to perform a hysterectomy, removing the whole uterus."

This is criminal, considering how easy it is to avoid and/or cure this common problem, and many unnecessary hysterectomies are carried out on young, childless women. Doctors rarely tell women that they have options, so they are terrified by the prospect that the fibroids may become cancerous.

Burton Goldberg states, "The deleterious effects of hysterectomy have obviously not prevented its widespread use. During a Congressional investigation in 1977, the American Medical Association (AMA), testifying on the reasons for the high rate of hysterectomy, stated that the operation was used for sterilisation and as a preventive method to forestall cancer of the uterus in later years. The truth is the operation is a big moneymaker. That aside, the AMA's justifications are unconscionable, given the serious consequences of the procedure."

Women are rarely warned about these consequences; a one year recovery period, emotional trauma, accelerated aging of the ovaries, and a seven-fold increase in heart attacks and angina. When the ovaries are taken also, pancreatic problems and adrenal weakness occur, along with vaginal dryness, headaches, mood swings, urinary tract problems, hair loss and fatigue. So many of the women attending Hippocrates tell us that one of the worst symptoms is that sexual fulfilment, after hysterectomy, is a thing of the past. All this for an unnecessary operation that could have been avoided by following the dietary rules in this book and using natural progesterone!

Uterine Cancer

Diet is a major risk factor in this, as in most cancers. It is well known that when women from developing countries emigrate to industrialised countries, their risks for uterine and breast cancer rise substantially. Eating lots of salads and shunning junk food offers protection, as does progesterone. Doctors Lee and Peat, who have been so helpful to me in my research, are not the only scientists who recommend progesterone. There are a great many more. For example, Neils Lauersen, MD, Professor of Obstetrics and Gynaecology at New York Medical College, and author of *PMS: Premenstrual Syndrome And You*. Dr Lauersen says, "No human cancer has been reported during progesterone treatment; quite the reverse, progesterone has been used in treating specific uterine cancers."

Fibromyalgia

Fibromyalgia, which we have been hearing a lot about in recent years, is a severe, debilitating, painful condition mostly affecting women. Although not strictly a hormonal condition, it is included here because its symptoms can mimic those of oestrogen dominance. It is commonly manifested by pain in the fibrous tissues of the body – the muscles, ligaments and tendons. Other common symptoms associated with fibromyalgia include fatigue, sleep disorder, cognitive impairments, numbness and tingling sensations, irritable bowel symptoms, and more. The symptoms are so close to the symptoms of oestrogen dominance, or progesterone lack, that it appears to be beyond coincidence. There have been anecdotal reports of women getting rid of all their symptoms by simply using progesterone.

It is interesting that the symptoms of fibromyalgia mimic those of oestrogen dominance – particularly when you consider that during pregnancy the placenta produces ten times more progesterone than is produced normally in an ovulating woman, and that many women have reported that the only time they have been free of symptoms was during each of several pregnancies. One woman who had suffered symptoms for 30 years reported that during her seven pregnancies the symptoms disappeared. She finally got the message, started taking natural progesterone, and has been well ever since.

As Raquel Martin, in **The Estrogen Alternative** says, "What great protection progesterone provides us during pregnancy! Could it also be critical for our good health?"

Unless it is in the early stages, however, management of this terrible condition is not as simple as merely using progesterone on its own. More about the effect adrenal exhaustion and hypothyroidism have on all aspects of health, including fibromyalgia, can be found in *Chapters 1* and *2*.

Menstrual Irregularities

Heavy, painful periods and PMS are easily prevented by faithfully adhering to a good diet. But I mean *really good* – follow the rules in this book and don't deviate for at least a month to give your body a chance to heal itself. If it doesn't, it would be wise to consult a qualified natural therapist about possible adrenal insufficiency and/or thyroid function. Your life may be so stressful that your adrenals can't cope, and your thyroid, which is crucial for all aspects of health, may have been inadequate since birth or, possibly, so injured by the wrong foods (such as soy) that it will need support (see *Chapter 1*, *That "Mystery Illness"* and *Chapter 2, Adrenal Insufficiency*). There are natural methods for improving these glands, such as homeopathics and acupuncture. And please don't forget your natural progesterone!

Oestrogen dominance, relative to progesterone, has a profound effect upon most aspects of female reproductive system health. PMS and problem periods are no exception, a fact attested to by so many prominent scientists that there isn't space to list them all.

Vaginitis

This unpleasant condition occurs more frequently among women who take birth control pills. These dangerous little pills prevent hormone-generated mucous from being produced. This mucous protects the vagina from infectious organisms. All of which proves, once again, that you can't play around with mother nature without consequences. Dr Lee says that natural progesterone will provide relief for this condition, but that it can take three to four months.

There are many causes of vaginitis: poor diet, bacteria, yeast overgrowth, parasites, nylon undies and pantyhose and tight clothing. Antibiotics bring quick relief, but they do not address the causes, and symptoms recur, leaving the patient with the problems antibiotics themselves cause. Loss of intestinal flora creates a perfect environment for vaginitis, so it is essential to get into the habit of taking an effective acidophilus.

Keep your immune system strong through careful diet, as it is needed to fight off infections. Do not use perfumed products near your vaginal area, and use warm water, not soap, which can be extremely irritating. Do not use tampons; the reasons are explained at the end of this chapter.

Alternative medicine can offer help for this condition, but if it is not effective, see a physician, as vaginitis can spread to other organs and cause serious harm.

Ovarian Cysts

Women tend to panic when diagnosed with ovarian cysts, and who could blame them? Many fear that cancer of the ovaries will be the next step, but in the majority of women this is not the case. It is wise, however, to have a medical examination to rule out this possibility. Burton Goldberg, in his helpful book, **Women's Health**, quotes the noted natural health specialist, Ralph Golan, MD, of Seattle, Washington, who says, "An operation need not be a first option unless the findings are suspicious for malignancy or there are other clear indications for surgery. Often the cysts shrink and disappear by themselves." If surgery is performed, the surgeon may remove the ovaries and even the uterus. This drastic measure will send the woman into premature menopause, with all the physical and emotional trauma that entails.

Several factors need to be identified and corrected; smoking, including passively, must be stopped. Correcting any thyroid insufficiency is essential, and diet must be improved, as what women eat can be both the cause and the cure for ovarian cysts. Dr Lee says that adding natural progesterone from day 10 to day 26 of the menstrual cycle will very likely shrink ovarian cysts and cause them to disappear without further treatment. The chance of avoiding an operation will be greatly enhanced by sticking faithfully to all of the above measures.

Urinary Tract Infection (UTI)

This miserable affliction occurs mostly in women, although men who have had urethral operations can develop it. Sometimes it develops slowly, with frequent urination and some degree of pain. Untreated, the infection is likely to escalate, with urination as frequent as every few minutes, accompanied by burning pain, and even a few drops of blood in extreme cases. I used to call it 'the kiss of fire', and had it several times a year. Once I learned how to eat healthfully, the attacks stopped.

Cystitis is bacterial, so physicians usually prescribe antibiotics, which stop the pain and mask the infection. These drugs do not, however, cure anything, and often perpetuate the problem, setting women up for chronic, lifetime cystitis and frequent antibiotic use. This occurs because antibiotic suppression drives the infection deeper into the body where it is less apparent and harder to correct, and reappears when the host is weakened.

As always, the best approach to any UTI is prevention; drink plenty of pure water and do not turn your intestines into a breeding ground for bacteria by eating junk food and drinking excessive alcohol.

Ingesting sugar has a profound influence on UTI. Sugars and grains, which rapidly break down into sugars, will fuel disease-causing bacteria in the intestine and are likely to infect the bladder.

Keep man-made fabrics away from your body and never wear pantyhose without cotton panties underneath. In cold weather, keep your nether regions insulated by warm undies. Avoid tampons.

Good hygiene is important, but be aware that most soap is toxic, and does not belong on delicate tissues. Very warm water will keep you clean. If you are not comfortable with that, Nancy Evans has a lovely, safe coconut soap, which is detailed in **Resources**. Bubble baths are filled with scary chemicals, talc is dangerous, and commercial douches contain extremely irritating chemicals. The anus is a source of contamination, so wipe from front to back after bowel movements.

Sexual intercourse, I am sorry to inform you, can cause severe irritation, thus the term 'honeymoon cystitis'. Cleanliness is essential, and remember that penetration without sufficient lubrication can cause small abrasions in the vagina that allow bacteria to breed. Wise women take care to drink plenty of water after intercourse. Tedious as this is, it sure beats a miserable bout with a UTI! Contraceptive creams, jelly and foam can irritate, as can spermicidal and/or lubricated condoms.

A particularly nasty chemical, *Nonoxynol-9* (N-9), is found in most vaginal gels, foams, creams, suppositories, and sponges, and is also used as a lubricant. According to British medical journal **The Lancet**, it should be banned, but of course has not been, and is still a danger. Beware of a product, advertised as "The answer to a woman's true sexuality", which contains *propylene glycol*, *methylparaben* and other must-avoid chemicals, in spite of being promoted as "safe and natural".

So, avoid all sexual 'aids' and lubricants as they all contain harmful ingredients, even when not listed on labels. All will increase your danger of contracting cystitis, or any of the other conditions mentioned in this section. Stick with pure coconut oil and Dr Peat's progesterone oil and know that you will be safe.

Constipation can be an underlying cause of frequent cystitis attacks. If you are not regular, increase your magnesium intake to establish healthful elimination. In order to keep your all-important immune system perking, make certain your thyroid is functioning properly.

Lactobacillus acidophilus helps to restore bacterial balance in the vagina and urinary tract, and can help prevent cystitis. I have heard good reports about 500mg of acidophilus vaginal suppositories, inserted twice weekly for two weeks, and once a month for two months.

Cranberry juice is a popular remedy, helping some, but occasionally aggravating the condition for others. It is necessary to hunt around to find an unsweetened, unpreserved juice. Don't drink it if you cannot find a pure one, because the sugar and additives will aggravate the condition. Cranberry capsules can be of help for some. Diluted pineapple juice can stop an attack, but it has to be caught quickly, and it is necessary to eat nothing until the urgency stops. In Australia all the pineapple juices are contaminated with unnatural vitamin C and other nasties, so avoid them. Pure juices are readily available in the US.

Parsley can be helpful, as a tea or just eaten raw. Steep a large bunch of parsley in two quarts of boiling water and allow to sit for 20-30 minutes. This is both a remedy and a preventative.

Some natural health practitioners suggest going entirely off solid food and drinking copious amounts of pure water. Some recommend eating nothing but watermelon for two days, and these remedies are often successful if started immediately symptoms appear.

Extreme stress can bring on a cystitis attack, as can anger and resentment which are suppressed. A woman I know was being stalked by a man who appeared occasionally and frightened her with his menacing appearance. Each time she encountered him she felt an immediate burning in the vagina, which led to cystitis. When the police were finally able to persuade the man to leave her alone, the cystitis attacks stopped.

Far and away the finest remedy we have found for a UTI is *D-mannose*. It works perfectly on the 90 per cent of cases that are caused by the E-Coli bacteria. Reports coming in to us have been conclusive; D-mannose acts both as a preventative, and as a cure that completely replaces the need to take dangerous antibiotics. This is a real find: women have been looking for this kind of help for centuries. See **Resources** for Australian and US sources.

D-mannose is a naturally-occurring simple fruit sugar (not to be confused with our old enemy, cane sugar) and is safe for young children, diabetics and the elderly. The container recommends only ½ teaspoon every three hours during an attack, but we have found that it's better to take a full teaspoon. I have had plenty of experience suggesting this remedy to women, and I can recommend it wholeheartedly, even for severe, long-term UTIs.

This is how D-mannose does its job: E. coli bacteria stick to mannose molecules present on the surfaces of the cells that line the bladder. When a person with an E. coli infection takes D-mannose, the 'loose' molecules of D-mannose surround and coat each E. coli bacterium, so they can't stick to the bladder. The next time the patient urinates, the D-mannose-coated E. coli are rinsed away. This treatment is quicker, and certainly safer than antibiotics.

This excellent remedy also helps some people who do not have an E. coli infection, but simply have to urinate more frequently than average. Somehow, it appears to relax the bladder and urethra. A mother, whose nine-year-old daughter had been plagued by cystitis for years, rang me in desperation. Her physician had just said he wanted to give the girl a triple dose of antibiotic – a huge dose of the medicine that had not worked for years, and would add to the girl's toxic load. I suggested D-mannose, and she was kind enough to ring me a month later to report that her daughter was finally well. Then, six months later, at open house at Hippocrates, she told me there had been no recurrences, and that her son also benefited. A real godsend!

D-mannose will not, however, cure *chlamydia*, *mycoplasma*, and other non-Ecoli infections. These are mainly caused via sexual contact and will require a trip to the doctor.

The safest approach to UTIs is to employ natural methods as quickly as possible before the infection takes hold. I recommend always having D-mannose on hand, just in case. If you do not have it, and if fasting proves unsuccessful, it is essential not to delay medical treatment, as UTIs can work their way up into the bladder, and even to the kidneys, causing a serious and painful illness. I'm advised that '*Triprim*' is milder and less dangerous than other antibiotics. It is only necessary to take one tablet per day for three to seven days, depending upon how quickly the pain and frequency are gone. But remember – it is essential to re-establish the intestinal flora after taking any antibiotics. Get the best acidophilus you can find and take it religiously to undo the damage.

Incontinence

Incontinence is a dilemma for many mature women. Symptoms can range from tiny 'urgency' drips to serious leakage. Before submitting to the knife, we advise trying two natural remedies that can be of help. One is a Celery and Juniper tablet, which can be found in pharmacies and health food stores. We have had favourable comments from women regarding this remedy.

Another method, which has been used successfully for half a century, is the Dr Kegel pelvic floor exercises. This takes time and dedication, and it is essential to do it properly. It is increases in intro-abdominal pressure that cause the pelvic floor and urethra to weaken, and these exercises were designed to strengthen them.

Because most women have not been properly instructed in how to do the exercises, they are not always successful, and word of mouth is that they don't work. But they do, if done properly. First, squeeze the vaginal muscles (the ones you use to stop the flow of urine) and hold for a count of 10 seconds. Relax for a count of five, then repeat. Do five sets, three times per day. Consistency is the key, and results are noticeable in three to four weeks. While doing the Kegels, do not contract your abdominal or buttock or thigh muscles at the same time you are contracting the vaginal area. Should you squeeze incorrectly, the problem will be aggravated.

My experience with D-Mannose is new, but I have reason to believe that it can help to relieve incontinence in some instances. A number of women have told me that their problems were eased. Please let me know your experiences with this effective, safe remedy.

Reproductive Illnesses

Prevention beats being carved up, and one of the most important measures women can take to protect themselves from *all* reproductive illnesses is to *shun tampons*, unless they are guaranteed to be made of pure cotton. Amazingly, governments permit manufacturers of these poison tubes to bleach them, using dioxin, a cancer-causing chemical that is toxic to the reproductive system. Fibres from tampons left behind in the vagina create a breeding ground for the dioxin, so male partners are affected as well, and the immune systems of both sexes are broken down over time. Even sperm counts can be lowered by this potent poison.

Manufacturers also use asbestos, which is permitted because, since asbestos-contaminated tampons are not classified as food, they are not considered dangerous. This is a clue to the intelligence (or could it be the corruption?) of our regulators. Why asbestos? Because it causes women to bleed more; therefore,

More Blood = More Use = More Sales = More Profits

for greedy companies.

These extremely dangerous chemicals are easily absorbed, through the delicate mucosa of the vagina, into the bloodstream. Because dioxins are endocrine disruptors they can create many life-threatening health problems, and seriously upset the hormonal balance necessary for female health. Seventy-five years ago, when these chemicals were not used, there were virtually no reported cases of endometriosis, versus five million in the US today. This is no coincidence.

If government 'watchdogs' actually did their jobs instead of supporting industry, these killers would be banned. Instead, manufacturers are permitted to do as they wish. They can only continue doing this if we cooperate. Complain.

Organise pickets. Warn your friends. It does take time to get their attention, but once their bottom line is affected changes will come. My optimism, unfortunately, is not based on experience with industry. Remember when the toxic shock syndrome was proved to be caused by dioxin-containing tampons? There was a hue and cry, and much PR about a safe tampon being produced. Nothing happened, and I don't understand it. After all, tampons are destined for an area where safety is paramount and beauty will go unobserved.

Useful Instrument

A scientific product which readers may find useful in helping to observe and understand their natural ovulation cycle better, is the *Arbor Test Microscope*. This instrument helps with birth control by using a saliva sample to display and interpret hormonal changes taking place. Details in **Resources**.

Coca Cola Does It Again!

Evidently this multinational company is not content with raking in billions promoting their heavily-sugared, chemical-laden, bone-debilitating old fashioned Coke, and their thoroughly discredited and despicable Diet Coke (see **Chapter 4**, *Excitotoxins*). They have now hopped on yet another money spinning bandwagon – a cholesterol-reducing orange juice, called *Minute Maid Premium Heart Wise*.

So, what is this magic ingredient that they claim will reduce the cholesterol our bodies need in order to manufacture essential hormones and keep our brains perking? In a word, PHYTOSTEROLS! And what will phytosterols do to our bodies? Simply put, they will create havoc. This is a quote from one of Coke's news releases:

> The product will contain plant sterols, an additive that has been used in cholesterol-fighting margarine and other food products. Plant sterols have been shown to cut bad cholesterol levels by about 10 percent when used consistently.

Right. Bear in mind that you are probably already getting a surfeit of plant sterols if you ingest any of the many manufactured foods and supplements that contain them. And what exactly are they? As my colleagues and fellow anti-soy activists, Valerie and Richard James of New Zealand, say, "Phytosterols are natural plant estrogens. Because of their reputations in folklore as abortifacients, menstrual cycle disrupters and ecbolic (hastening labour or miscarriage) agents and are known to stimulate uterine tissue and have hormonal influences on the reproductive tract, the World Health Organisation sponsored a huge study to investigate 'Nature's Contraceptives'. This can be accessed through the April and May 1975 issues of the *Journal of Pharmaceutical Sciences* including *Farnsworth et al 1975a*, and *Farnsworth_et al 1975b*."

The study concluded that, **"If one inspects the structures of the estrogenic sterols, one can see a striking similarity of the skeletal structures of these compounds with the structure of the synthetic estrogen diethylstilbestrol."**

That's *DES*, which those of you with good memories may remember as the drug given to millions of women so they would not miscarry. What these unfortunate women didn't know, and wouldn't discover for years, was that taking DES condemned their female children to early death from cancer. And now Coca Cola wants to target a new generation in the same way. As the James' say on their website, "Soyonlineservice is appalled and horrified that Coca Cola would target children with such compounds for profit. We are even more appalled that this is occurring in the same year that the European Commission experts calculated that daily exposures could be way beyond twice a safe amount *(http://europa.eu.lnt/comm/food/fs/sc/scf/out192_en.pdf)*."

We at Hippocrates Health Centre are appalled and horrified as well, but not surprised, considering the track record of the food processors. Watch out for this government-sanctioned poison. Warn your children. Warn your friends. "They" are trying to kill us all!

Hold the presses! Shortly before this book was due to go to the printer, a reader sent me a box of pure cotton tampons, made by a company that does not use dioxin. The box says "100% Natural Cotton. No synthetics, no dyes, no chemicals. Hypo-allergenic. Be natural." They make a full line of sanitary products and are sold all over Australia in supermarkets and in chemists. Information can be found on their website, www.cottons.com.au. You can also reach them on 1-800-814-792. The company is called COTTONS.

> "Your hysterectomy is your doctor's Mercedes payment."
>
> (Said by millions of women – when it was too late.)

> "She who speaks the truth needs a fast horse."
>
> (Ancient proverb - gender changed.)

11

The Menopause

There <u>are</u> safe alternatives to the heavily-touted aids and treatment, such as HRT, which do more harm than good

Let me tell you a sad story of medical neglect... mine. Starting with my first menstrual period, one week out of every month was a misery of pain, flooding and huge clots that made school, and later, work, difficult, to say the least.

Inevitably, I had severe anaemia from the blood clots and was given toxic iron tablets. No physician, and I saw a few, had anything to offer me other than dilation and curettage (D&C) which did absolutely no good and, of course, left poisons in my liver from the anaesthesia. Then, 40 years ago, two gynaecologists told me that I absolutely had to have a hysterectomy if I wanted to survive. By then I knew what that meant, so I told them they would have to catch me first, and instead I learned how to eat properly.

Two weeks after going on a strict diet, I had my first normal period and, from then on, breezed right through. I guess you can imagine that I was disillusioned by the medical profession, and regretful about all the unnecessary suffering I was put through because no one told me that if I ate properly I would have been spared years of misery. It is so simple: those heavy, painful periods were nature's way of ridding my body of the rubbish I was putting in it. Once I learned that, I never took another bite of unhealthy food. It wasn't worth it. And on the subject of medical malfeasance, I want to tell you another sad story.

This one is about an American heroine, Frances Kelsey, a pathologist who practiced in Washington, DC. This brave woman single-handedly kept *Thalidomide* out of the USA because she suspected it was dangerous, and she nearly lost her position, because the pharmaceutical companies put pressure on her and on the Food and Drug Administration to force her to back down. She was actually told she would be fired, so she gave a press conference, spilled the beans, and the FDA had to relent. Of course, you all know the end of that story. She saved millions of American children from deformity.

Heinous Crime

A story such as this gives you an idea of the corruption endemic in the agencies that are supposed to protect us. They don't – they protect the multinationals. It's no different in Australia and we have to educate and protect ourselves and our families.

When the scandal broke, in my naivety I assumed that Thalidomide would be permanently removed to protect the pharmaceuticals from damage payouts. Imagine my amazement when I learned that this drug is still being sold, this time as a 'treatment' for AIDS, leprosy and as a tranquiliser. Men and women are asked to promise not to conceive children while ingesting it. Terrific.

Thalidomide can be transmitted to the foetus by both mother and father, and it is unknown how long it remains active in the body. To compound this outrage, the same horrible defects are being passed down to second and third generation children, who never used the drug. Oh, yes, and it is being sold over the counter in some Third World countries!

How is it possible that any organisation could commit so heinous a crime? Who are these fiendish men and women executives who make such decisions, casually condemning innocent children to lives of misery? And how is it possible that 'civilised' people can be so evil? There! I'm glad I got that off my chest.

Now that I've had yet another dig at the multinational pharmaceuticals, back to hysterectomies. Dr Kelsey was chief pathologist for Washington DC and Maryland, and it was her job to examine every sample of tissue from women who had had hysterectomies, to see if they were cancerous.

Some time after the thalidomide scandal, Dr Kelsey gave another press conference, during which she stated that an amazing 89 per cent of hysterectomies were unnecessary! Now I'm not saying that the majority of doctors are venal. But you would be wise to remember that your hysterectomy pays for your doctor's country club dues or Mercedes payment.

British medical journal, *The Lancet*, declared, "Women who have hysterectomies after the age of 60 increase their risk of developing incontinence by 60 per cent."

Dr William Campbell Douglass wrote, in *Second Opinion*, "Since incontinence may not occur until years after a hysterectomy, patients are not likely to associate it with the previous operation. That is rarely mentioned at the time of the surgery. How many surgeons are going to say, 'Oh, by the way, you may frequently wet your pants or lose control of your bowel movements in 10 – 20 years as a result of this surgery'?

Scare Tactics

There is, in my opinion, absolutely no excuse for a doctor to employ scare tactics that result in a woman having her organs removed. Most symptoms that can lead to hysterectomy can be corrected by sticking faithfully to a prudent diet. But remember, prevention is infinitely better than damage control once symptoms become serious. And, if you neglect your health until cancer invades your female organs, a hysterectomy may be your only option. Speaking of such things, a woman who attended the Hippocrates program told me the following medical horror story. Her physician told her she had breast cancer and uterine cancer and had to have a hysterectomy and one breast removed. When she awoke from the anaesthesia, the doctor said he had good news for her – the biopsy showed she hadn't had cancer after all. And she didn't even sue the bastard!

So, ladies, before submitting to the knife, get several opinions, and try to find an honest doctor and an efficient laboratory. And remember that, according to Dr Raymond Peat, "Spotting, breakthrough bleeding and abnormally long periods are often caused by hypothyroidism. In the light of this knowledge, I feel that a physician who advocates removal of the uterus for excessive bleeding, without first trying thyroid therapy, is not practicing medicine properly."

They are not always easy to find, but there *are* thousands of doctors with good motives, and many innovative physicians who have embraced natural healing. But they are sometimes vilified and even forced out of the profession by their medical associations, and/or their governments. We should never forget the example of Dr Ignacz Semmelweiss who, during the 19th Century, had the effrontery to suggest that childbirth fever might be caused by doctors going straight from the autopsy room to the delivery room, without washing their hands. His fellow physicians were infuriated by this slur and the poor man was ruined, barred from practicing medicine again. This sort of outrage is still happening, sometimes to doctors who have found natural methods to cure so-called incurables. Many of these physicians have been forced out of the US, and have established clinics across the border, in Mexico.

The bottom line is that we must all choose our practitioners with care, ask questions, must not accept the cop-out diagnosis, "It's all in your head" and, most important of all, live so that we do not fall into the clutches of the bacteria-filled hospitals and drug cartels. They will kill you if you give them a chance.

Fifty Lung Diseases

For example, *The Australian, August 31, 2000*, reported that the first World Congress on Lung Health and Respiratory Diseases, which was held that month in Florence, heard that "...hundreds of drugs supplied for disorders including high blood pressure, allergies, rheumatism, infections and cancer can cause lung diseases... French physician Phillippe Camus, of the University Medical Centre in Dijon, told the congress he had found at least 50 lung diseases and syndromes – including coughs, breathlessness, pleurisy and acute respiratory failure – that could be caused, or aggravated by, common medicines. He said 310 drugs had so far been identified as affecting the lungs... Professor Camus' team has created a website, www.pneumotox.com, which lists drugs according to the number of reports of adverse lung events made about them." A few of the drugs mentioned were beta-blockers, ACE-inhibitors, antibiotics, non-steroidal, anti-inflammatory painkillers and anti-depressants.

On the subject of drugs and the pharmaceutical cartels, in 1966 *oestrogen* suddenly appeared and was touted as the miracle that would keep women young forever. Gynaecologist Dr Robert Wilson wrote *Forever Feminine*, a runaway bestseller (on which you can read my 'caustic commentary' elsewhere) that promised to save women from what he termed "The tragedy of menopause, which often destroys their character as well as their health." He also referred to menopause as 'living decay', turning what is a natural life passage, welcomed by women in primitive societies, into a disease to be treated and 'cured'. And probably to even be ashamed of. He actually referred to menopausal women as "vapid cows."

Conveniently, he failed to disclose that his Foundation received millions of dollars from the very laboratories that manufactured the hormone he so enthusiastically recommended. He was, apparently, unconcerned about the dismal lack of research to prove its safety and long-term effects.

Mass Murder

The publicity campaign was so vivid and relentless that I remember it well. As Professor Raymond Peat, the father of progesterone therapy, said, "Advertising gets a bad name when it can't be distinguished from mass murder." And, make no mistake, this was the mass murder of millions of women who, advised by their doctors and persuaded by the advertisements, jumped on the oestrogen bandwagon and took what is now called 'unopposed oestrogen'. Which means that, in spite of the research, progesterone was not given along with oestrogen in order to keep the oestrogen from causing cancer. Which it did, in alarming numbers.

It was prescribed that way for about fifteen years before doctors finally bowed to the research, accepted the danger (many were sued and didn't have any choice) and started prescribing progesterone as well. Except it wasn't really progesterone, which is natural and protective against cancer. It was a synthetic version, laboratory-made, which actually promotes cancer.

But what about those ill-informed women who took oestrogen before progesterone was thought important? And what about the millions of women who are still on the synthetic oestrogen/progesterone combination? In the opinion of the scientists we trust, they would be well-advised to discontinue these dangerous drugs, slowly and carefully, and with the help of a qualified professional. Some researchers claim that women who do this return to a normal risk of cancer after two drug-free years, which is encouraging. I hope this is true.

The drug companies named these imitation progesterone time bombs 'progestins' and 'progestogens'. Those of us with suspicious natures cannot help surmising that they were so named in order to confuse doctors and patients into thinking they were progesterone – the real thing. And this is, of course, exactly what happened. Further, the drug companies cleverly maligned natural progesterone so that women, and even their doctors, do not realise that they are taking a product that does not provide the full spectrum of natural progesterone's biological activity.

As John R. Lee, MD, the physician who, using Dr Raymond Peat's research, pioneered the use of natural progesterone, says in his best-selling book, **What Your Doctor May Not Tell You About Menopause**, "The synthetic progestins now being heavily promoted in hormone replacement therapy have undergone molecular alterations at unusual positions. As these strange, not-found-in-nature molecules travel down the hormone pathways, they occupy progesterone receptor sites, create actions different from natural progesterone, cannot be used as precursors of other hormones (as progesterone can), and are difficult for the body to metabolise and excrete. These molecular alterations carry a heavy burden of potential undesirable side effects. This, however, does not seem to deter the marketing of them."

To illustrate what can happen to women who are given a synthetic version of progesterone, this is what happened to Lesley Cook, from Russell Island in Queensland, who was given a prescription for tablets which are described in the Consumer Product Information slip as "...similar to, but not the same as, the natural hormone progesterone". Lesley told me she became sicker each day she took the tablets, and her eyes started stinging badly, and then she could no longer see to read – having had perfect sight until taking the tablets. She quit after only three days, but it was too late – her eyes had been ruined. The side effects listed on the product information slip were long, with "blindness and death" listed last. Since when are these "side effects"?

By the time Lesley telephoned me she had been unable to read for eight months, and her eyes were still stinging badly. As it happened, I was able to suggest an old remedy, which has been used for centuries, which she tried. I'm delighted to report that after a few days the pain was gone and her sight was restored. You can read more on this in **Remedies**.

Frightening Side Effects

Synthetic progesterones are not all alike, and people are not all alike, and some will have obvious, immediate bad effects, while others will have delayed reactions, making 'pinning it' on the progestogen/progestin impossible.

It is always wise to read the Consumer Product Information slips which are inserted in the packaging of medicine. Some of the side effects are so frightening that it is enough to drive even the most devoted junk food junkies to natural healing!

It is not difficult to understand why some women have adverse reactions to synthetic versions of progesterone. The following is from Dr John Lee's book, **Natural Progesterone: The Multiple Roles of a Remarkable Hormone**:

> To appreciate the scope of progestin side effects, it is instructive to review the **Physicians Desk Reference** (PDR) pages for medroxyprogesterone acetate. An abbreviated list from the 1993 PDR follows:
>
> **POTENTIAL SIDE EFFECTS OF MEDROXYPROGESTERONE ACETATE**
> *Warnings:*
> - Increased risk of birth defects such as heart and limb defects if taken during the first four months of pregnancy.
> - Beagle dogs given this drug developed malignant mammary nodules.
> - Discontinue this drug if there is sudden or partial loss of vision.
> - This drug passes into breast milk, consequences unknown.
> - May contribute to thrombophlebitis, pulmonary embolism, and cerebral thrombosis.
>
> *Contraindications:*
> Thrombophlebitis, thromboembolic disorders, cerebral apoplexy, liver dysfunction or disease; known or suspected malignancy of breast or genital organs, undiagnosed vaginal bleeding; missed abortion; or known sensitivity.
>
> *Precautions:*
> - May cause fluid retention, epilepsy, migraine, asthma, cardiac or renal dysfunction.
> - May cause breakthrough bleeding or menstrual irregularities.
> - May cause or contribute to depression.
> - The effect of prolonged use of this drug on pituitary, ovarian, adrenal, hepatic, or uterine function is unknown.
> - May decrease glucose tolerance; diabetic patients must be carefully monitored.
> - May increase the thrombotic disorders associated with estrogens.

Adverse Reactions:

- May cause breast tenderness and galactorrhea.
- May cause sensitivity reactions such as urticaria, pruritus, edema, or rash.
- May cause acne, alopecia and hirsutism.
- Edema, weight changes (increase or decrease).
- Cervical erosions and changes in cervical secretions.
- Cholestatic jaundice.
- Mental depression, pyrexia, nausea, insomnia or somnolence.
- Anaphylactoid reactions and anaphylaxis (severe acute allergic reactions).
- Thrombophlebitis and pulmonary embolism.
- Breakthrough bleeding, spotting, amenorrhea, or changes in menses.

When taken with estrogens, the following have been observed:

- Rise in blood pressure, headache, dizziness, nervousness, fatigue.
- Changes in libido, hirsutism and loss of scalp hair, decrease in T3 uptake values.
- Premenstrual-like syndrome, changes in appetite.
- Cystitis-like syndrome.
- Erythema multiforme, erythema nodosum, hemorrhagic eruption, itching.

Why do you reckon physicians prescribe these drugs when natural progesterone is available and does not have these side effects?

The following, reprinted with permission from Dr Lee's ***What Your Doctor May Not Tell You About Menopause***, shows how vital natural progesterone is to your wellbeing.

Functions of Progesterone

- is a precursor of other sex hormones, including estrogen and testosterone
- maintains secretory endometrium (uterine lining)
- is necessary for the survival of the embryo and fetus throughout gestation
- protects against fibrocystic breasts
- is a natural diuretic
- helps use fat for energy
- functions as a natural antidepressant
- helps thyroid hormone action
- normalises blood clotting
- restores sex drive
- helps normalise blood sugar levels
- normalises zinc and copper levels
- restores proper cell oxygen levels
- has a thermogenic (temperature-raising) effect

- protects against endometrial cancer
- helps protect against breast cancer
- builds bone and is protective against osteoporosis
- is a precursor of cortisone synthesis by adrenal cortex

It is important to stress that Dr Lee is referring to *natural progesterone*, not the synthetic progestins or progestogens which are so frequently prescribed.

We women have an American law, passed in the late 1800s, to thank for this disquieting situation. At that time the US Congress ruled that *medicines could be patented only if they were not natural substances.* On the surface this seems a good idea, as it would appear to protect herbs and other natural medicines. In practice, however, it created an atmosphere of suppression, as the drug companies, becoming more and more powerful, suppressed natural remedies, even causing some (such as hemp) to be banned, and made synthetic versions of the ones they perceived as profitable. They learned to isolate and transform the 'active ingredients' in herbs, and these new derivatives could then be patented.

Aspirin is just one of many evil examples of this process. It has multiple side effects, hospitalises 30,000 and kills more than 6000 people each year in the United States, and causes bleeding in the intestines and stomach. Aspirin is synthesised from willow bark, which works as well and is safe. But willow bark cannot be patented, so it has been forgotten.

No Easy Explanation

The greatest scientists in the world cannot explain exactly how hormones do their complex jobs in our bodies. They make a pretty good stab at it, and perhaps one day they will work it out, but for now, there is an alarming reliance on guesswork. So how can I, a novice and potential victim of the medical/pharmaceutical complex, hope to explain this intricate interaction to others? The answer, of course, is that I cannot. But the one thing I do know for certain is that hormones fabricated in a laboratory are unnatural and dangerous. The only people who benefit from these synthetic hormones are the drug companies that push them on to an unwary and often trusting public, and rake in countless billions.

Apparently they ignored or suppressed information that Dr Raymond Peat published in 1972: "I have found that estrogen induces cellular conditions that resemble those produced by X-rays and carcinogens, and which probably reflect the production of superoxide or other radicals." And, of course, it is common knowledge that X-rays cause cancer.

The oestrogen patch is reputed to be less dangerous than oestrogen pills, because it is thought to be gentler on the liver. That may be but, according to

Dr Brian Henderson, the patch produces higher levels of *oestradiol*, which is the most potent form of oestrogen. This form is even more potent than *Premarin* (the urine from pregnant mares) which would seem to negate any liver-saving the patch may afford. Dr Henderson states, "The effect of that should be to make one's breast cancer risk go up substantially more on the patch than on Premarin."

One of the most persuasive arguments doctors use when prescribing oestrogen is its supposed prevention of cardiovascular disease. According to Dr Lee, this is misinformation that was based on one study only, and it was hopelessly flawed and manipulated. Since that study, there have been many others that have found that oestrogen has no coronary benefit; on the contrary, its use increases risk of stroke, bleeding from a brain artery and the risk of cardiovascular disease. These studies, unfortunately, have received (as you might expect), little media coverage. Dr Peat wrote in his *Newsletter*, "By the 1940s estrogen was known to produce excessive blood clotting, miscarriage, cancer, age-like changes in connective tissue, premenstrual syndrome, varicose veins, orthostatic hypotension, etc... Estrogen affected the liver's production of clot-regulating proteins, and it also relaxed large veins, allowing blood pooling that slowed the blood sufficiently to give it time to form clots before returning to the lungs... Progesterone, by opposing estrogen, is universally protective against vascular and heart disease."

Idiocy or Subterfuge?

"So far," Dr Peat continues, "the rule in most estrogen/progesterone research has been to devise experiments so that claims of benefit can be made for estrogen, with the expectation that they will meet an uncritical audience. In some studies, it's hard to tell whether idiocy or subterfuge is responsible for the way the experiment was designed and described, for example when synthetic chemicals with anti-progesterone activity are described as progesterone. Since one estrogen-funded researcher who supposedly found progesterone to be ineffective as treatment for premenstrual syndrome practically admitted to me in conversation an intent to mislead, I think it is reasonable to discount idiocy as the explanation for the tremendous bias in published research. With the vastly increased resources in the estrogen industry, resulting from the product promotion 'for the prevention of heart disease', I think we should expect the research fraud to become increasingly blatant. **Rather than being heart protective, estrogen is highly heart-toxic, and it is this that makes its most important antagonist, progesterone, so important in protecting the heart and circulatory system.**"

The following quotes are taken from an article of Dr Peat's which appeared in the ***Townsend Letter for Doctors and Patients***, *January 1997*:

"In the 1940s, Alexander Lipshuts demonstrated that a continuous, weak estrogenic stimulus was immensely effective in producing, first fibromas, then cancer, in one organ after another, and the effect was not limited to the reproductive system...

"The concept of a 'protective estrogen' is very similar to the idea of 'protective mutagens' or 'protective carcinogens,' though in the case of estrogens, their promoters don't even know what the normal, natural functions of estrogen are...

"Pharmaceutical misrepresentations regarding the estrogens rank, in terms of human consequences, with the radiation damage from fallout from bomb tests and reactor leaks, with industrial pollution, with degradation of the food supply -- with genocide, in fact."

Risky Business

Thousands of other scientists agree with the unpopular stand taken by Doctors Lee and Peat. But there isn't any real point in considering the so-called heart protection of oestrogen. If all of these scientists who think for themselves, rather than accepting the pharmaceutical industry's assurances, are wrong, and even if oestrogen *does* protect the heart, would it be worth it? If you are still on the fence, consider the following excerpts from long advertisements that were placed in many publications by *Wyeth-Ayerst*, a company that manufactures and promotes oestrogen:

WHEN ESTROGENS SHOULD NOT BE USED: during pregnancy; while breast feeding; if you have had any heart or circulation problems; if you have had undiagnosed vaginal bleeding; if you have had cancer.

DANGERS OF ESTROGEN: cancer of the uterus; cancer of the breast; gallbladder disease; abnormal blood clotting; heart disease; excess calcium in the blood.

Side Effects

In addition to the risks listed above, the following side effects have been reported with estrogen use:

- Nausea, vomiting, pain, cramps, swelling, or tenderness in the abdomen.
- Yellowing of the skin and/or whites of the eyes.
- Breast tenderness or enlargement.
- Enlargement of benign tumours of the uterus.
- Breakthrough bleeding or spotting.
- Change in amount of cervical secretion.
- Vaginal yeast infections.
- Retention of excess fluid. This may make some conditions worsen, such as asthma, epilepsy, migraine, heart disease, or kidney disease.
- A spotty darkening of the skin, particularly on the face; reddening of the skin; skin rashes.
- Worsening of porphyria.

- Headache, migraines, dizziness, faintness, or changes in vision (including intolerance to contact lenses).

- Mental depression.

- Involuntary muscle spasms.

- Hair loss or abnormal hairiness.

- Increase or decrease in weight.

- Changes in sex drive.

- Possible changes in blood sugar.

This is potent stuff, and has motivated many women to quit. If you are one of them, doctors say it is not wise to stop taking HRT 'cold turkey'. Because I am not a physician, I am not permitted to give medical advice on how to stop taking any drug. The US-based internet site, www.how.to/takemaca, prepared by physicians, carefully details the way to gradually stop, by replacing with Peruvian Maca, a wonderful natural remedy about which you will find more at the end of this book.

Let's take a moment to sort out some of the confusing technical terms that have been bandied about so much in the past decade: *oestrogen dominance, estrone, estradiol, estriol, xenoestrogens, phytoestrogens, isoflavones*. If you cannot define these words, you are not alone, and I think it is a scandal that we women are left to grapple with these confusing and crucial health issues ourselves. But what can we do? Our doctors have neglected their homework and turned their brains over to the pharmaceutical giants.

Complex Subject

In a way, I can understand this cop-out. After many gruelling years in medical school, learning what the drug companies decree (after all, they *do* finance the med schools) most doctors do not have the stomach for further research. They have demanding practices to run, lives of their own to live, and it is so much easier to sit back and believe the glossy, drug-pushing brochures the 'detail' people so obligingly deliver to their surgeries. There is no way a busy doctor could take the time to pore over the huge stacks of research papers and books that are necessary in order to understand this complex subject. Nor would they be willing to wade through and throw out the obvious propaganda and bedevil biochemists and physicians in other countries for information on just this one subject. I'm only able to do this because I'm retired and able to devote myself (more than) full time. And, please do not misunderstand me; I do not set myself up as an expert. I am just a cantankerous woman who wants to know the truth and trusts precious few scientists to tell it.

I'll start with *'oestrogen dominance'*, which is not a term you will read in the newspapers and magazines which extol the virtues of HRT and the many 'cure-alls' for what supposedly ails mature women. If you believe this propaganda on HRT, you will be convinced that oestrogen is all we women need to be fulfilled, have strong bones and pliable vaginas. According to Dr Lee, this is *not* what we need, because oestrogen dominance, common to women in industrialised countries, *is* the problem, not lack of oestrogen. In Dr Lee's book, he lists the following causes of oestrogen dominance:

1. Estrogen replacement therapy
2. Premenopause (early follicle depletion resulting in a lack of ovulation and thus lack of progesterone well before the onset of menopause)
3. Exposure to xenoestrogens (cause of early follicle depletion)
4. Birth control pills (with excessive estrogen component)
5. Hysterectomy (can induce subsequent ovary dysfunction or atrophy)
6. Postmenopause (especially in overweight women)

These factors are exacerbated by the tendency of some doctors to prescribe oestrogen to symptomatic women ten, even fifteen, years before menopause, when they are suffering from oestrogen dominance. While certain symptoms may be alleviated by HRT, what these women are really suffering from is lowered progesterone, not lack of oestrogen! And, had they been given natural progesterone when symptoms first appeared, rather than HRT, their toxic oestrogen load would have lessened.

The following, from Dr Lee's *What Your Doctor May Not Tell You About Menopause*, is a list of symptoms that can be caused or made worse by oestrogen dominance:

- Acceleration of the aging process
- Miscarriage
- Allergies
- Osteoporosis
- Breast tenderness
- Premenopausal bone loss
- Decreased sex drive
- PMS
- Depression
- Thyroid dysfunction mimicking hypothyroidism
- Fatigue
- Fibrocystic breasts
- Uterine cancer
- Foggy thinking
- Uterine fibroids
- Headaches
- Water retention, bloating
- Hypoglycemia
- Fat gain, especially around the abdomen, hips, and thighs
- Increased blood clotting (increasing risk of strokes)
- Gallbladder disease
- Irritability
- Infertility
- Memory loss
- Autoimmune disorders such as lupus, erythematosus, thyroiditis and possibly Sjogren's disease.

It is important to remember that, when oestrogen becomes the dominant hormone while progesterone is deficient, oestrogen becomes toxic to the body. So, clearly, oestrogen dominance is something to avoid.

Oestriol *(or **estriol**)* is the oestrogen that is said by many physicians to be the safest and is frequently used in vaginal suppositories to counteract vaginal dryness and thinning skin. Yet Dr Peat states, "When administered subcutaneously, estriol induced abortions and stillbirths... When added to long-term culture of human breast cancer cells, estriol stimulated their growth, and overcame the antiestrogenic effects of tamoxifen, even at concentrations hundreds of times lower than that of tamoxifen. The data do not support an anti-estrogenic role for estriol in human breast cancer." At Hippocrates many have stated that these suppositories have given them vaginitis.

Phytoestrogens are plants with oestrogen-like activity. They are weaker than the oestrogens in our bodies, and compete for the same oestrogen receptor sites throughout the body. They are also known as '*isoflavones*', and are deceptive, because they are touted as 'safe' vegetable forms which can be used in place of artificial hormones.

But before you start dosing yourself with these heavily advertised menopausal aids, (soy products, red clover, black cohosh, ginseng, coumestrol, anise, dong quai, etc.), consider what Dr Peat has to say about these 'safe' plants:

> "Women who have cancer fail to eliminate estrogens, including phytoestrogens, at a normal rate, and so are retaining a higher percentage of the chemicals consumed in their diets... They (phytoestrogens) suppress the detoxifying systems of the body... The estrogens in clover have been known for several decades to have a contraceptive action in sheep, and other phytoestrogens are known to cause deformities in the genitals, feminisation of men, and anatomical changes in the brain, as well as functional masculinisation of the female brain... The isoflavones (many of which are now being promoted as 'antioxidants' and 'cancer preventives') are toxic to many organs. They have clear estrogenic effects. They are not only immediately active in the mature individual, when they are present prenatally, they cause feminisation of the male genitalia and behaviour, and early maturation of the female offspring, with the tissue changes that are known to be associated with increased incidence of cancer."

Most damning of all, Dr Peat wrote, "The phytoestrogens pose a risk to the breast, and uterus, the liver, colon, and pancreas, which isn't surprising, **since estrogen is known to be carcinogenic for every tissue**."

This blanket condemnation of the phytoestrogens, or isoflavones, *includes* the slickly advertised and hugely promoted soy products, which Dr Peat has studied extensively and considers extremely toxic. You can learn more about their dangerous effects in ***Chapter 9,*** *Soy – The Abominable Bean.*

The search for a drug-free treatment for relieving the hot flushes and some other unpleasant symptoms of menopause has led many women to take black cohosh. Because it was herbal, they presumed it was safe. Here are just two instances from impeccable sources, which indicate that, on the contrary, it is very dangerous.

In the **Medical Journal of Australia**, *2002 177 (8): 440-443*, three eminent researchers from Brisbane's Princess Alexandra Hospital reported on their investigations into clinical, biochemical and histological evidence of severe hepatitis. Peter W Whiting, MB BCh, BAO, FRACP, Gastroenterology Fellow, Department of Gastroenterology and Hepatology; Andrew Clouston, MB BS, PhD, FRCPA, Histopathologist, Department of Anatomical Pathology, and Paul Kerlin, BA, MD, FRACP, Senior Visiting Gastroenterologist and Hepatologist, gave details of cases of liver damage, including one where "One patient required urgent liver transplantation for fulminant hepatic failure after the brief use of black cohosh."

And in July 2003, researcher Vicki Davis of the Mylan School of Pharmacy at Duquesne University in Pittsburgh, told a meeting of the American Association for Cancer Research that black cohosh may make pre-existing cancer more likely to spread. Research teams at Duquesne and in Canada fed black cohosh to female mice bred so that they are prone to breast cancer. They gave them the daily equivalent of 40mg of the supplement, the amount normally recommended for menopausal symptoms.

They found that although mice were not any more likely to develop breast cancer in the first place, those that did develop it were more likely to see a deadly spread of the cancer. Results showed that 27 per cent of mice fed black cohosh had the cancer spread to the lung, compared to 11 per cent of the mice that did not eat the herb.

While the findings do not prove that using black cohosh could endanger a woman with undiagnosed breast cancer, Davis said it would be risky to take it. She said that women who have breast cancer – or any other form of cancer – may need to be especially wary.

Beware these "Menopausal Aids"

<u>**Promensil,**</u> widely advertised as a menopausal aid, is a phytoestrogen or isoflavone extract of red clover. It is known that permanent infertility has occurred in sheep grazing on red clover in Australia. Their abnormalities were similar to other animals that were neonatally exposed to oestrogens. Further, *coumestrol*, which is found in red clover, is *six times more potent* than isoflavones. In trials with breast cancer cells it was found that the cells responded identically to red clover as they did to *estradiol,* a known cause of cancer. Yet another reason to shun extracts of red clover, which is in many herbal products.

According to expert New Zealand anti-soy activist Richard James, "Each [*Promensil*] pill contains 40mg of contraceptive isoflavones found in soy bean and red clover. This dose has been proved by a US Federal Government Laboratory to cause goitre and thyroid abnormalities, and has been designated as a thyroid carcinogen. Yet, it is being pushed by Novogen as a tonic for women."

In late 2000, Novogen mounted an elaborate and expensive advertising campaign for this product. One of their ads featured an impressive two-page colour spread in *The Australian Magazine*, *December 2-3 2000*, extolling the virtues of their menopausal aids, Promensil and Rimostil – which would have cost an enormous amount of money. I just wish I could afford such impressive ads to warn people *against* their products, as well as the many other dangers lurking at our chemists, supermarkets, health stores and in our medicine cabinets.

Remifemin, a heavily-advertised menopausal product, is derived from black cohosh, another phytoestrogen. According to the brochure, it "…contains 50% alcohol by volume," and the "…medium of extraction is ethanol 60% by volume, as well as "… isopropyl alcohol 40% by volume." These are petroleum products and are well known to be extremely detrimental to our health.

Kordel's Phyto-Femme, another so-called menopausal aid, is definitely one to shun. It contains scary quantities of the very same isoflavones we need to avoid. This manufacturer has also been taken to task by a government authority over the claims made for its product. Annette King, New Zealand's

Those 'Trusted Names'…

Novogen actually claimed in some of their advertisements, that the prominent Professor Alistair MacLennon, head of the Gynaecology Department of the University of Adelaide, and editor of *Climacteric*, endorsed Promensil. The professor did not in any way endorse this product, and asked Novogen to cease using his name. Surprisingly, they continued, even after being warned by Professor MacLennon's solicitors. He then complained to the Therapeutic Goods Administration (TGA), who took action against Novogen. Leading gynaecologist and obstetrician Dr Rodney J Baber, MRCOG, FRACOG, of Sydney's North Shore Private Hospital, wrote in a professional journal on *2 May 2000*, "… as a result of Alistair's complaints, the TGA found against Novogen and instructed them to withdraw their advertisement. This was reported in the lay press here in a fair and honest way, and I hope the same will be the case in New Zealand."

Unfortunately, this has *not* been the case. As Richard James reported, "Promotions that the Australian panel condemned are still being aimed at New Zealand women not only by Novogen, but by Blackmores, Herron and Sanitarium."

Health Minister, declared on February 18 2003, that the Ministry of Health "…agrees that the Kordel pamphlet breaches the Medicines Act by making therapeutic claims to regulate the menstrual cycle, regulate and correct hormone imbalances, relieve muscular cramps and spasms and improve circulation. The

Ministry will send a warning letter to Kordel's with a timeframe for response. Prosecution will be considered if the response is not satisfactory."

**Revival** is yet another isoflavone-based menopausal aid, recommended by its manufacturer to be taken at a dosage rate of 150mg per day. Are they not aware that it only takes 32mg per day of isoflavones to depress thyroid function sufficiently to cause enlargement of the gland, which can lead to goitre? Do they care? And why does a well-known women's health 'expert' continue to use and enthusiastically endorse it despite having been diagnosed with hypothyroidism herself?

**Evista**, a '_Selective Estrogen Reuptake Modulator_', actually tends to increase hot flushes, causes severe leg cramps, and boosts risk of serious blood clots in the legs, eyes and lungs of sedentary women.

**Vagifem** (oestrogen used vaginally) is supposed to reduce vaginal dryness, but causes irritation, headache, vaginal pain and abdominal pain.

**All Menopause Aids**, other than the few recommended in this book, are fraudulent and dangerous in my opinion and in the opinions of all the scientists and doctors I trust and respect.

Xenoestrogens

This brings me to the term '_xenoestrogens_', a major cause of oestrogen dominance. We have the chemical multinationals to thank for the calamity of petrochemical pollution we are forced to live with. Not only food, but most of the products we use, day in and day out, are contaminated with these chemicals which, combined with the other risk factors listed above, create oestrogen dominance. Read what Dr Peat wrote about xenoestrogens in _**The Townsend Letter for Doctors and Patients**_:

> "Pollution of the environment and food supply by estrogenic chemicals is getting increased attention. Early in the study of estrogens, it was noticed that soot, containing polycyclic aromatic hydrocarbons, was both estrogenic and carcinogenic. Since then, it has been found that phenolics and chlorinated hydrocarbons are significantly estrogenic, and that many estrogenic herbicides, pesticides, and industrial by-products persist in the environment, causing infertility, deformed reproductive organs, tumours, and other biological defects, including immunodeficiency. In the Columbia River, a recent study found that about 25% of the otters and muskrats were anatomically deformed.

> "Estrogenic pollution kills birds, panthers, alligators, old men, young women, fish, seals, babies, and ecosystems. Some of these chemicals are sprayed on forests by the US Department of Agriculture, where they enter lakes, underwater aquifers, rivers, and oceans. Private businesses spray them on farms and orchards, or put them into the air as smoke or vapours, or dump them directly into rivers. Homeowners put them on their lawns and gardens.

> "Natural estrogens, from human urine, enter the rivers from sewage. Many tons of synthetic and pharmaceutical estrogens, administered to menopausal women in

quantities much larger than their bodies ever produced metabolically, are being added to the rivers.

"In the same way that weak estrogens in the environment may become hundreds of times more estrogenic by synergistic interactions (J.A. McLachlan, et al., *Science, June 7, 1996*), combinations of natural, medical, dietary, and environmental estrogens are almost certain to have unexpected results."

Dr Peat is a scientist of world renown and his opinions are well worth heeding. It should be blindingly obvious to anyone who bothers to read the research done by the biochemists who are not employed by the multinational drug companies, that oestrogen replacement is chiefly what we do ***not*** need! What we need is to find ways to avoid oestrogen dominance by limiting our exposure to environmental and drug xenoestrogens, to at least partially diminish their deadly effect upon our bodies.

The combination of vaginal dryness and thinning skin is one of the most irritating symptoms of menopause. I faxed my favourite biochemist, Dr Peat (who I'm sure will be thrilled if I ever finish researching and leave him in peace) for information on this subject. At the same time I had the gall to ask him to answer two pages of medical questions. Incredibly, he took the time to reply, faxing back four dense pages of invaluable information. I quote here one paragraph:

"Vagina: vitamin A and E: Thyroid, progesterone and vitamin A all have important anti-atrophy effects, and vitamin A is known to be essential for maintaining the activity of mucus-producing cells in mucus membranes. When retinol is added to vitamin E (in coconut oil or cocoa butter) and applied topically, it often has the desired effect of increasing the function of the mucus-secreting cells."

Nothing daunted, I faxed back suggesting that Dr Peat formulate a suppository of his natural progesterone (the only one we recommend) along with coconut oil and vitamins A and E. Unfortunately, he isn't interested in manufacturing vaginal suppositories, which is a pity but understandable. Through my network of women throughout Australia I learned that many are using 500 units of vitamin E (capsule form) inserted in the vagina each night. It does appear to help - several women have reported success after only a few weeks. The best results, however, are achieved after two months of faithful use. It's a bit messy, and it's necessary to wear a pad. But it certainly is preferable to using oestriol suppositories and taking a chance of cancer. A word of caution when using vitamin E capsules: all are made from the dregs of soy oil processing and can be dangerous for susceptible people.

Skin Test First

One woman reported that this practice led to an annoying bout with cystitis. She was positive, because she gave it two tries, several months apart, and each time she got cystitis several days after inserting the capsules. She described herself as "...unusually delicate in that area."

When I got this report, I faxed Dr Peat and asked him about using the vitamin E capsules for this problem. He replied, "I don't think people should use any capsule for applying things to vaginal membranes; some people get good results using suppositories containing vitamin A and E. Anything that is taken orally or intra-vaginally should be tested first on the skin; after testing it on the arm, a drop can be put on the edge of the lip. Any allergic reaction will probably reveal itself there."

Judging by Dr Peat's reply, it seems the culprit causing cystitis was the capsule material, not the vitamin E. Perhaps simply puncturing vitamin E and A capsules and inserting that bit of oil would not produce any problems, and might help the condition. A health professional should be consulted before trying this remedy, and if anything is inserted into this very delicate area, it must be immaculately clean!

The remedy for vaginal dryness and thinning of the skin most often prescribed by physicians is oestriol suppositories. These suppositories do alleviate symptoms, but many women have reported toxic reactions and vaginitis from their use.

Many health professionals claim that oestriol is the least dangerous of all the oestrogens. Some say that if used as a suppository, oestriol is not absorbed through the vaginal tissues and into the bloodstream. A female American doctor who should have known better, wrote, "This means that you can safely use estriol vaginal cream to help restore your vaginal and urethral tissues even if you've had breast cancer or another estrogen-sensitive condition."

Carcinogenic

Because Dr Peat has repeatedly written that oestriol is dangerous, I faxed him to clear up the absorption issue. His reply was as follows: "Estriol is very well absorbed by vaginal membranes; in rabbit studies, for example, its contraceptive action was clear when applied vaginally. In proportion to its estrogenic actions, estriol is just as carcinogenic as estradiol." I trust Dr Peat implicitly and wouldn't dream of using oestriol for any condition, nor would I ever recommend its use to other women, no matter how dire their symptoms. Natural remedies for this condition must be tried.

If you need a sexual lubricant, do not use any of the commercial products. Their ingredients read like a chemistry lesson, and these potent chemicals have no place on delicate membranes, which will absorb them into the bloodstream. In addition, do not allow your partner to use a lubricated condom, as the ingredients are carcinogenic and immunosuppressive. A pure olive oil or coconut oil may be used safely for this purpose, but under no circumstances use a commercial coconut oil. They are all dangerous! Yes, even most from health stores.

Natural Progesterone

The first time I heard Dr Peat's name mentioned was at a lecture given in Australia by Dr Lee. For those of you who are unfamiliar with Dr Lee's work, he is the man who alerted the world, through his writing and many lecture tours, to the danger of giving synthetic oestrogens and, even more deadly, giving them without the cancer-mitigating progesterone. Dr Lee said that he first learned about progesterone from the pioneering work of Dr Raymond Peat, and according to Dr Lee, most of what he knows about progesterone, he learned from Dr Peat's research.

It is well known that an excellent way to deliver natural progesterone is through the skin. The medical profession denied that this was possible for years, and only gave in when it was proved that the oestrogen patch was an efficient way to get oestrogen into the body. But what is not well known is that western women are being ripped off by poor quality progesterone creams. These contain wild yam, extracts of fenugreek, black cohosh and various other herbs that contain steroid precursors of progesterone. The advertisements make these products sound good, but the human body does not have the necessary enzymes to convert these vegetable steroids into progesterone, and the actual amount of progesterone in the creams is insignificant.

As if this isn't bad enough, some creams contain chemicals which no woman with any sense would want *on*, much less *in*, her body. And don't be fooled by the labels that have only benign ingredients listed. Every time I have insisted upon being given the exact ingredients in writing, I have been shocked by the discrepancy between the label and the facts. Or, the companies in question have refused to disclose ingredients. And, it's important to remember that these creams are designed to break through the skin barrier. This means that, along with the safe ingredients, dangerous chemicals are carried through into your body and bloodstream.

Some of the progesterone creams made at compounding pharmacies, by prescription only, do contain the correct kind of progesterone in the proper amounts, but we have had several reports of vaginitis from women using the vaginal creams, and miserable, itching rashes and wild mood swings by women using the rub-on variety. We assume that these creams must contain allergens, but the pharmacists have refused to disclose ingredients when I have told them of problems and asked for them. When I had one of these creams that caused vaginitis tested on an AcuBase computer, I was told it was semi-poisonous! I know for a fact that most contain *methyl paraben, propyl paraben* and other dangerous chemicals.

Some women on the over-the-counter creams do experience substantial relief from their hot flushes. These creams, however, do not contain enough of the correct kind of progesterone to help build bone, which is much more urgent than dealing with hot flushes.

For many years after Dr Peat's research was done, other people formulated and sold progesterone creams in the USA, reaping the benefits of his work. He was not satisfied by the quality of these creams, did not approve of the way the progesterone was derived, nor of the amount in the creams, which in many instances was not adequate for bone building. He also disapproved of the toxic chemicals in the creams.

Natural Antioxidant

Finally, only a few years ago, Dr Peat developed his own system for delivering progesterone, which fitted right in with what we think is right: he put a 10 percent solution of progesterone in vitamin E oil, and designed it to be put on the gums, one of the most absorptive areas of the body.

This allows the progesterone to enter the blood almost instantly, from the oral membranes. Because vitamin E is a natural antioxidant, artificial preservatives are unnecessary. Dr Lee rates this oil the most effective one he has tested. Further, it is the most economical of all the progesterones. Information on ordering Dr Peat's patented *Progest E Complex*, together with careful dosage instructions, will be found at the end of this chapter. (Please do not attempt to call me or Hippocrates Health Centre for advice on progesterone, since there is nothing we can add to Dr Peat's own directions, which are printed on pages 180-181 of this book).

Importantly, natural progesterone can be beneficial in treating ailments that are not specifically hormonal in nature. As Dr Peat writes, "For topical treatment of arthritis, osteoporosis, tendinitis, bursitis, varicose veins, sun-damaged skin, acne, wrinkles, etc., progesterone oil can be applied directly to the affected area. To speed absorption it is best to apply a few drops of olive oil [*or coconut oil*] to the area, and then to rub the progesterone-vitamin E solution into and around the affected area. Some of the progesterone will be absorbed systemically, but the highest concentration is sustained in the local area, helping to correct the problem locally."

Experiments have shown that progesterone relieves anxiety, improves memory, protects brain cells, and even prevents epileptic seizures. It promotes respiration, and has been used to correct emphysema. In the circulatory system, it prevents bulging veins by increasing the tone of blood vessels, and improves the efficiency of the heart. It reverses many of the signs of aging in the skin, and promotes healthy bone growth. It can relieve many types of arthritis, and helps a variety of immunological problems.

Not all products with labels stating that they are derived from wild yam extract or soy actually contain any progesterone. In *What Your Doctor May Not*

Tell You About Menopause, Dr Lee writes "Progesterone is obtained by extracting specific components from plants (e.g., *diosgenin* from wild yams or soybeans) and then converting them to actual progesterone in the laboratory. .... Now, with the success of progesterone supplementation, many companies are producing products listed as containing wild yam extract, but they actually contain no progesterone." The process of making the kind of natural progesterone we need is complex and usually not done by makers of over-the-counter creams.

One aspect of Dr Peat's progesterone that concerned me was that it is derived, through this complicated laboratory process, from wild yam, or the dreaded soybean. Since he dislikes soy as much as I do, I faxed him, asking him how much soy is left in the oil after processing. This is the answer I received from his assistant: "As you know, the two main sources of progesterone are wild yam and soybeans. We have used both sources and there is no detectable difference. By the time it is the molecule progesterone, there is nothing left of the original plant. I've heard Dr Peat use the following illustrative example when asked about this: 'You can made vodka from potatoes, but there is no vodka in potatoes.' An issue that is important is purity, and the sources we use are always USP progesterone."

Few physicians are aware of an article on progesterone published in the ***British Journal of Cancer***, reporting the results of a twenty-year study that tracked every woman having surgery for node-positive breast cancer in three major London hospitals. At the time of surgery these women's hormone levels were recorded. It was found that the survival rate after 18 years for those with normal progesterone levels was 75 percent. The survival rate for women with low progesterone at the time of surgery was only 30 percent. Yet, most doctors don't know about these landmark, life saving studies! Is this not shameful?

Dr Lee believes that, had these women been on progesterone, they wouldn't have developed the breast cancer in the first place! He says that when he first started prescribing progesterone it was for women who had had breast cancer or endometrial cancer, and because of this could not take HRT. He then started giving it to *all* of his mature patients, and nineteen years later, not one had died from breast or uterine cancer!

An American study followed 40,000 women for eight years to determine who died from cancer of the ovaries. Published by ***The Johns Hopkins Journal of Epidemiology***, the conclusion was that the only fatalities from this malady were among the women who were on unopposed oestrogen.

Heart Health

The protection from heart attacks mature women get from progesterone has been amply documented, in study after study. One example is an experiment using unfortunate Rhesus monkeys. First, the animals were given oestrogen and then heart spasms were provoked. All died. Then the same experiment was tried, first giving the monkeys natural progesterone before provoking heart spasms. The scientists found that it was not possible to produce heart spasms in the monkeys who were protected by the progesterone.

Premenopausal women, and even young women, can benefit from natural progesterone if they are experiencing problem periods. Even infertility can be reversed with progesterone. It is important to stress, however, that often a dramatic improvement in diet can completely reverse problems that may have been blamed on hormones. Certainly, no young woman should play around with even this natural hormone unless she is absolutely certain that she is deficient, and the way to determine this is *not* through blood serum tests.

These conventional tests measure only the hormones that are being sent to the liver for excretion. According to the scientists I respect, saliva tests are more relevant because they reflect the amount of biologically active hormones in the bloodstream. That is the important measurement. The World Health Organisation has adopted the saliva hormone assay, rather than the serum assay, for that reason. Further, the samples last longer, can be handled less delicately, and remain accurate longer. If your health professional cannot or will not organise this test for you, find one who will.

Recently I have been listening to audio tapes of talks Dr Lee has given. The exasperation in his voice is clear when he describes the obstinacy of his fellow doctors who insist that artificial progesterone is identical to natural progesterone. He says that all of the biochemical books agree with him, but that he cannot convince most other doctors.

Frustration

He vehemently insists that it has been proved that we women can be protected from breast cancer, endometrial cancer, and ovarian cancer by using progesterone. In the tape, he says, in frustration, "What are they *waiting* for? If we get all women on progesterone, they will have to commit suicide to die!"

Dr Lee's frustration is understandable – I had the same feelings while originally researching this book and realising that 'establishment' medicine was using its power and wealth to label us 'dissenters' as unscientific ratbags. Then, almost three years after my first edition appeared, the results of an HRT study called the **Women's Health Initiative** hit the front pages of most newspapers. Millions of women, all over the world, were stunned and terrified by the findings.

Sponsored by the National Institutes of Health, the study followed 16,000 women who were on HRT to determine its safety and efficacy. What the study found demolished *Wyeth Pharmaceuticals'* claims that HRT is protective. On the contrary, HRT was found in this study to cause increases in heart attacks, strokes, blood clots and breast cancer. It was also proved that HRT did not protect against Alzheimer's or decrease the risk of bone fractures, as Wyeth claimed. In other words, it finally proved that Wyeth spread 'scientific' lies in order to rake in billions, over the bodies of women whose doctors fell for their propaganda.

Wyeth stock fell 24 percent after the report was made public, and it couldn't have happened to a more deserving company. It's undignified, I know, but excuse me while I gloat!

Our phone lines were clogged after the news hit. Hundreds of women told us they had thrown away their pills without even consulting the doctors who had prescribed them. Predictably, Wyeth didn't offer suggestions to women about the safe way to quit – slowly and carefully, with the guidance of a qualified professional. And unfortunately, most of the 'qualified professionals' didn't have a clue, either.

Purveyors of 'safe phytoestrogen menopausal aids' leapt eagerly on the bandwagon and stepped up their advertising campaigns, hoping to snare millions of terrified women. Those who had quit HRT were easy pickings – many had incapacitating symptoms and were desperate for safe substitutes. We warned all the women who rang, and hundreds of women at my lectures, that these money-spinners are all dangerous, and will be discredited eventually, as HRT is today. There are no exceptions. The only good that can come from taking these products is to the bank balances of the companies that flog them. In May 2003, the National Institutes of Health released yet another damning report on HRT – this time showing it was responsible for an alarming number of cases of dementia, especially Alzheimer's Disease. Wyeth's immediate response was firstly to claim that the 4000 women tested, who had been on HRT for years, were "older than the age group at which the treatment was aimed", and then to announce that they would produce a lower-dosage version of their medication! They don't miss a trick do they? And Wyeth isn't the only "ethical" pharmaceutical company to turn a negative report into a new marketing opportunity. As ***What Doctors Don't Tell You*** reported on *July 31, 2003*:

> "The pharmaceutical industry has lost one of its best money-spinners after HRT therapy was so thoroughly trashed by the influential Women's Health Initiative trial. But the pharmaceuticals didn't get where they are today by being anything other than resilient (and creative). They are already suggesting that a powerful antidepressant could be a suitable replacement for HRT.

> "Specifically they have been testing paroxetine (Paxil), a selective serotonin reuptake inhibitor. They tested it on 165 menopausal women who had been complaining of hot flashes-and, compared with a placebo, it seems to be effective over a six-week period.

In fact, the researchers conclude, Paxil could well be a good alternative therapy to HRT.

"This breakthrough discovery may lose its edge a little if we now reveal three facts: Fact 1: Paxil is manufactured by GlaxoSmithKline. Fact 2: three of the four researchers are full-time employees of GlaxoSmithKline, and the fourth is a consultant to the company. Fact 3: GlaxoSmithKline paid for the research.

"The employees (sorry, researchers) may also have been diffident to talk about adverse reactions to the drug. That's a pity because Paxil is not well tolerated, with around 16 per cent of users having to discontinue treatment. The more common reactions include sweating, tremor, dizziness and insomnia (Aren't they supposed to be menopausal symptoms? -EH), headache, sleepiness, constipation, and female genital disorders. Serious reactions have included hypertension, tachycardia, pain, ulcers, arthritis, osteoporosis, delirium, hallucinations, grand mal, asthma, conjunctivitis, eye hemorrhage, breast atrophy, and kidney malfunctioning."

Should Be Banned

Advertisements for 'safe' hormone creams were also increased to take advantage of the hysteria after the original Women's Health Initiative report appeared.

We reminded women then that all the bases in these creams are dangerous, as detailed earlier in this book. Many are in *Sorbeline*, which is a dreadful petrochemical product that does not belong on our highly-absorbent skin. It should be banned; please throw it out if you have any. Some are in bases of macadamia or other safe-sounding oils, but contain some of the nastiest preservatives known to man – even when not listed on the labels; they will go into your body along with the hormones. Compounding chemists who make them have been known to lie about ingredients or refuse to disclose them. See page 179 for a compounding chemist who makes products to my specifications.

I wish I could tell you exactly how to negotiate your way safely through the hormone minefield. But I cannot, because we all have different needs, and it will be necessary for you to discover for yourself which hormones, if any, are appropriate for your body. Education is your best, and possibly your only, defence.

A good place to start is to learn the difference between –

Natural And Synthetic Hormones

If testing proves that you are low in a hormone and you are offered a natural hormone, which closely mimics your own hormone structurally and chemically, would you prefer it to a man-made derivative of a hormone that has been altered so a drug company could patent it?

The answer seems obvious, yet even now, after all the publicity about the dangers, many doctors are still cavalierly prescribing these tiny troublemakers, seemingly oblivious to, or uninterested in, the difference between *physiologic* (natural) and *pharmacologic* (synthetic) doses. Physiologic (which means they are equivalent to your normal body function) hormones, prescribed properly, and carefully monitored, do not promote abnormal (cancer-causing) actions in the body. These natural hormones are identical in molecular structure to the hormones your body produces. They cannot be distinguished from inborn hormones, even though they are synthesised in a laboratory.

Pharmacologic hormone doses, on the other hand, are much stronger than normal production and suppress natural hormone production, often leading to serious health problems. They interfere with normal hormonal receptors, and create deficiencies of the body's own natural hormones, because our bodies do not have receptors for synthetic hormones. Taking them is tantamount to throwing a monkey wrench into delicate machinery.

For example, as Dr Peat wrote in *From PMS To Menopause*, "Medroxyprogesterone acetate (synthetic progesterone) causes cancer, impairs circulation to the heart, causes birth defects and suppresses the production of progesterone. I feel that the involvement of the various government agencies in the promotion of this poison, and the suppression of information about natural progesterone, has been conspiratorial and deliberately criminal, and those involved should be identified as criminals."

I'm with you, Dr Peat, and I hasten to add that several women have told me that they were blinded by synthetic progesterone. Small wonder, when you consider that blindness and death are listed at the very bottom of the long list of side effects enclosed in the synthetic progesterone container.

Natural progesterone has no adverse side-effects, yet most doctors continue to prescribe the deadly synthetics.

You will need to protect yourself from your doctor in another way –

Learn That Cholesterol is Good

Do not allow an uninformed doctor to persuade you to go on an extreme cholesterol-lowering diet, nor put you on cholesterol-lowering drugs (see *Chapter 6, Oils and Fats*). Judging by the way most physicians have embraced the cholesterol-is-evil propaganda, they never learned, or have forgotten the following:

All of the sex hormones are derived from cholesterol. All of the steroid hormones, which help us deal with stress, inflammation and injury, are derived from cholesterol. Stick to the low-fat diet favoured by most doctors and you will deprive your body of the raw materials that enable it to make hormones you badly need.

And please do not be spooked by what doctors refer to as 'bad' LDL cholesterol. As Dr Peat says, "LDL is extremely good because it is used as a source for producing progesterone and DHEA." Many scientists concur, and research has proved that low cholesterol, particularly LDL, is strongly associated with death from cancer and shortened lifespan in elderly people (see **Chapter 6, Oils and Fats** for details). Of course, this contrary research is not widely circulated, because it would cut into the revenue of the companies that sell cholesterol-lowering drugs and polyunsaturated oils. The last thing the multinationals want you to do is educate yourself so that they cannot poison you and shorten your life, while making billions.

You will also need to –

Protect Yourself From Surgeons

Beware the scalpel-wielding man or woman in white. Hang on to your uterus and your ovaries: you need them, and a hysterectomy is never necessary unless a woman has cancer. Live by the rules in this book and you should be able to overcome all female problems, if you haven't waited too long. If you are considering surgery, rush to the library or bookstore and get **What Your Doctor May Not Tell You About Menopause**, by John R Lee, MD. What he says about hysterectomies is a real eye-opener. If it's already too late you will need natural hormones to make up those lost because your uterus is gone.

Next, you need to know –

About Precursors

Hormones don't just spring up in the body, one by one. First, they are created by cholesterol, as mentioned earlier. Then, precursors get into the act. Simply speaking, a precursor is a substance that is the source of another substance. In other words, once cholesterol has worked its magic, and created the crucial hormone *pregnenolone*, the pregnenolone becomes a precursor for other hormones, as shown in the following diagram:

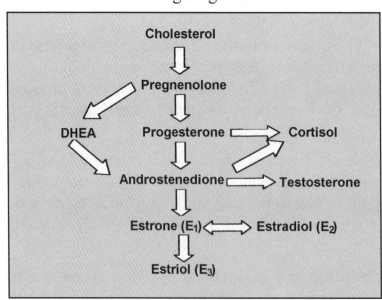

Take Control of Your Health and Escape the Sickness Industry

As the diagram illustrates, end-stage hormones are dependent upon the proper production of precursor hormones. Study the diagram and you will see that pregnenolone creates progesterone and DHEA, and that progesterone creates other hormones. So, although the fact seems to have escaped many health professionals, the crucial hormones are pregnenolone and progesterone, because often it is not necessary to take any other hormones – some of which can be dangerous. Further, and this is comforting, after about fifty years of medical use, *no toxic side effects have been found for natural progesterone or pregnenolone.*

There are so many compelling reasons to take these two hormones, if you are suffering a deficiency, that an entire book would be needed to list them all, and to explain their beneficial effects upon the human body. Dr Peat's paper on pregnenolone is very informative, and he has kindly given me permission to reprint it in the section, ***In Other Words…***. Please read it in full – you will get lifesaving information that will enable you to become your own expert.

There is a lot about progesterone in the pages of this book, so you should be well-informed about this invaluable hormone. But pregnenolone may be new to you, and it is important to understand that it is considered the 'mother hormone', because it is the precursor to all of the adrenal hormones. Levels of this hormone decline dramatically with age, and replacement doses can achieve near 'miracles', such as noticeably stronger muscles, greatly improved digestion and energy levels. Arthritis, memory loss, depression and moodiness can also be helped.

As Dr Peat explains in ***From PMS To Menopause***, "Normalizing the stress hormones with pregnenolone often seems to have the effect of correcting the function of the thyroid gland, probably because it is suppressed by stress. Since pregnenolone is the precursor for progesterone and DHEA (and all the other steroid hormones) it often has the same effects as progesterone or DHEA, and it has the advantage that it allows the body to *produce just an optimum amount of those hormones, without creating an excess.*" (My italics).

Your Body Understands

Your body is an incredibly complex, sophisticated computer, and it is wiser than you are, and understands your needs better than any doctor can. If you provide it with the right kind and amounts of progesterone and pregnenolone it will very likely be nudged into making its own DHEA and any other hormones needed for its wellbeing. Based upon my limited experience with friends, women who have attended the Hippocrates program, and myself, I believe that the best way to start a natural hormone replacement program is by taking these two safe precursor hormones. After a few months, you will discover if they are going to do a good job of regulating your other hormones.

If they do not, you will then have to depend upon a doctor for advice, and this can be tricky. Your first hurdle may be to convince her or him to order saliva hormone tests for you. The World Health Organization is on your side; for years it has recommended saliva tests as much more accurate and cheaper than blood tests.

Next, if your tests reveal a lack of DHEA or testosterone, your doctor is likely to prescribe doses that are way too high. Dr Peat says that at the age of 50, about 4mg of DHEA per day will usually restore the level of DHEA to a youthful level. He says that it is important to avoid taking more than needed, because it is easy to overdose, thus feeding into oestrogen pathways. Large amounts of those sex hormones can disturb the function of the thymus gland and the liver. Women have reported that they were prescribed 15 and 20mg per day and had bad side effects (swollen, painful breasts and anxiety) that indicate that, as Dr Peat warns, the DHEA turned into oestrogen and/or testosterone. He advises that, if DHEA is needed badly, it must be carefully monitored, even though the high levels that are normally present in healthy people would suggest that replacement doses, to restore those normal levels, would not be likely to produce toxic side effects. Women have reported to me that they were prescribed 100mg per day, and that's foolhardy, in my opinion. I wouldn't chance taking any more than the 4mg per day Dr Peat says is safe.

Natural testosterone can have even worse effects: debilitating headaches, sore muscles, sore throats, usually starting on the first day, and continuing until the testosterone is discontinued. One woman told me she had never had a similar headache, and described it as "pumping." All the women I've interviewed told me that the worst of the symptoms lessened the first day off testosterone and each subsequent day improved, with total cessation of symptoms after three or four days. All this for a substance that is supposed to make us feel better!

All the women had very sore breasts, as if they were about to have a period – a symptom of oestrogen overload. I was one of them. In the interests of experimentation, I had the hormone salivary test done. When it was found that I was low in DHEA and testosterone, I tried replacement first on one, then on the other. The DHEA, which was prescribed as a natural USP DHEA capsule, 15mg, had to be discontinued after three days because of the above symptoms of oestrogen overload. Had I insisted upon Dr Peat's recommended dose of 4mg, (I'm embarrassed to admit that I'd forgotten), my experience might have been better. Next, I tried a testosterone cream in a safe base, and the oestrogen overload symptoms kicked in after the second application, so I quit before any other side effects could rear their ugly heads.

The question is – am I, and my friends and the women who attend the Hippocrates Centre, super-delicate, or have we simply been prescribed excessive doses, or are these substances better left alone? I don't pretend to know, and most certainly do not consider myself an expert – and, in any case, all the 'experts' have differing convictions. I do know that progesterone and pregnenolone do not appear to have anything but beneficial side effects, and these are the hormones I recommend and take myself. Perhaps next time I have a salivary test, the results will indicate that the pregnenolone I have been taking will have persuaded my DHEA and testosterone to find levels that are appropriate for my body. If not, perhaps I will find the courage to try the DHEA and testosterone in tiny doses.

In the final analysis, we must all listen to our bodies, and with help from qualified professionals, decide which hormones to take. But pay close attention to symptoms, and if your breasts get tender, or if you have other unpleasant symptoms, that will be an indication that you are on the wrong track.

I tried for years to locate a compounding chemist in Australia who was willing to make up hormone creams that are 100% natural and 100% organically certified. Finally, I found one and he went to great lengths to use pure macadamia oil and a plant preservative I trust. He also has a safe porcine thyroid vegi-cap without preservatives. He is able to ship abroad, with a prescription from a registered Australian doctor, which is a big help to overseas readers who cannot find safe creams locally. You'll find more details in **Resources**.

The only way women can learn about these life saving substances is through what Dr Lee calls 'the women's network' – which is one of the reasons I have written this book. I am alerting you. Each one of you can then alert ten friends, to tell them how to get the correct progesterone from Dr Peat in the USA. Then they alert their friends. The women's network is a powerful weapon, and it's the only one we have to use against the hugely powerful, immensely wealthy multinational drug companies, who are unconcerned about the damage they are doing to women in the name of the bottom line.

Six years ago I was grappling with the problems many women face in menopause when, just as my friends and I needed it most, I discovered *Maca*, a health-giving cruciferous root vegetable which grows only in the High Andes of Peru. Used for over 10,000 years, this ancient remedy has proven to be of great benefit in dealing with both female and male ailments, and as a general aid to wellbeing and good health. Rather than attempting to describe it myself, I strongly recommend you read two interesting and informative articles describing the history and benefits of this truly amazing vegetable (taken in powdered form), which the magazine *Nature and Health* has kindly agreed to allow me to reprint in the *In Other Words* section.

To conclude, I'd like to quote the words of famous anthropologist Margaret Mead on mature women: *"The most creative force in the world is the menopausal woman with zest."*

True. But we are not going to have zest if we permit the menopause/osteoporosis industry to turn this natural, liberating change into a shameful condition to be fought every inch of the way, and treated with devastating drugs.

How to Order and Use Dr Peat's Progest-E Complex

A patented formula containing 10% natural progesterone in natural vitamin E oil
28ml (2,800mg per ounce)

Prices (subject to change)
1 to 2 bottles: $US24.00 each
3 to 4 bottles: $US23.00 each
5 to 6 bottles: $US21.00 each
7 to 11 bottles: $US20.00 each
12 or more: $US18.00 each
Plus Shipping

For non-USA buyers:
If you are willing to have your order take a little longer, Kenogen will ship up to 3 bottles using Global Priority Mail for about US$8.75. This class of mail is uninsurable, which is why Kenogen doesn't use it for orders of 4 or more.
   Shipping 4 to 10 bottles is now US$26.50 and this is insurable.

IMPORTANT: Please do not telephone Hippocrates Health Centre to order progesterone oil. We do not, and cannot, import this product – we merely recommend it. You must order it yourself from the USA.

To Order, fax Dr Peat's company, *Kenogen*, in Eugene Oregon. If faxing from Australia, dial 0011 first, to get out of the country. Then, dial the USA code, which is 1, followed by 541-485-8781. Alternatively you can e-mail them at kenogen@efn.org. Kenogen accepts Visa and Mastercard; they need your credit card number, the expiry date, the number of bottles you want, and your name and address printed carefully. If you do not have a fax or a credit card, we suggest you ask a friend. Do not expect Kenogen to acknowledge your fax or answer any questions or return phone messages. They merely fill orders when they arrive by fax or email.

Ordering eight bottles at a time is economical: the shipping charge of approximately US$20 is the same for one bottle as for eight, so many of our readers club together to save money. A bottle should last between three and five months. It is wise, if ordering lots of bottles, to ask Kenogen to put several names on the package so Australian Customs will understand that the import is for several people, and for personal use only. Resale is not permitted. Kenogen gives a small discount to my readers, so be sure to mention this book, or Hippocrates Health Centre, when you order.

To repeat: *please do not phone us for any other information on Progesterone*. We are being flooded by calls and cannot handle them, as we are overwhelmed by orders for this book. Absolutely everything we have learned about progesterone, from many scientists, is in this book.

Here are Dr Peat's instructions for using his progesterone oil.

For general purposes, it is most economical and effective to take progesterone dissolved in vitamin E orally, for example taking a few drops on the lips and tongue, or rubbing it into the gums. (It is good for the general health of the gums.) These membranes are very thin, and the progesterone quickly enters the blood.

When it is swallowed, the vitamin E allows it to be absorbed through the walls of the stomach and intestine, and it can be assimilated along with food, in the chylomicrons, permitting it to circulate in the blood to all of the organs before being processed by the liver.

Preferred storage is to refrigerate after opening (However, this is not necessary for daily use. And if the product is refrigerated, it will increase the amount that is in one drop. Please adjust your dosage accordingly).

Women's needs and symptoms vary, so each must find her own dose. Overdosing may produce a feeling of euphoria, but is not dangerous. The oil should be used in sufficient quantity to make symptoms disappear.

Menstruating women should time its use so that the cycles are not disrupted: apply the oil 14 to 15 days before the period is due, and quit when it starts, or the day before it is due.

Postmenopausal women should use the oil for 14 days of each month, allowing "time off" for the pituitary to remain active. If symptoms are severe, increase by individual drops, as often as needed, for the entire month if necessary, cutting back to two weeks per month once symptoms clear. Alternatively, one half the normal dose may be used for the second two-week period. Once the system has regained equilibrium, the aim is to use the oil for only two weeks each month.

A must-read for all women

Awaken the Warrior

By Dr. Karen Coates and Master Coach Vincent Perry

This book compliments TAKE CONTROL OF YOUR HEALTH AND ESCAPE THE SICKNESS INDUSTRY. Dr. Coates and Mr. Perry make it easy to understand the bio-chemistry of the body and the way stress affects it in so many terrible ways. Their book provides sound advice on how to avoid the seemingly inevitable decline into illness as we age, and provides a roadmap to follow. It is a practical guide that includes a unique exercise program and proven methods for regaining optimal health at any age.

Details for purchasing and information on their training seminars can be found at www.pumma.net, or by telephoning (07) 5536-7464 within Australia.

"Doctors see breasts as sacks of money to be milked, rather than fountains of nourishment for the nation's babies, and lovely symbols of the feminine gender."

"Breast cancer therapy is a failure, but no one wants to own up to it."

- William Campbell Douglass, MD

12

Breast Health

Why prevention, not surgical mutilation, is the way to go; how to avoid becoming a cancer statistic

1: WHAT YOU CAN DO

√ Get On a Healthful Diet and Stick With It

There have been innumerable studies linking breast health with the plentiful consumption of vegetables and fruits. These studies have been so impressive that the evidence is impossible to refute. For example, the late Dr John Lee, quotes a study which found 48 percent less breast cancer among enthusiastic vegetable and fruit eaters. *The International Journal of Cancer* reported a significantly reduced risk of breast cancer among those on high potassium diets. Apricots, bananas, avocados, figs, raisins, almonds, pistacios, pumpkin kernels and tomato paste all have extremely high levels of this important mineral.

There are, of course, other factors involved. People who eat lots of fresh food are less likely to pig-out on junk food, and that will substantially lessen their likelihood of getting breast cancer, or any other cancers.

The *Journal of the American Medical Association* reported a study proving the link between overweight and breast cancer risk. It was conclusive, so eat those healthful vegies and fruits, and shun the junk, fattening foods.

√ Apply a Natural Progesterone

The natural progesterone oil specially formulated by Dr Peat, *Pro-Gest*, will protect your breasts and all your other female organs from cancer if used faithfully. Dr Lee, in his *Newsletter*, *February 2000*, wrote the following interesting paragraph: "I believe that progesterone is a potent protector against the 80 percent of breast cancer that is hormone-related. My colleagues and I have asked thousands of women the following question: 'Of all the women you know who got breast cancer, how many were using natural progesterone?' Except for a handful who by coincidence (or intuition) started using it a few weeks or months before their diagnosis, we haven't found any. I would like to pose the same question to you. If you know of a woman using natural progesterone who has gotten breast cancer, please e-mail me at *info@johnleemd.com*, or send a letter to P.0. Box 3527, Santa Barbara, CA 93130." (Since Dr. Lee's death, there are people who are continuing his work and will answer e-mails.)

√ Live a Tranquil Life

There is a profound connection between stress and breast cancer. If you find it difficult to cope, you may well find it worthwhile to learn meditation.

√ Make Exercise a Rule of Life

Take a daily walk. If it's raining, don a raincoat and boots, or use a rebounder indoors if you have one. If not, walk smartly in place in a well-aired room, while breathing deeply.

Take Control of Your Health and Escape the Sickness Industry

√ Sun Yourself Regularly

Get out in the sunshine regularly, without sunscreen, to absorb the crucial vitamin D that will protect your breasts. Read why in *Chapter 8*, *Bone Health II*.

√ Take a Selenium Supplement Daily

The value of this important mineral is explained in *Chapter 8*, *Bone Health II*. There is now a liquid selenium available in Australia, called Selenosol, made by Nutrition Care Pharmaceuticals. All countries with high concentrations of selenium in the soil have low cancer rates; in Senegal the soil has the highest concentration of selenium in the world and the population has the lowest death rate from cancer of any place on Earth.

√ Drink Pure, Fluoride-free Water

F. Batmanghelidj, MD, in his book, *Your Body's Many Cries for Water*, says that chronic dehydration contributes to the development of breast cancer. "The breast," he explains, "is a water-secreting organ... If a woman already has breast cancer, drinking plenty of water will assist with any therapy by flushing out toxins... If you want to prevent metastasis from occurring, it is urgent that you drink enough water. If you don't, your breast may suffer horribly because of its unique role in supplying fluids."

√ Wear a Soft Brassiere – or None at All

Fifty years ago a top-rated breast specialist shocked me. "Persist in wearing boned brassieres," he said, "and you will substantially increase your likelihood of breast cancer." I quit. Subsequently, I learned that he didn't go far enough, and that he should have warned me against wearing all bras.

Have you ever noticed how red the areas around your breasts are after removing your bra? This is a sign that the bra has slowed the lymph flow, which is crucial for filtering out the toxins that naturally collect in the breast. Without this lymphatic drainage, your breasts cannot keep themselves healthy. There have been some exceedingly persuasive studies that concluded that the more hours each day you wear a bra, the likelier you are to suffer from breast cancer. Some women actually sleep in their bras, and their risk is the highest.

As you know, boned bras were replaced by wired bras years ago, and they are even more dangerous because of the way the wires dig in and compress the flesh. My advice is to go bra-less as much as possible. When you must wear a bra remove it as soon as you get home, and only wear soft ones.

√ Try Iodine

William Campbell Douglass, MD, writing in *Wise Traditions*, makes this suggestion: "Take one drop of *Lugol's solution* (iodine) daily in a glass of water.

Iodine is excellent for breast health. A few people are allergic to iodine – observe closely for rash after the first dose. An even more effective treatment with Lugol's solution (also known as APF) is to paint the cervix with it. Often the breast lumps will disappear before the patient leaves the doctor's office." I have never encountered this therapy before, but I like the old-fashioned, non-invasive sound of it, and I invite feedback from readers. Many doctors recommend that women take 3–8 drops of Lugol's Iodine per day, half in the morning, and half in the evening, for breast health. (See page 20 for instructions.)

√ *Breastfeed*

Breastfeeding is not only best for babies; it also protects their mothers from breast cancer.

2: *WHAT YOU MUST AVOID*

✗ *Soy – and Everything Made From It*

Avoid the *Abominable Bean* in all its forms! *Chapter 9* explains why this insidious killer is to be shunned. Never forget that the US Department of Energy Health Risk Laboratory has published research showing that isoflavones in soy act in the same way as the outlawed insecticide *DDT* to cause breast cancer cells to multiply.

✗ *Dental Amalgam Fillings*

Don't let your dentist inflict them on you. If you have any – get your dentist to remove them. They contain mercury, the second most hazardous thing on Earth. If your dentist won't co-operate, find one who will. See also *Chapter 17, Dental Health*.

✗ *Excessive Alcohol Intake*

Keep your alcohol consumption to a bare minimum. All alcoholic beverages contain some carcinogenic elements which could increase your susceptibility to breast cancer.

✗ *The Beauty Parlour*

Beauty parlours and hairdressing salons are filled with hazards for breast health. Hair dyes are a witches' brew of cancer-causing chemicals, all of which are easily absorbed through the scalp. Shampoos and conditioners are filled with a shameful array of dangerous petrochemical substances. Even if you don't have ceramic nails put on, some silly woman in the same room will, and the pungent odour from that is enough to make some people faint on the spot. Others complain of searing pains in their lungs when exposed to these toxic chemicals, which should be against the law. Refuse to patronise salons where they are used. Eventually the message will get across.

Cosmetics are chock-full of cancer-causing chemicals (see *Chapter 25, The Banned List*). Choose carefully and don't be taken in by the slick ads. Consider switching to pure coconut oil for cleansing and moisturising. I use nothing else. Refer to *Resources* for some cosmetics that are safe.

✗ Flax Oil

Don't be influenced by the flax oil enthusiasts; they are as misguided as those who beat the drum for soy. It is always rancid, and even if it were fresh it would still, like soy, be oestrogenic due to the isoflavones they both contain, which can contribute to cancer, or make existing cancer worse.

✗ 'The Pill'

A number of studies over the past few decades have shown that the chance of getting cancer increased by about 25 percent in women who used oral contraceptives compared to those who have not. In March 2002, Australia's *ABC News* reported the findings of a major ten-year Norwegian study involving over 10,000 women, which not only confirmed those earlier findings, but also concluded that for women aged over 45 who take the pill, the risk of breast cancer is doubled.

If you have been taking the pill, my suggestion is to quit and become serious about your diet to overcome the damage. The body is very forgiving and will reward you.

✗ Pollution

Living near nuclear plants, hazardous waste disposal sites, chemical plants and sources of electromagnetic radiation contribute to breast cancer, as well as all other cancers. Living in the US puts women at a higher risk than does living anywhere else in the world – and the farther northeast, the greater the risk. There are many variables involved in this statistic, but certainly the degree of pollution is a significant factor.

✗ Sugar

I know it's hard, but, ladies, please eliminate or at least substantially reduce your sugar intake. Next time you're tempted to tuck into that 'irresistible' treat, consider the findings of an important study reported in *Medical Hypotheses, July 1983*, based on a comparison of breast cancer deaths in 21 countries. The study found that the higher the sugar consumption, the higher the death rate. For example, in the UK, where sugar consumption is 145gm per person per day, there were 23 breast cancer deaths per year, per 100,000. In Japan, where daily per capita sugar consumption is only 57.4gm, there were only 6.8 breast cancer deaths annually per 100,000. Data from other countries provided comparable results, and there have been many other studies with similar findings, too numerous to include here. Trust me, they all point the finger at

White Death as a major cause of breast cancer. Get the sugar monkey off your back, and look forward to a longer, healthier life in all ways.

And don't switch to artificial sweeteners instead; they are infinitely worse – see ***Chapter 4,*** *Excitotoxins*.

X *Polyunsaturated Fats*

Polyunsaturated fat is another substance you must avoid in order to protect your breasts. But the good news is that you won't have to deprive yourself of the delicious, old-fashioned fats our forebears ate with relish and in robust health. These fats – coconut oil, olive oil and meat and butter from animals that graze on grass and are organically raised – are protective of your breasts.

But you *must* keep away from the highly-promoted polyunsaturated oils that have been conclusively implicated as major causes of the huge increase in breast cancer. If the proponents of polyunsaturates thought about them logically they would understand that they cause cancer. These fats have been used for decades to suppress the immune systems of transplant patients. In other words, when an organ is transplanted, the immune system tries to expel it. The polyunsaturates are so immuno-suppressive that they are utilised in emulsions to stop the immune system from doing its job. This is fine for a transplant patient, but the rest of us want our immune systems to be as strong as possible. Without a well-functioning immune system, we have no defence against breast cancer or any other diseases. How the medical system can recommend a substance for the 'health' of our hearts, and then use the identical substance to render inactive the immune system of a transplant patient, is both mysterious and amazing.

And what about the 'essential fatty acids' that are so heavily promoted as crucial for our health? According to Dr Peat, this fad originated due to faulty interpretation of certain tests performed on rats in the 1930s. He says, "It is now known that polyunsaturated fats interfere with thyroid hormone in just about every conceivable way – and they have a strong estrogen-promoting action." And oestrogen is known to contribute to breast cancer. "Consumption of these fats leads directly to the development of such degenerative scourges as cancer, diabetes, heart disease, arthritis, osteoporosis, and connective tissue disease," says Dr Peat.

Study after study has found that trans-fatty acids, from partially hydro-genated vegetable oils, contribute to cancers of organs that are rich in fat tissues, such as prostate glands and breasts. These mechanically altered oils are used in most processed foods, and avoiding them takes dedication. Healthy traditional people never had these oils and still do not consume them. Prior to the 20th Century, they were rarely used in industrialised countries. Since then, polyunsaturates have taken over, and so have breast cancer, lung cancer, and many other scourges. So, please, shun all these man-made, plastic oils, along with sugar, and your overall health will benefit enormously. There's more on this in **Chapter 6,** *Oils and Fats.*

✗ Smoking

Don't get the idea that you can simply avoid sugar, the 'bad' oils and the other no-nos listed above, and keep breast cancer at bay while continuing to smoke. According to Professor Samuel S Epstein, MD, this killer addiction "...represents the greatest source of breast-cancer-causing radiation in consumer products. It brings toxic levels of radioactive lead and polonium into the lungs of smokers as well as second hand smoke recipients... What is most disturbing is that the risks of breast cancer are highest among those who start smoking heavily in adolescence... One study found that very young smokers raised their lifetime risk by a remarkable 80 percent."

A Canadian study found that women who start smoking as teenagers are 70 percent more likely to develop breast cancer than non-smokers. Those are not good odds, and it's hard to feel pity for anyone stupid enough to take up this deadly habit, considering the evidence. I do, however, feel sympathy for those of us unfortunate enough to be exposed to selfish individuals' second-hand smoke, which contains "... up to 150 times higher levels of carcinogens than smoke directly inhaled by cigarette smokers," according to Dr Epstein. Don't allow your friends to expose you to breast cancer!

✗ Milk

There is a great deal of persuasive evidence that all milk products are breast cancer risks. The purveyors of soy 'milk' point to the low breast cancer incidence in China, which is one in 10,000 women, compared to one in 12 women in Australia and England, and one in nine in the US. But this huge difference is not due to soy consumption, which is much lower in China than the multinational propagandists would have us believe. In China, the women who have been seduced by Western food, due to their financial and social status, are the ones who contract breast cancer. Milk products, and the other Western foods and drugs they ingest, are to blame.

Dairy herds in industrialised countries are kept in deplorable conditions, and the milk they produce, in abnormally large amounts due to drugs, is subjected to various chemical processes which are in themselves hazardous to health. The poor cows are pumped up with dangerous chemicals and dosed regularly with antibiotics. They are subjected to growth hormones to increase production, and these hormones create havoc in women's breasts. This is all done in the name of profit; tremendous profit. And of course, the drugs the cows are given go into the milk. This is self-evident. Don't doctors warn lactating women to avoid certain foods and drugs because they will affect their breast milk? They should also warn women to avoid the drugs in commercial milk!

So, my advice is – ignore the fear-mongers who warn that we must guzzle milk and eat cheese and yogurt for the sake of our bones; their claims are now thoroughly discredited.

✗ Oestrogen

A Harvard University research team reported that oestrogen feeds cancer, while progesterone inhibits it. There are hundreds of other equally convincing studies implicating oestrogen as a cancer risk. So, if your physician doesn't want you to go off HRT, or is pressuring you to go on it, point him or her in the direction of the *Journal Of The National Cancer Institute*, *June 3, 1998*, for enlightenment. Or at least show him or her *Chapter 11*, *The Menopause*, in this book.

✗ Constipation

This common complaint is an enemy of breast health, so keep your bowels open. This also holds true for fibrocystic breasts, which is not a disease, but a benign condition present in almost all women to some degree. The sometimes painful, lumpy breasts connected with this condition can be frightening, but do not lead to cancer. According to Dr Lee, progesterone solves this problem.

There is also a correlation between caffeine consumption and these breast lumps, and good diet, with special emphasis on regular elimination, will go a long way toward clearing up the symptoms. In constipation, food moves slowly through the colon, causing excess waste to pass into the bloodstream, creating a toxic environment, which is bad for all aspects of health. Don't let this happen to you – taking magnesium to bowel tolerance will cure the worst cases of constipation. Use magnesium chloride, never the excitotoxin magnesium aspartate.

✗ Anti-perspirants

There is evidence that anti-perspirants can lead to breast cancer. They prevent perspiration, which is one of the means the body uses to purge poisons, a safeguard for our breasts. If these poisons remain in the body, they do not go elsewhere to be eliminated; they become deposited in the lymph nodes. The lymph nodes are located in the upper outside quadrant of the breast area, which is the location of most breast cancers. It is postulated that ordinary deodorants are safe, provided they do not contain aluminium, because they merely control odour and do not suppress perspiration. So far as I know there haven't been any studies on this. Who would fund them?

To avoid offending, spread a bit of bicarbonate of soda, slightly dampened, in your armpits.

3: Q: WHAT ABOUT THE 'PREVENTION' DRUGS RECOMMENDED BY DOCTORS?

A: They Don't Work!

And they're dangerous. The drug *Tamoxifen* has shown a slight decrease in breast cancer risk in the women who have taken it. The very serious risks, however, associated with Tamoxifen preclude its use: a 700 percent increase in fatal blood clots, serious risk of liver and uterine cancer and hepatitis, corneal opacities and damage to the retina. Dutch investigators who studied more than a thousand women found that those who had taken Tamoxifen for two years or more had a greater risk than previously reported of dying from endometrial cancer.

When the patent on Tamoxifen expired, three companies came up with new versions: Novartis is flogging *Femara*, AstraZeneca has *Arimidex* and Pharmacia is pushing *Aromasin*. The public relations campaigns promoting these drugs are first rate, but the side effects include nausea, bone pain, fatigue, thinning hair and arthralgia. These are the short-term effects. Since these new drugs are very similar to Tamoxifen, the long-term effects are probably going to prove to be similar as well. After years of raves in the press and wholesale prescribing of Tamoxifen, it was discovered that long-term use caused blood clots, severe gynaecological problems and uterine cancer.

And for what? These drugs are aimed at women who do not have breast cancer, but have a family history of it. How about explaining to women how to live so that they will give their immune systems every weapon to fight back? Does it not occur to the physicians who prescribe these 'preventatives' that 'family history' includes common diet and other habits?

Watch out for 'new improved' versions; there is one thing you can count on from the pharmaceuticals – new drugs will always come along, followed by little-publicised side effects, often followed by quiet removal from the market, frequently followed by lawsuits and out-of-court settlements. Drugs for 'protection' from non-existing breast cancer are no exceptions. They are, however, more immoral than the usual drug puffery, because these drugs are incredibly dangerous, they don't cure anything, and women use them as a substitute for learning about and practicing the prudent life.

4: SELF EXAMINATION

"... better off examining your thumbs"

Women in the industrialised world have been whipped into a state of near-hysteria by the cancer industry. They have been urged to examine and rush to the doctor if a lump is felt. The industry neglects to mention that breasts are composed of glandular tissue and are naturally lumpy, some more than others. They also don't mention that by the time a lump can be detected by palpation, it has been there a long time and contains millions of cells. It should not be disturbed. As Dr Douglass says, "If the cancer is the extremely malignant 'eating' kind, the patient is already doomed. If it is a slow-growing tumor, then finding it early will make no difference, except it will usually lead to unnecessary armpit surgery as well as removal of the breast. The armpit surgery (removal of the lymph nodes) is likely to spread the cancer if the armpit has already been invaded by cancer cells; if it hasn't been invaded, then the surgery is unnecessary."

The tendency to panic is understandable, and I fully empathise, having been there myself. Years ago, I was caught up in the self-examination routine and found a lump. The specialist I consulted uttered the dreaded "I don't like the feel of that," and turned his back on me, leaving me to hyperventilate while he fiddled with something on a table. Then, without a word, he advanced upon me, brandishing a syringe that would have been excessive even for a horse doctor. I backed up, holding up my hands for protection, feeling that he was planning to assault me. Which is precisely what he intended; if I had allowed that cowboy to plunge a long needle into my breast, he would have sent millions of cancer cells into my body, had the lump been cancerous. If the biopsy proved it to be benign, he would have no doubt urged a lumpectomy, a disfiguring and usually unnecessary, sometimes dangerous, procedure. As it happened, it was a simple clogged milk duct, which a second specialist diagnosed simply by palpation. Had it been more sinister, I would not have submitted to the "cures" of Cancer Inc. I would have blitzed my body with detox and wheatgrass juice.

In February of 2003 big cancer news was reported – finally it had been proved that Breast Self-Examination (BSE) was not only useless, it could be dangerous. 266,064 women in Shanghai were divided into either a BSE instruction group or a no-instruction group. The women received periodic instruction and were followed for ten years. The number of breast cancer deaths was nearly identical in both groups. BSE, however, did detect more benign breast lesions, prompting authorities to warn that BSE increases a woman's chances of having a benign breast biopsy. BSE may seem harmless, but causes anxiety for many women, and has a high rate of false positives. As Susan Love, MD, wrote in the *New York Times* when this news broke, "It is time to entirely rethink the question of early detection of breast cancer."

Dr Douglass tells of a friend "...who lived in a state of constant anxiety, bordering on terror, because she has lumpy breasts and was always examining them. She had suffered through five operations, all negative. She would have been better off examining her thumbs."

5: MAMMOGRAMS AND OTHER OPTIONS

Mammogram Madness

For decades, the mammogram industry has been scaring women into having regular mammograms to 'prevent' breast cancer. Their government-supported public relations campaigns have been so successful that women have the idea that 'mammograms prevent cancer'. The truth, however, is that *mammograms can cause breast cancer*. There are at least two reasons for this – radiation and physical compression – both integral parts of the procedure. It seems to have been forgotten that radiation was the first proven cause of cancer, and, if you have ever been subjected to a mammogram, you know that they squeeze the breasts tightly in a vice before shooting radiation through them. The danger is exacerbated due to the fact that breasts are more susceptible to radiation than other tissue.

In 1996 John W Gofman, MD, PhD, revealed in his book, ***Preventing Breast Cancer: The Story of a Major, Proven, Preventable Cause of This Disease***, that past exposure to ionizing radiation – primarily medical x-rays – is responsible for about 75 percent of the breast cancer problem in the United States.

What the proponents of mammograms fail to tell us is that, after all this squeezing and squashing and possibly spreading cancer cells, an all-clear on a mammogram is not a guarantee that there is no cancer developing. Not only do they miss 10 to 15 percent of all cancers, but interpreting them is far from an exact science. There is a high risk of false negative and false positive findings.

A further problem with mammograms is that they may help spread an existing mass of cancer cells. The compression during testing, according to pathologist Lorraine Day, MD, can cause existing cancer cells to metastasise from the breast tissue. If there are cancer cells, they are more likely to spread to other parts of the body, because cancer cells are now circulating in the bloodstream.

University of Illinois' Emeritus Professor Samuel S Epstein, MD, points out that "Since 1928, physicians have been warned to handle cancerous breasts with care – for fear of accidentally disseminating cells and spreading the cancer. Nevertheless, mammography entails tight and often painful breast compression, particularly in premenopausal women, which could lead to distant and lethal spread of malignant cells by rupturing small blood vessels in or around small undetected breast cancers."

Dr Charles B Simone, former clinical associate in immunology and pharmacology at the (US) National Cancer Institute, concurs. "Mammograms increase the risk for developing breast cancer and raise the risk of spreading or metastasising existing growth," he states.

According to Dr Douglass, "One animal study found that the number of metastases will increase by 80 percent if the tumour is manipulated. A human study reported in the **British Medical Journal** confirms these ominous findings. They discovered that there were 29 percent more deaths from breast cancer in women who had had mammography."

All this disturbing and reliable information, unfortunately, does not filter down to the people who need it most, women. Mammograms are big business! The last thing the industry will admit is that they can cause cancer, and are not even accurate.

There has been a huge increase in breast cancer during the past twenty years and, as the **New York Times**, *January 24 2002*, reported, regular mammograms have contributed to them. And for what? As the late Dr Lee wrote in his newsletter, "For a breast cancer cell to become large enough for detection by palpation, the cancer has to have been growing for about 10 years. If found one year earlier by mammography, the cancer has been growing for about nine years, which is plenty of time to spawn metastases if the cancer is prone to do that. The one-year difference between palpation and mammography detection is ultimately of little importance."

No Way of Knowing

Dr H Gilbert Welch, senior researcher from White River Junction, Vermont, discovered that in women who die from other causes, 40 percent have had common lesions that showed up on mammograms. According to Dr Welch, no expert is capable of knowing which of these will develop into cancer, and which will remain dormant.

Biopsies of a suspicious lump found in a mammogram do not improve survival rates, because cutting into the lump invades the protective pocket that helps keep it from spreading. Research in Germany showed that women who had not had biopsies lived longer than those who did. Surgeon Emeritus George Crile, from the Cleveland Clinic in the US, says, "It gives credence to what our patients already think and tell us – that cutting into cancer spreads it and makes it grow."

If your physician is nagging you to have yearly mammograms, I strongly recommend you refer him or her to the following public statements made by two world authorities with intimate knowledge of the procedure.

At a meeting of the British Royal Society of Medicine in 2002, Professor Michael Baum said that screening for breast cancer should be scrapped, because it caused hundreds of healthy women to undergo risky, mutilating and unnecessary treatments even when they may never develop the disease. An eminent breast surgeon and researcher, Professor Baum's statement drew considerable attention because he was one of the physicians who helped set up the UK's £50-million-a-year breast-screening service.

And on the other side of the Atlantic, similar views are held by Samuel S Epstein, MD, Chairman of the Cancer Prevention Coalition and Professor Emeritus of Environmental and Occupational Medicine, University of Illinois School of Public Health, Chicago, who adds, "Screening mammography poses significant and cumulative risks of breast cancer for premenopausal women. The routine practice of taking four films of each breast annually results in approximately 1 rad (radiation absorbed dose) exposure, about 1,000 times greater than that from a chest x-ray. The premenopausal breast is highly sensitive to radiation, each 1 rad exposure increasing breast cancer risk by about one percent, with a cumulative 10 percent increased risk for each breast over a decade's screening. These risks are even greater for younger women subject to 'baseline screening'."

Far more preferable to this uncomfortable and hazardous treatment are two relatively new diagnostic tools now gaining wide acceptance; *CRT-2000*, which uses computer technology, and *Digital Thermal Imaging (DITI)*, a 15-minute non-invasive test. In an article entitled **Thermography vs Mammography** published in the **Townsend Letter for Doctors and Patients**, *January 2000*, Rose Marie Williams, MA, of New Paltz, New York, gave the following clear description of CRT-2000:

How CRT-2000 Works, and Why it is a Marked Improvement on Previous Technologies

Using a heat sensitive instrument wired to a computer, the CRT-2000 takes quick measurement of 112 point locations on the face, torso and arms. The body is then exposed to cool ambient temperature for ten minutes and the procedure is repeated, taking about 30 minutes for the entire scan, performed by a trained technician.

Descriptive medical literature explains how the mechanism relies upon the interface of the autonomic nervous system and the cutano-visceral circuit – since 70 percent of the thermoregulation of the skin is modulated by the locally underlying organs and tissues. When the skin is exposed to cool air, a capillary constriction usually occurs, while the body shunts blood to the head. The response phenomenon to cold as reflected in skin temperature is controlled by internal organs such as the liver, pancreas, breast, or teeth. (CRT-2000 is also useful for dentists who choose to practice in a holistic manner).

Because this scan is a direct measurement of the Autonomic Nervous System it is considered a vital key for physicians to approach the underlying disturbance mechanisms of disease and health. CRT-2000 is not the infra-red thermography of decades ago which resulted in false positives and was ultimately abandoned by the medical community.

The scan offers a more complete revelation of the patient's 'vitality' and ability to 'regulate' or adjust to stress from different vital organs. Additionally, it determines the integrity for detoxification, creating a picture of the 'global' health status. CRT facilitates information about early cellular and metabolic dysfunction which often lead to disease. Dr Beilin brought it through the FDA for marketing approval, and he testified to a Congressional Committee with NIH and NCI interest and enthusiasm.

In use by over 1,500 physicians in Europe, the CRT-2000 scanning device is used to compile physiological information that may be as valuable as MRIs or X-rays. For seeing dysfunction in tissue integrity in its earliest stages, it may be a most important adjunct to X-ray or MRIs.

CRT truly offers the possibility of early detection, even before degeneration such as a malignancy is manifested, offering practitioner and patient the opportunity to implement physiological and lifestyle changes that reinforce a healthy immune response. Follow-up scans can easily chart the patient's progress in health promotion, or suggest another approach may be indicated.

My friends in the US tell me that the top health professionals are using this machine. People are becoming increasingly aware of the dangers of X-rays, and this technology from Germany has proved to be a popular way to avoid radiation and still get a correct diagnosis. Up until now it has not been available in Australia, which is not surprising, considering how backward-thinking many of our physicians are. So, when I read the above article, I rang Rose Marie Williams in New York to learn what I could about distribution. To my delight, she put me on to Jenny Burke, Laboratory Director of *Australian Biologies* in Sydney, where they are now using this machine. At present, as far as I know, there are only three other professionals using it in Australia – in Victoria and Perth (see *Resources*), and I would be interested to hear of any others. The machine is amazingly inexpensive, when you consider how valuable it is, and I think we should all nag our health professionals to invest in them.

The second innovative diagnostic tool is *Digital Infrared Thermal Imaging (DITI)*, which involves a 15-minute non-invasive test (see *Resources*). There is no contact with the body of any kind, no radiation and the procedure is painless. DITI detects the subtle physiological changes that accompany breast pathology, whether it is cancer, fibrocystic disease, an infection or a vascular disease. Utilising infra-red technology, thermal imaging technicians capture a digitised image of the breasts in the form of an infra-red thermogram, or heat picture. The resultant data is stored in a computer and can be printed on high-resolution colour printers, or sent electronically to a doctor for analysis.

The doctor then compares the thermal patterns in each breast. Any significant asymmetries, or any specific blood vessel patterns in one breast that do not appear in the other, indicate a physiologic abnormality. This may be pathological, or it might indicate an anatomical variant. A positive thermogram should be a wake-up call for further monitoring and serious preventative measures.

All thermograms are kept on record and form a baseline for future routine evaluations. I have been told that this technology can detect abnormalities two to five years ahead of palpation and mammograms.

Magnetic Resonance Imaging (MRI)

This is a diagnostic tool that uses "…powerful, but harmless, magnetic fields and radio-waves". Perhaps one day it may become known that MRI is not as harmless as they claim, but for now it is considered effective and safe, according to studies in three prestigious medical journals. It's still in its infancy in Australia; it is expensive, and there is no Medicare rebate at this printing.

6: MEDICAL INTERVENTIONS

Slash, Burn, Mutilate, Poison – Take Your Pick

Dr Douglass offers this unequivocal advice: "If you develop a large lump in the breast, do not submit to more surgery than a simple lump removal and do not allow them to cut into the lymph nodes in your armpit... Pass on the radiation and chemotherapy. Radiation is highly destructive of not only tissues, but the immune system, which then makes you more susceptible to all diseases. It is usually a terrible price to pay for a temporary shrinkage of a tumor."

Keep in mind that when hundreds of oncologists were sent questionnaires asking if they would submit to chemotherapy, 80 percent said they would not. They know, from gruesome experience, what chemotherapy does to people, but they keep recommending it. One reason for this is financial, of course, but I think the main motivation is that chemotherapy, radiation and surgery are the only approved 'cures' for cancer, and physicians can get in trouble with their medical boards if they do not push the 'big three'.

This is tragic and evil, when you consider that there are many natural detoxification procedures for cancer which medical associations and governments suppress. The latest 'buzz' therapy for metastatic breast cancer is bone marrow transplants and high-dose chemotherapy. The women who have undergone this procedure have suffered horrendously. The American Society of Clinical Oncology has discredited a study purporting to prove the effectiveness of this therapy. The Society revealed that questionable data produced by the University of Witwatersrand in Johannesburg, South Africa, indicated that this procedure was more effective than it is, and that the university fired the researcher, Dr Werner Bezwoda, when they discovered he had faked this data. Yet, despite this, the Society has not abandoned the procedure, and advises women to undergo it "only if they are enrolled in a clinical trial." In other words, if they are willing to be guinea pigs.

Is Chemotherapy as Bad as they Say?

No. It's worse. Somehow the medical profession and the pharmaceuticals decided it would be a good idea to inject poison into the veins of desperately ill people to kill cancer cells. It was conveniently ignored that the poison also kills good cells, has terrible long-term effects and can destroy hope for recovery.

A new study confirms that women with breast cancer who receive chemotherapy (in addition to surgery and radiation) have a 28 times greater chance of developing leukaemia than those who avoid such drugs. *The Townsend Letter For Doctors And Patients, December 2000*, reported:

> French doctors looked at over 3000 breast cancer patients treated between 1982 and 1996. Ten developed acute leukemia and all ten of these had also received chemotherapy. In comparison, women who received no chemotherapy had no increased risk (*J Clin Oncol 2000; 18:2836-42*). The increased risk was especially apparent in younger women who received the drug mitoxantrone (*Novantrone*). "In women with early breast cancer and potential long survival, short term beneficial effects of mitoxantrone should be weighed against possible long-term threatening side effects," the researchers concluded.

Here is yet another reason that we should spare no effort to find truly non-toxic alternatives to chemotherapy.

The following appeared in the *Gold Coast Bulletin*, Queensland Australia, *July 14-15, 2001*:

> Chemotherapy given to women with early-stage breast cancer causes their bone density to decline at a faster rate than previously known, increasing the risk of osteoporosis, say US researchers.

> Scientists led by Dr Charles Shapiro at Ohio State University said they were surprised to find that 35 premenopausal women treated with chemotherapy experienced up to an 8 percent loss in bone density after 12 months of treatment.

> The bone loss in the patients treated with chemotherapy was so significant that the study was halted to allow the women to seek care from their own doctors.

What About Surgery?

We've commented elsewhere on the 'adverse incidents' endemic in the hospital system. Again, from the *Gold Coast Bulletin*, *February 1 2003*, comes another example of such an 'isolated incident' with particularly disturbing relevance to the subject of this chapter:

Hospital Admits Dual Breast Removal Error

> A 46-year-old American woman who was told she had advanced breast cancer had both breasts removed, only to learn doctors had given her another patient's diagnosis. "There was an accidental switch. Two patients' slides were switched. It was a once-in-a-lifetime mistake," said Terri Dresen, a spokeswoman for United Hospital in St Paul, Minnesota.

Linda McDougal, an accountant from Woodville, Wisconsin, was diagnosed in May 2002 with an advanced stage of breast cancer and had both breasts removed three weeks later. Two days after the surgery, her surgeon informed her that biopsy results showed she did not have cancer. "It has taken me seven months to be able to talk about this," McDougal, a mother of three, told the *Pioneer Press,* a local Washington newspaper.

"This is an isolated incident. We're talking here about an exceptional doctor who is distraught about what happened," Dresen said. "We're truly sorry."

McDougal is still being treated at the same hospital for infections she developed after undergoing reconstructive plastic surgery. She plans to sue the hospital for damages.

I should hope so!

For those women who elect to have breast cancer surgery, the following statement by Dr. Johnathan Collin in the **Townsend Letter for Doctors and Patients** is of the utmost importance:

A study published in November in the journal **Cancer** concluded that women who have breast cancer surgery in the first 10 days of their menstrual cycle had a worse long term outcome than women who had their breast cancer surgery in the latter two weeks of their cycle. This theory was bantered around in the 80s with some researchers claiming exactly the same theory; repeated studies were unable to confirm it. Surgeons were divided but primarily considered menstrual cycle irrelevant in scheduling breast surgery. Intriguing as the research was, too many surgeons considered the improbability of such a theory; how could the timing of surgery play any role in determining the long-term survival of a cancer patient? The answer appeared to be hormonally-related. The early phase of the menstrual cycle is estrogen dominant, the latter phase is progesterone-dominant. Conceivably breast cancer surgery done while estrogen hormone is elevated may permit rogue cancer cells a better chance to implant in distant tissues metastatically; progesterone hormone elevation may block such implantation and theoretically prevent metastasis from occurring. The theory is unproved; all the scientists have is evidence distinguishing breast cancer patient outcomes between two groups – those having surgery early in their cycle versus those having surgery later in their cycle. If estrogen-versus-progesterone dominance is not the deciding factor, what other explanation could there be for different survival outcomes based on timing of surgery?

Such is the paradox in examining women's health. As rational as we may be in seeking answers with clinical trials, there are times when treating women may require more than science. Not all healing is surgery, antibiotics and vitamins. Neither is it listening and hugs. Sometimes healing only comes forth from deep within the female mystique and we healers need to pay attention to its demands.

If your surgeon refuses to cooperate with this timing, I suggest you find one who will. Remember two things; it is your life at stake, not the surgeon's, and you are employing him or her, not the reverse.

7: QUESTIONS TO ASK YOUR DOCTOR

If You've Been Given a Breast Cancer Diagnosis

Some oncologists only tell the patient what should be done after a positive diagnosis. The *Newsletter of Alternative Medicine Research Foundation* has published a list of questions you are entitled to ask, and a review of what the answers indicate, which can be viewed at *http://topica.com/lists/altresearch*.

Some Herbs are Dangerous!

As mentioned elsewhere in this book, it is of concern that many women assume that "natural" is safe, when the opposite is often the case. Some herbs are known to cause breast cancer cells to proliferate. For example, it has been found that don quai caused a human breast cancer cell line to grow 16-fold, while the use of ginseng increased the cell growth 27-fold. (Menopause, 2002; 9:145-150)

Even the popular black cohosh has shown a tendency to spread breast cancer, and there are warnings that it should not be used for longer than six months, or used at all if there is a history of breast cancer in the family. (VL Davis, et al. Amer Assoc Canc Res Annual meeting, July 11-14, 2003, Washington DC abstract R910).

Women who want to replace the drug oestrogen with herbs, often substitute one type of hormone replacement with another. In a study, plants were tested for their ability to compete for progesterone and estradiol in human breast cancer cells. It was found that soy, red clover, liquorice, verbena, hops, thyme and tumeric all acted as tumour promoters. (Proc Soc Exp Biol Med, 1998; 217: 369-78).

Scary information, especially considering how freely some therapists give out these potent herbs.

> Men occasionally stumble over the truth, but most pick themselves up and hurry off as if nothing had happened.
>
> *- Winston Churchill*

> "Whose bread I eat,
> His song I sing."
> (Ancient Proverb)

Male Sexual Dysfunction

Causes, Remedies, and
Why You Should Avoid the
Unkindest Cut of All

Most prescription drugs and even over-the-counter nostrums contribute to sexual dysfunction in both men and women. They can damage the vascular system, the nerves and the endocrine system. And endocrine problems lead straight to low serum testosterone, which leads straight to impotence.

Hundreds of men have asked me if it is true that Maca powder is a natural, safe substitute for *Viagra*. My answer is that doctors in Peru and the US say that it is, provided, and this is crucial, provided the man is not taking drugs to lower cholesterol, or to lower blood pressure. These drugs can have such a damaging effect upon erectile function that nothing, not even Maca, can revive it.

In these cases, the only hope I can offer is that men who have been given virtual death sentences by their cardiologists recover by embracing the Hippocrates Health Centre program. Even men who have been told they would die if they didn't have triple bypasses! They can often discontinue these libido-dampening drugs, *but only under medical supervision.* It is, as I'm sure you'll agree, preferable to get your dietary act together before your physician tells you the end is near.

According to a report in the ***Journal Of The American Medical Association)***, *Prozac* (the anti-depressant) causes sexual dysfunction in 75 percent of the patients who take it! If you were depressed prior to taking Prozac, think how much worse you would feel if it caused you impotence. So, men, stop thinking every problem can be solved by a pill and look to your medicine cabinets and lay the blame where it belongs – with a medical profession that hands out drugs like jellybeans, and often does not warn men about this dreadful side-effect, and wouldn't know the right diet if they fell over it.

It's up to you. Go over your kitchen with a critical eye and accept responsibility for your condition. Be resolute when tempted and remember that artery disease contributes to impotence, as the result of atherosclerotic disease of the vessels that supply blood to the penis, and to the nerves that make erection possible.

Is that chocolate mousse *really* worth such a sacrifice? Are those highly promoted plastic oils (which are in nearly all manufactured food and which have been clogging your arteries) so delicious that you are prepared to lose your masculinity? Re-read **Chapter 6**, *Oils and Fats*, and resolve not to become yet another victim of the oil cartels. *They* don't care if you become impotent, or have a killer heart attack, and most doctors do not know that the very oils which are wrongly touted as heart-friendly are deadly for your arteries.

If you are considering a vasectomy, think again. The first bad news to surface when they became popular was that arthritis sometimes is a side-effect of the snip. More pertinent to the subject at hand, there is persuasive evidence that vasectomies can lead to impotence. William Campbell Douglass, MD, in **Second Opinion**, *January 2000*, tells of a study run at a Well-Man clinic in London, which reported on 445 men who complained of impotence. A 'marked reduction' in testosterone levels was found when more than 10 years had elapsed since the vasectomy. Dr Richard Petty, who runs the clinic, said, "Men contemplating a vasectomy must take a calculated risk and accept it could have an erosive effect on testosterone levels. I would not have one myself." Dr Petty said there is no explanation why testosterone levels go up following vasectomy surgery and then, years later, drop off.

Dr Peat says, "When impotence occurs after vasectomy, a few small doses of progesterone, about 5 or 10mg per day [*there are three mg of progesterone in each drop of Dr Peat's progesterone oil*], will often restore normal potency in just two or three days. This is because damage to the vas deferens can specifically, but temporarily, suppress progesterone production. This is one of the situations in which I recommend the use of supplemental progesterone for men. The others include arthritis, epilepsy, dementia, stroke and some other circulatory problems, migraine, and cancer."

Dr Douglass says, "I have always maintained that a man cannot escape harm from a vasectomy any more than a woman can escape harm from a tubal ligation. In both cases a natural channel is being blocked. Where does the sperm go? Where does the blocked egg go and what effect does this blockage have on hormone levels in males and females?"

In other words you can't, at least you shouldn't, mess around with Mother Nature. For example, Viagra can have unpleasant side-effects, including blindness and death, and cannot overcome impotence when erectile-dampening drugs and a hopeless diet are contributing factors. It's better and safer to look to natural methods, such as magnesium, zinc, boron, Co-enzyme Q_{10} and Maca powder when problems arise. But Maca is not suitable for men with prostate cancer.

Approximately one-third of all cases of impotence occur due to endocrine problems. According to physicians in Peru and the US, Maca helps alleviate impotence because it regulates and supports the endocrine glands. It will not, however, overcome the deleterious effects of powerful drugs, and it is not recommended for men with enlarged or cancerous prostates.

Pharmacological testosterone replacement, as opposed to natural, through injections, tablets, implants and patches, is widely used in the US and Europe, as well as in Australia. This therapy may give a temporary improvement in function, followed by problems you don't even want to think about. Except in cases of documented testicular degeneration, this potent hormone should not be taken in pharmacologic doses.

Dr Michael Colgan explains that testosterone production can be improved by melatonin, seligiline, DHEA and acetyl-carnitine, but do not attempt self medication here. Just remember, prevention is much better than a chancy 'cure', and your very first effort should be to follow the rules in this book. If, after a fair trial, your manhood does not come bouncing back, sterner measures may be warranted, such as studying Dr Colgan's book (see **Resources**) and then taking it to a knowledgeable physician.

Are you confused? Then you are not alone. I'm confused, most physicians are confused, if not downright dangerous, because of their sketchy understanding of what occurs in the body when one pharmacological hormone, such as testosterone, overwhelms the others. This field is in its infancy and should be approached with great care, and only if you are convinced, beyond a shadow of a doubt, that your physician knows exactly what he is doing.

And, if you find one who does, and if you have a satisfactory long-term result, please let me know so I can advise other men.

"Your doctor might recommend surgery. But that's easy for him to say – he doesn't have to wear the diapers."

- Dr William Campbell
Douglass

14

The Perils of Prostate

What can happen to the prostate gland, and what you can do to make sure it doesn't happen to yours

Normally the size of a walnut and situated at the base of the bladder, the prostate gland forms a vital part of the male reproductive system. Hormonal changes after middle age can cause it to become enlarged, and subject to a number of conditions ranging through varying degrees of discomfort, inflammation and cancer.

In 1995, a British survey reported in *The Times* revealed that most men were largely unaware of the significance and potential health dangers relating to the prostate. Some 89 percent of men surveyed didn't know where the prostate is located, while 62 percent of them mistook it for the bladder itself.

Although it appears that men today are becoming more aware of the possible health implications resulting from neglect or abuse of this important part of their anatomy, many misconceptions still abound. Most 'problems' are quite preventable and certainly not inevitable, particularly if a sensible diet is followed, and many men live to enjoy a ripe old age untroubled by the natural changes to their metabolism. On the other hand, painful conditions such as prostatitis, an inflammation of the prostate caused through infection, can affect both young and old.

Since 1973 the incidence of prostate cancer has risen by 50 percent. As far as I am aware, no studies have been done to ascertain the reason for this huge increase. Studies cost millions of dollars, and there's no grant money available for finding ways to prevent illnesses – only billions available for studies to discover new moneymaking drugs, or to perfect more intricate surgery to 'correct' problems. I have done a study of my own. It has cost nothing and was merely the result of meeting hundreds of men and talking to them. This was the conclusion, and I pass it on free of charge; men who eat *really* well, do not smoke and do not drink alcohol to excess or take legal or illegal drugs, do not contract prostate problems. It's as simple as that – *men, you are doing it to yourselves!*

Physicians have concentrated upon treatment of prostate enlargement, infection and cancer, rather than giving a bit of thought to the rise of our junk food culture, which corresponds directly to the soaring rate of prostate problems. It's the same old story – there isn't any money to be made by prevention, but there is a pile to be made in treating and operating on terrified men.

Dr William Campbell Douglass, an invaluable source of sound information and advice on medical problems affecting men and women, has this to say on the Perils of Prostate: "It is absolutely vital that you get your diet, nutritional needs, and hormone levels in balance. If you don't, getting rid of the cancer will be a temporary fix. You'll need to work with an alternative-minded doctor to do so.

"The thing men over 60 dread most is not prostate cancer, not a heart attack, not a stroke – it's prostate enlargement. Not being able to urinate naturally and always worrying about a bathroom being close at hand is a truly humbling way to live. While prostate enlargement is not related to prostate cancer, it causes symptoms in one-fourth of men by age 80, and nearly all show signs of 'Benign Prostatic Hypertrophy' (BPH) by the age of 85. If you have early symptoms of BPH – frequency of urination, a burning feeling at the pubic area after urinating, and a stream that isn't what it used to be – take saw palmetto, one capsule twice daily."

Throw Out the Junk

So, what else can you do if you already have – or want to avoid –problems with this essential little gland? For a start – throw out all the junk food in your kitchen; attend Hippocrates Health Centre if possible, for a serious toxaemia cleanout; quit smoking this minute, and avoid passive smoke, stop drinking and eliminate all grains from your diet. And, yes, I do mean pasta, bread, and all the grains that are in vogue and considered healthful by misguided professionals. Hard as it is, at least give it a fair try. You will probably find that shunning these indigestibles will ease symptoms and make you feel much better. Wean yourself, with professional help, from any drug dependence you may have – legal or illegal. According to the UK magazine *What Doctors Don't Tell You*, "Many medicines, including antihistamines, decongestants and anti-depressants, can turn a partly obstructed prostate into a fully obstructed one." On this point, be particularly wary of HCB *(Hexachlorobenzene)*, as it is known to cause prostate cancer.

So many natural remedies are offered for prostate problems that it would be impossible to swallow them all, and I certainly don't suggest you try. My suggestion is to find a natural practitioner with first-rate credentials and with his or her help decide which of the many recommendations that follow will suit your particular circumstances. And remember – prevention is always preferable to cure!

WHAT YOU SHOULD TAKE

√ *Selenium*

The mineral selenium should be at the top of your must-take list for prevention and for alleviating existing symptoms. Selenium is one of our best safeguards against cancer of any kind. For example, a Finnish study of 10,000 people found that those with low levels of serum selenium were six times more likely to suffer from fatal cancer. As Robert Jay Rowen, MD, reported in his *Second Opinion Newsletter*, "In 1996 Dr Larry Dark, of the University of Arizona, published startling data suggesting that prostate cancer could be reduced by as much as an amazing 60 percent by supplemental yeast-derived selenium, 200mcg per day. Selenium is a powerful antioxidant that participates in key and crucial detoxification and free-radical scavenging enzymes. His work is being confirmed in other ongoing studies." In effect, selenium actually provokes cancer cells into committing suicide. See *Resources* for a reliable source.

√ *Zinc*

Chronic prostatitis patients usually suffer from low levels of this mineral, which is crucial for prostate health. But it isn't enough to pop zinc tablets. Phytates in soy products interfere with zinc absorption, so it is important to stay entirely away from soy, and that includes lecithin, soy oil and soy flour. Many drugs also interfere with zinc absorption: diuretics, corticosteroids, *Tagamet, Zantac, Pepcid*, etc. Stay away from drugs, soy and junk food if you value your prostate, and I'm sure you do, and take a zinc tablet for prevention and/or to ease the pain and reduce the swelling of existing prostate illnesses. But do not overdose, because a high intake of zinc can reduce calcium absorption if your calcium intake is low. Jonathan V Wright, MD, recommends zinc picolinate or citrate, "…at a dosage of 30 milligrams three times daily to start, tapering down slowly as symptoms recede."

When grappling with protocols for prostate problems, it is wise to remember that people don't die from a deficiency of any of the recommended herbs. What does kill, however, is a deficiency of essential nutrients. The zinc and fatty acids that are needed for your prostate are also needed for all of your tissues and organs. Unroasted pumpkin seeds and sunflower seeds are great sources of essential fatty acids and zinc. But please be sure to soak them overnight to remove the anti-enzyme actions. Then, if you prefer, you can put them in a food drier (no higher than 38 degrees Celsius or 100 degrees Fahrenheit) or in your oven, turned to the lowest possible setting for a while, to make them crunchy. Zinc also occurs in other seeds and nuts, oysters, liver, meats, poultry, raw egg yolk and wheatgrass juice. Food sources are ideal for prevention, but if your prostate is already in strife, more extreme measures should be adopted.

√ Boron

Dr Rex Newnham, leading expert on boron (see **Resources**), told me that this mineral contributes to prostate health. As it is scarce in most soils, it is crucial for those of us who are not able to grow our own food organically. See **Chapter 8**, *Bone Health II*, for further information.

√ Tomatoes

Eat lots of tomatoes, for the *lycopene* they contain. A recent study found that men with early prostate cancer who took lycopene showed signs of decreased malignancy. Lycopene produces the red colour of tomatoes, and it is a natural antioxidant. The trials quoted in the study used lycopene supplements, not tomatoes, because one would have to eat about a kilo per day to get the same therapeutic result. Lycopene tablets and capsules are sold in health stores. A tomato-rich diet would be of benefit to everyone, as other studies indicate that it appears to protect against colon, rectal, oesophagus, stomach, mouth, throat and cervical cancer, as well as prostate cancer.

√ Saw Palmetto

The herb favoured by Dr Douglass and most recommended by alternative practitioners is saw palmetto, said to block the formation of dihydrostestosterone, which is believed to be responsible for prostate enlargement. **What Doctors Don't Tell You** reported, "In one double-blind trial of 100 men with benign prostatic hypertrophy (BPH) the herb decreased night-time urinary flow rate by more than 50 percent, and reduced by 42 percent the amount of urine left in the bladder after urination."

In **Second Opinion**, *January 2000*, Dr Douglass advised, "If you have a prostate problem, make a strong tea out of saw palmetto berries (weak at first to test your sensitivity, then gradually increase the strength), or make an infusion (prolonged soaking in water). Keep refrigerated and drink the tea or the infusion, one cupful, three times a day. This simple treatment is supported by a great deal of scientific evidence." Even the AMA recommends it.

√ Pygeum Bark

This natural remedy, botanical name *Pygeum Africanum*, has been used in France, with good results claimed, although some adverse effects have also been reported.

√ Cernilton

A pollen extract used in Sweden, cernilton produced an improvement in nearly 70 percent of patients in a controlled study. The conclusion of the trial's authors was that cernilton is of benefit when treating mild to moderate BPH (**British Journal of Urology 1990**, *66:398-404*).

√ Citrus Pectin

Traditional Chinese medicine offers citrus pectin (MCP). Michael Broffman of Pine Street Clinic, San Anselmo, California, has found that his patients with prostate cancer remained stable or improved on this treatment, and metastases stabilised in some.

√ Epilobium

A high-profile herb highly recommended by many people. Ron Gellatley, ND, writing in **Nature and Health,** *June/July 2000,* described it as "...a botanical miracle for anyone with prostate problems, and a specific for helping the bladder to empty properly. I take it in tincture form." He credited many things – Cat's Claw, Pau D'Arco, Astragalus and the homeopathics *Carcinosinum, Cancer, Thymus* and T_4 for helping him in his successful fight against inoperable prostate cancer. He recommends having a qualified homeopath make up your specific constitutional remedy.

√ Quercetin

Occurring naturally in tea, onions, leafy vegetables and apples, quercetin disarms *androgens*, which fuel prostate cancers, and causes dramatic reduction in the Prostate Specific Antigen (PSA). It is also available in supplement form, and practitioners recommend taking 400mg three times daily, for prevention.

√ Stinging Nettle Extract

Readily available and highly recommended by Dr Jonathan Wright for relief from an enlarged prostate. Milk thistle and turmeric (curcumin) are also natural supplements that help the prostate.

√ Vitamin E

Most therapists recommend taking vitamin E, claiming that, especially when combined with selenium and vitamin D, it will lower the risk of prostate cancer, because it inhibits Androgen Recepton (AR) activity in the prostate cancer cells. The reason for this is that vitamin E regulates, or even halts, the genes responsible for prostate cancer growth. While I most certainly recommend selenium, due to its lack in so many soils, I do not recommend taking 'natural' vitamin E capsules, and most certainly not the synthetics. Stick to food sources for your vitamin E, and you will benefit greatly (see **Chapter 15**, *Dietary Supplements*, for details).

√ *A Daily Dose of Sunshine*

Sunlight is important; researchers in the US found that prostate cancer mortality declined with increasing sunlight intensity. It is known that vitamin D_3 inhibits the growth of tumours, and that UV light is needed for synthesis of D_3 in the body. This means exposure without sunscreen, at least three times each week. If you live in an area with little intense sunlight, be sure to supplement with vitamins A and D, as advised in **Chapter 8**, *Bone Health II*, and **Chapter 15**, *Dietary Supplements*.

√ *Progesterone*

Dr Joseph Mercola, director of the Optimal Wellness Center in Schaumburg, Illinois, wrote in **The Townsend Letter For Doctors And Patients,** *December 1998*, "As a male ages, his progesterone level decreases just like it does in women... When progesterone levels decrease, the male's 5 alpha reductase converts the testosterone to dihydrotestosterone, which is useless at removing the prostate cancer cells that estradiol stimulates. Estradiol also stimulates the enlargement of the prostate. This allows the prostate gland to swell and enlarge and in many cases transform into prostate cancer... All cells, with the exception of brain and muscle cells, multiply continuously. The genes which regulate this cell growth are *p53* and *bcl2*. If the gene bcl2 dominates, the opposite will occur and the cell growth is controlled and the cancer does not occur... *Estradiol turns on the cancer gene bcl2*, and *progesterone turns on the anti-cancer gene p53*! Standard chemotherapy, using poisons to stop cell hyperplasia, do not work, as they kill normal cells easier than cancer cells."

According to Dr Mercola, progesterone inhibits 5 alpha reductase far more effectively than the drug *Proscar* and saw palmetto (mentioned previously), which are often used to treat prostate problems by conventional and alternative medicine.

Dr Raymond Peat is a leading authority on progesterone, so I faxed him a list of questions regarding prostate problems and impotence. He faxed back, "In benign prostatic enlargement, a little progesterone can help to shrink the gland, but the important thing is to keep estrogen low with adequate protein and thyroid. *Pregnenolone* [see **Chapter 27**, *In Other Words*...] is easier to use than progesterone, since a person who isn't very familiar with his physiology is likely to have trouble interpreting his reactions to progesterone, which antagonises both testosterone and estrogen.

"Progesterone would seem to be a logical part of treating prostate cancer, but the dose would depend entirely on the particular situation. For example, in large doses, it can help to control pain. The right way for a man to maintain normal progesterone levels into old age would be to eat a high protein diet with the lowest possible level of polyunsaturated fats, and a moderately low level of iron."

Dr John R Lee, in *What Your Doctor May Not Tell You About Menopause,* wrote, "Men with a lack of progesterone, such as men castrated either surgically or chemically, will experience accelerated osteoporosis within two to three years. Since there is no evidence that progesterone is a risk for men with prostate cancer, I would hope that a clinical trial of progesterone would be offered to protect their bones in conditions of testosterone deficiency." Regrettably, I feel that to be unlikely, since the pharmaceuticals can't make money from natural progesterone.

Dr Mercola, again writing in *The Townsend Letter For Doctors And Patients,* said, "The dose of natural progesterone for men is 10 to 12mg per day. Men do not need time off like women and can take the progesterone daily." Because the dose needs to be as precise as possible, please consult a qualified therapist when using this natural hormone. It is essential to use the right progesterone – see *Resources* for the only one we recommend. **Do not touch the pharmaceutical versions, progestogen and progestin**.

Bent Formby, PhD, from Sansum Medical Research Institute in Santa Barbara, California, uncovered further evidence that progesterone may help men with prostate problems. Dr Formby found that progesterone inhibits the growth of prostate cancer cells – and that estradiol and DHT accelerate prostate cancer cell growth.

New Zealand doctor, Earl Conroy, for whom I have great respect, also believes that men need progesterone as much as women do, both for prevention and cure of prostate problems. This hormone counteracts the high oestrogen in our environment which is creating hormonal havoc in both men and women. Maintenance of the thyroid gland, according to Dr Conroy, is also exceedingly important, as is sticking faithfully to a good diet and cutting all polyunsaturated oils out of your life.

√ *Co-enzyme Q*$_{10}$

Wayne Martin, a natural health advocate with encyclopaedic knowledge, wrote in *The Townsend Letter For Doctors And Patients, December 1999,* "...results of trials have been so good that there is an indication that if every prostate cancer patient were maintained on co-enzyme Q$_{10}$ from day one of discovery, death from prostate cancer could drop to near zero." He advises buying the brand made by *Bio-Tech* (see *Resources*), although it is costly for Australians.

According to scientist Karl Folkers, an expert on Q$_{10}$, it is necessary to take it the following way so it can be assimilated: get a cup of hot tea or water and put a teaspoon of pure coconut oil in it. Then empty a capsule of Q_{10} on the surface and watch it melt. Drink it hot.

It is not advisable to flood the body with a wide assortment of herbs, no matter how highly touted. Combining the right ones, chosen carefully, with the diet and detoxing program at the health centre, or strict adherence to the rules in this book, is ideal.

√ *Hyperthermia*

Dr William Campbell Douglass, in his **Second Opinion Newsletter, February 2001**, reported on the latest treatment for prostate cancer, hyperthermia. It is a long report, so only the pertinent sections are quoted here.

> There are currently two types of hyperthermia being used. One uses microwaves and the other uses radio waves. The microwave treatment hasn't seen the success the radio-wave therapy has, and it burns both cancerous and non-cancerous tissue alike. In prostate-cancer patients, the microwaves cause agonising urethral pain, which has caused many doctors to abandon the treatment altogether. The radio-wave treatment, on the other hand, seems to have a much greater success rate and doesn't cause urethral pain.

> The radio-wave technique has two ways it can heat the cancer: locally (which hits only the affected region) and whole body. Both types require heating the body to a temperature of 107-111 degrees Fahrenheit. With local treatment, the heat is directed straight at the cancer by passing electromagnetic waves from a transmitter through the patient to a receiving plate. Cancer tissue is more dense than normal tissue and radio waves are more readily absorbed by denser tissue, so the heat is concentrated in the tumour, killing it.

> The whole-body treatment is used with cancers that have spread beyond the organ, which is oftentimes the case with prostate cancer. Early diagnosis of prostate cancer is very difficult, so by the time your cancer is found, it has probably spread beyond the prostate. In some cases, many doctors will use both the whole-body and the local treatment together.

> How does hyperthermia work? High temperatures kill cancer in several ways… damaging the membranes, proteins, and enzymes of cancer cells, making them much more vulnerable to anti-cancer agents. That means almost any treatment currently used to treat cancer, whether it be chemotherapy, radiation, herbs, or nutritional agents, will be more effective if used in conjunction with hyperthermia. Many studies have shown that cancer cells succumb to chemotherapy and radiation much faster after being exposed to high levels of heat.

> In my opinion, chemotherapy for prostate cancer is malpractice and will be so viewed some day, even when used in conjunction with hyperthermia. Radiation by itself is a desperate measure, offering temporary relief, but at a terrible price due to immune depression. It might be useful when used with hyperthermia, but I think the nutritional approach is a better way to fight a tumour.

> As I said earlier, most of the doctors in the US are using the microwave form of hyperthermia. I don't recommend this type of treatment for prostate cancer because of the pain it causes in the urethra. In order to get radio-wave hyperthermia, you'll

probably have to go to Europe. The treatment has been approved by the FDA, but doctors in the US have been slow to make the move.

Dr Douwes, who cured my friend Ellis using hyperthermia, told *Alternative Medicine* magazine that 'killing malignant tumours is usually not difficult, and a synergy of treatments works best for that. The biggest challenge comes about afterward, to keep tumours from coming back once patients leave the clinic and resume a normal lifestyle. To prevent their reoccurrence, one must keep the immune system strong with diet, exercise, nutritional supplementation, and especially a positive mental attitude.'

These are the same things you need to do in order to prevent the cancer from developing in the first place.

Hyperthermia is not readily available, and is too expensive for many, but Dr Robert Jay Rowen has discovered another option, a budget heating device called the *Delwa-Star Rectal/Vaginal Heater*, which he says has an 80 percent success rate in chronic prostatitis. As Dr Rowen says, this device, "...may have far-reaching preventive and immune stimulating effects against cancer-causing pathogens." In other words, it is likely that it will assist in management of cancer, but no one dares make that claim for serious ethical and legal reasons. Please see *Chapter 26*, *Remedies*, (Pages 316 and 317) for more on this device, which can also help women's ailments, and *Resources* for ordering details.

√ *Magnetism*

Dr Earl Conroy says, "For serious prostate problems, I always have patients buy a magnet they can sit on for a couple of hours a day. This relieves inflammation of the prostate." See *Chapter 26*, *Remedies*, for details.

√ *Herbal Tincture*

As well, Dr Conroy has developed a herbal spray tincture which contains a crucial configuration of herbs – traditional, Ayurvedic and Chinese, to maintain optimal prostate function. He believes, as do many first-rate scientists, that "oestrogen dominance" (caused by xeonestrogen pollution) has contributed mightily to our epidemic of prostate illnesses. *Prolactin* (a pituitary hormone) is another contributing factor, as it can cause enlarged prostates. These enemies of your healthy prostate are triggered by the excessive oestrogen mentioned above, as well as by low DHEA and low progesterone. Dr Conroy's tincture is designed to address these risk factors.

√ *Action to Take*

Dr Douglass makes these recommendations for those in the US who are diagnosed with prostate cancer; they may also be helpful to readers elsewhere.

• Do not submit to surgery

- Contact the North American Hyperthermia Society at 630-571-2904, or www.thermaltherapy.org. Alternatively, contact the European Society for Hyperthermic Oncology (ESHO) at www.cv.ruu.nl/radiotherapy/esho.

- You can also contact Dr Friedrich Douwes directly at the Klinik St. Georg, Rosenheimer Str. 6-8, 83043 Bad Aibling, Germany. Telephone: 49-8061-398-0; e-mail: Prantseck@t-online.de; www.klinik-stgeorg.de.

WHAT YOU SHOULD AVOID

X *Flax Oil*

The next time you are impressed by a glossy ad for flax oil, or a naturopath raves on about how important it is for your general health, and especially for your prostate, remind him or her that flax (linseed) has never, until recently, been a human food or medicine. *Martindale's Pharmacopoeia* categorises it as an emetic for cattle, a contraceptive/abortifacient and a modifier of the menstrual cycle in India. Now, suddenly, it is being heavily promoted as a 'health' food, in the same manner as soy, with similar catastrophic results, due to the effects of phytoestrogens which both contain. Please bear in mind that flax is known to destabilize the thyroid and is highly oestrogenic. Men, do you really want that female hormone in your body?

Lots of well-credentialed health professionals are now singing the praises of flax oil, and those of us who are warning about it are dramatically outnumbered. But consider this, from Charles E Myers, MD, medical oncologist and former Director of the Cancer Center, University of Virginia, Editor-in-Chief of *The Prostate Forum*, and founder of the American Institute for Disease of the Prostate in Charlottesville, Virginia: "Nine published studies have analyzed the impact of Alpha Linolenic Acid (ALA) – one of the very substances in flax seed that is thought to be healthful for most people – **and have found that it can increase your risk of developing prostate cancer or speed the progression of an existing condition**."

If that isn't scary enough, the Harvard School of Public Health did a study involving more than 15,000 physicians and found that the men with the highest level of ALA had nearly a 300 percent increase in their risk of developing metastatic prostate cancer. "I've done some laboratory research of my own," says Dr Myers, "and I found that ALA more than doubled the growth rate of human prostate cancers. In fact, it was a greater stimulus than testosterone."

Dr Myers says that people need the omega-3 fatty acids for prostate health, but should get it from cold-water fish, not flax oil. He and Dr Joseph Mercola both stress that the fish (salmon, herring and sardines) must be harvested from the ocean, not from fish farms. Farmed fish do not have sufficiently high levels of vital EPA and DHA due to the artificial diets they are fed, rather than the naturally-occurring algae on which they feed in their natural habitat.

A trial from the Registro Nacional de Cancer, Montevideo, Uruguay, found that the two major risk factors associated with prostate cancer are a family history of prostate cancer and the intake of alpha-linolenic acid (from flax oil).

A recent study of about 47,000 men, reported in the **American Journal Of Clinical Nutrition** (July 2004 80 (1); 204-216), found that the ALA omega-3 fatty acids stimulate the growth of prostate tumours. The researchers found that men who were suffering from advanced prostate cancer had higher quantities of ALA from non-animal, as well as meat and dairy, sources. Scientists also found that EPA and DHA could reduce the risk of total and advanced prostate cancer.

Dr. Mercola, commenting on this, said, "Most anyone interested in nutrition has heard that omega-3 fats reduce the rate of cancer. Many early adopters of this information applied this to the plant-based sources of omega-3 (ALA). One of the highest sources of ALA is in flax seeds, so flax oil in the 90s gained widespread attention in the health community as an important source of nutrition. Ten years ago I was certainly caught up in that hype and had many of my patients take it. I rapidly found, though, that most people did not tolerate it well and I rapidly advised my patients to stop taking it. Now it is very clear that only a small percentage of the omega-3 in flax is converted to EPA and DHA. It is actually EPA and DHA that do the heavy lifting for cancer prevention, not ALA.

I'm surprised at the results of this study. I never suspected that high amounts of ALA would actually increase prostate cancer, but this appears to be the case. At worse I would have guessed that it had little influence on prostate cancer. ... It is very important to realise that cod liver oil is the ideal source of EPA and DHA for prostate cancer prevention, as it is loaded with vitamin D, which may be even more important than EPA and DHA in prevention of prostate cancer." For more information on flax oil, see page 71.

X Flax Seeds

Yes, seeds ground fresh daily are indeed an improvement on flax oil, as at least the rancidity problem is solved with that treatment, provided it is eaten before oxidation sets in. But flax seeds contain the highest concentration of lignans of any other food, and like the soy isoflavone genistein, can bind to oestrogen sites and produce oestrogenic activity. That is bad news, but even worse news for the flax seed enthusiasts, is that these lignans contain alpha linolenic acid (ALA) and will deliver a dangerous dose of the very chemical that many scientists have proved to dramatically increase the risk of prostate cancer. More on lignans on Page 221.

X Soy and Soy Products

Swimming against the tide again, my strong recommendation for prostate health is a total avoidance of all soya products. The same practitioners who are pushing dangerous flax oil are also pushing soy, in spite of the huge amount of evidence that it is a killer. Most don't appear to know, care, or have forgotten, that soy strips zinc from the body – and zinc is essential for prostate health. Further, few practitioners bother to warn men that soy, like flax oil, is highly oestrogenic, and does not belong in the body of a male.

Consider the conclusions of a definitive scientific study *(Santti R and others: Developmental estrogenization and prostatic neoplasia; Prostate 1994;24(2):67-78)*, into the effects of soy ingestion on developing males:

> "Evidence indicates that estrogen exposure during development may initiate cellular changes in the prostate which would require estrogens and/or androgens later in life for promotion of prostatic hyperplasia or neoplasia.

> " The critical time for estrogen action would be during the development of the prostatic tissue. We further suggest that estrogen-sensitive cells may remain in the prostate and be more responsive to estrogens later in life or less responsive to the normal controlling mechanisms of prostatic growth."

In other words, exposure of the developing male child to phytoestrogens in soy may make him more susceptible to prostate cancer later in life.

X Gelatin Capsules

The material used to produce these little containers is contaminated with xenoestrogens and present a danger to your prostate. Do not take them. Oestrogen pellets are put under the ear skin of cattle in some countries. These ears, along with other inedible body parts, are sent to rendering plants and used to make gelatin for capsules. Only accept vegetable capsules, or remove the contents from gelatin capsules before use.

X Sugar

Sugar should be completely eliminated from the diet of any man who has prostate illnesses, or who wishes to prevent them. Stay away from this poison. Study labels, or better still, do not buy manufactured foods. Read the section in this book on *Sugar* and start taking your health seriously by shunning one of the most dangerous substances in our food supply.

X Polyunsaturates

All polyunsaturated oils must be completely eliminated from your diet. Stick to triple virgin olive oil, pure coconut oil and butter. Re-read the information in *Chapter 6*, *Oils and Fats*, and follow the suggestions carefully, since most oils used today in practically all prepared foods and bakery goods are dangerous for your prostate health, as they are for your general health.

X Calcium Supplements

Don't take them, because calcium suppresses the synthesis of a form of vitamin D that inhibits prostate cancer.

X Synthetic Oestrogens from Plastics, Pesticides and Household Chemicals

Be vigilant in avoiding these pollutants, as your body can absorb them, and they are a causative agent in prostate cancer.

X Mercury Amalgam Fillings

Mercury poisoning from amalgam fillings is a primary cause of cancer. Get them out. See **Chapter 17**, *Dental Health*, for important details.

X Drugs

Be wary, and remember that all drugs have side effects. The FDA approved *Hytrin* and *Proscar*, yet Hytrin can cause fainting spells, nausea, dizziness, blurred vision and heart palpitations, and outright impotence can be a result of taking Proscar. I've seen and heard many reports and case histories and have only bad words to say about them; they work only occasionally, and have a list of horrible side effects. Look to natural methods first.

X PC-SPES

It has been discovered that a Chinese botanical formula, PC SPES, which was credited with fighting prostate disease, is contaminated with three pharmaceuticals: cancer-inducing DES, the pain killer indomethacin, and *Warfarin* (a blood thinner). Avoid it – but don't allow this to put you off natural remedies. They are infinitely safer than anything the pharmaceuticals can come up with, in spite of a few bad apples.

X Chondroitin Sulphate

Chondroitin sulphate must be avoided by men with prostate cancer. According to prostate expert Charles E Myers, it can cause prostate cancer to "explode and spread widely." Several researchers have reached the same conclusion. Chondroitin sulphate is often combined with glucosamine for osteoarthritis relief. Dr Myers says that there is no evidence that the glucosamine aggravates prostate cancer, so it is safe to take. Further, it isn't necessary to combine it with the dangerous Chondroitin for a therapeutic effect.

X Cadmium

The *March 1996* issue of **What Doctors Don't Tell You** contained a report on how cadmium levels in men's bodies stimulate the growth of human prostatic tissue. "Enamels containing cadmium compounds are still used as an internal coating for quite a large number of kitchen casseroles. When these are heated, small quantities of cadmium oxide may be formed and released into the food being cooked. Another common source of high cadmium levels is tobacco smoke (both by smokers and innocent bystanders). Draining the cadmium homoeopathically … should correct that." So, avoid tobacco smoke like the poison it is, and cook only in glass and stainless steel.

✗ Cereals

Ross Horne, in his book, **The Health Revolution,** makes a strong case for eliminating all cereal products for prostate protection, and replacing them with fresh fruit. He mentions one case, among others, "... in which two years on the *Pritikin* regression diet failed to correct the man's prostate trouble, but when he stopped eating cereals the problem was eliminated in about two weeks." We have observed similar improvements on the diet at Hippocrates Health Centre.

✗ Oestradiol

Oestradiol is a hormone which has contaminated US meat products, and is the rationale behind the French ban on US meats. Those canny, romantic French are carefully guarding their prostates!

So, unless you have faith that your government does not permit hormones in cattle feed and in pellets to be implanted in cattle, shun meat and poultry, which is also contaminated, or eat only organic and join the French in protecting your prostate. Oestradiol is a potent, gene-damaging, cancer-causing oestrogen, which is blamed for a 190 percent rise in prostate cancer, a 120 percent rise in testicular cancer and a 55 percent rise in breast cancer. All in the name of profit by a meat industry so rich and powerful that the US regulatory agencies don't even *try* to control them!

✗ Milk

Milk is also a danger to your prostate, as the calcium in dairy may inhibit the absorption of vitamin D, and thereby promote the growth of prostate cancer. According to the Physician's Health Study, men who consume more than 600 mg per day of dietary calcium had a 32 percent higher risk of prostate cancer than those who consumed 150 or fewer milligrams per day. (From the Moss Reports Newsletter 11/29/03).

Remember, when tempted by yogurt, cheese, ice cream or a glass of cold milk, what Dr Robert Jay Rowen wrote in **Second Opinion**, *December 2001*, "A study documented 1012 cases of prostate cancer among 20,885 men, and found that those with the highest milk consumption had a 30 percent increase in the incidence of prostate cancer."

When you consider the obscene things that are now done to what used to be a pure food, it is not surprising that it causes so many health problems. To make this statistic even more worrying, the study was conducted prior to the widespread use of Monsanto's Bovine Growth Hormone (BGH). I shudder to think what the long-term dangers of that money-spinner will be.

WHAT ABOUT SURGERY?

It is a popular truism that men, on the whole, will do anything rather than visit a doctor. Well, maybe, they have a point! Dr Douglass, no fan of prostate surgery, says, "Autopsies done on men in their eighties show that many of them, up to 70 percent, actually had some form of prostate cancer that they were unaware of and never required treatment for, since all the men died of other causes. Early prediction of prostate cancer leads to unnecessary treatment, anxiety, and a decrease in quality of life for many men. All of this hassle for a 'problem' that may never have impacted their lives."

Dr Michael Colgan, in his book, *Hormonal Health*, has encouraging information for men: "...benign prostatic hypertrophy (BPH) eventually leads to prostate cancer in most men. But they never know. The prostate cancer remains localised lifelong, without symptoms. The majority of men with prostate cancer die from other causes."

At least they did before the Prostatic Specific Antigen test (PSA) arrived on the scene. This test ferrets out cancers so tiny they can barely be seen under a microscope, and leads to operations that are totally unnecessary and kill men, make them impotent, or make sex too painful to bear. Since this test was developed it has frightened so many men into having their prostates removed that prostatectomy operations went up 600 percent in the US! This wouldn't be so bad if cures increased correspondingly but, according to the *Journal Of The American Medical Association*, radical prostatectomy fails to prolong life by even one month, over men who have refused the operation. Since most of the surgeons who perform these operations are men, it seems unconscionable that they would inflict such misery on their fellow males. But then, their fees of $37,000 per operation, in the US, tend to blunt conscience.

"But," you may ask, "my doctor says I should have PSA screening every year. Won't that protect me?" I'm sorry to say it won't; and according to countless doctors and scientists you will be worse off. Furthermore, you will be confused because, as Dr Rowen says in his *Newsletter*, many men with 'normal' PSA results have prostate cancer, while many whose PSAs are elevated, don't have cancer at all. This lack of precision frequently leads to unnecessary operations, which, in turn, can lead to tragic side effects. As Dr Rowen says,

> *"No conventional therapy has shown any value for prostate cancer over doing nothing."*

So many prestigious physicians agree with this opinion that it would be repetitious to quote them all. Lending further support to the 'leave well enough alone' protocol, this information comes from the Dr Fred Hutchinson

Cancer Research Centre in Seattle; after carrying out extensive research on the reasons for the huge surge in prostate cancer, they found that it was due to PSA testing. And, no, it was not the test that was dangerous; it was the inexact reading of the test, and the chance of over diagnosis. If the PSA levels are found to be high, physicians do not want to risk doing nothing, even though elevated PSA levels alone don't indicate the presence of cancer. Physicians are afraid of being sued, and with good reason, and at the very least will no doubt recommend a biopsy, which frequently comes back negative. That should bring a surge of relief to the patient, but often does not, because prostate biopsies are not risk-free – infections and bleeding often follow.

Professor of medical oncology at Winship Cancer Institute of Emory University, Dr Otis Brawley, says, "The concept that every cancer that can be found early can be cured is a faulty concept... By the time a dangerous cancer is detected, whether in the breast, prostate, or elsewhere, chances are great that it has already spread." Doctors Brawley and Rowen both say that they will not have a PSA test done.

As Dr Colgan says, "The PSA and other tests have become a fixture of annual physicals. And at the first hint of trouble, men are led to surgery like lambs to slaughter." The same way they lead terrified women to hysterectomies. He adds, "External beam radiation therapy and hormone therapy, the other two main treatments, have an even worse outcome than surgery. More than 50 percent of all radiation patients become impotent. With hormone therapy impotence is virtually certain."

The *January 2003* issue of **What Doctors Don't Tell You** reported remarkably similar findings from a number of impeccable professional sources:

> Prostate cancer is often a slow-growing condition that is not necessarily life-threatening. Other types of tumours, such as sarcomas, are also generally slow to grow.

> Unfortunately, doctors are often ill-equipped to discriminate between slow-growing, less aggressive cancers and those that are aggressive and life-threatening. This is the 'X factor' that prompts doctors to advise regular screening programmes and, on detection of a potential cancer, swift treatment with chemotherapy and radiation treatment.

> These slow-growing – and sometimes non-growing – tumours look the same as life-threatening ones under the microscope; they only behave differently in the body. The latest evidence suggests that regular screening is most likely to pick up these slow-growing, non-lethal cancers and lead to over treatment that may actually increase death rates rather than reduce it. *(Arch Intern Med, 2000; 160: 1109-15; Lancet, 2001; 385:1340-2, 1284-5)*.

> Chaos and clinical controversy rage at hospitals worldwide over the best way to treat prostate cancer. Doctors are unsure whether to treat, and those who do take positive action are uncertain about the type of treatment. *(Br J Urol, 1997; 79: 749-55; BMJ, 1998; 316: 1919-20; Med J Aust, 1998; 168: 483-6)*.

Prostate cancer is very slow-growing and doesn't spread; two studies have shown that 86 percent of patients with prostate cancer survive 10 years after diagnosis and, in two-thirds of cases, the cancer hadn't spread. *(N Engl J Med, 27 January 1994; JAMA, 22-29 April 1992).*

If nothing else, all the above surely point to the fact that medical science still doesn't know the answers – but that nature, as is so often the case, is quite capable of looking after things if allowed to do so without interference and abuse.

Impotent Victims in Diapers

So what about Trans-Urethral Resection Protocol (TURP)? Surely that's safe? OK – most doctors say it is. But then they would, wouldn't they? Here's how it works: a quarter inch pipe is inserted into the penis, to just below the bladder. This is used to fry your prostate with a hot wire loop. A year later, according to studies, 41 percent of victims will be in diapers, and 88 percent will be impotent. Do you still think quitting polyunsaturated oils, sugar and all junk food is "just too hard"?

Dr Douglass has a little good news: "Men have, in their lifetime, a 15 percent chance of being diagnosed with prostate cancer, but only a three percent chance of dying from it. In other words, leaving it alone is safer than submitting to the knife and/or radiation and chemotherapy. Prevention, as always, is the way to go."

More Scary News on Lignans/Flax

Men, I have a prediction to make – soon you will be bombarded by propaganda about the latest prostate-saving chemical. It will be brought to you by those neat people at Archer Daniels Midland (ADM), who are right up there, high on my list of despicable companies, nearly neck-and-neck with Monsanto Chemical. ADM grows immense amounts of soy and pushes it relentlessly, as does Monsanto, fully aware how dangerous their products are.

Now they have a licence that gives them "exclusive world-wide rights to produce and sell a flax lignan complex for use as an active ingredient in functional foods, nutraceuticals, pharmaceuticals, animal feed additives and veterinary products," according to a puff piece written by Bernard M. Collett, PhD., and printed in Townsend Letter For Doctors, who should have known better.

Pity the poor animals, not to mention the poor men who will be advised and propagandised into taking this "cure-all" phytoestrogen (female hormone) for their ailing prostates.

Men, you'd better duck! (See more on flax/lignans on pages 71, 214 and 215).

Leave Them the Hell Alone!

Dr Colgan says that in Sweden they have "...the best approach to microscopic or localised prostate cancers – they leave them the hell alone." He, like so many health professionals, recommends saw palmetto and pygeum, zinc picolinate, pyridoxine and silica, as they help prevent prostate overgrowth. "By this simple action, I and my colleagues intend to take our prostates to the grave untrammeled."

I'm with you, doc – at least I would be if I were a man!

> ### *So Sue Me!*
>
> To those manufacturers of dietary supplements who may feel the urge to take me to court for telling the truth about their products – please do. I would welcome the opportunity to bring this truth to the attention of the general public. My address is in this book.
>
> Go for it!
>
> *- E.H.*

15

Dietary Supplements

The good, the bad, the so-so and the downright dangerous

Everyone wants a magic bullet. I'd love one myself, if only I could find it. I'd also like a good-tasting snack food to have handy when I'm busy and need a quick pick-me-up, or to carry in the car. I thought I'd found one when I was introduced to the *Brain Garden* products. The following exchange of e-mails will serve to explain my disappointment:

Sent: Wednesday, 3 July 2002 15:36
To: chris@thebraingarden.com.au
Subject: carob bits

Dear Sirs,
Could you please tell me the ingredients that are in the small bits of carob that are in the Carob Pulse? They taste quite sweet and I need to know if they contain any sugar or anything other than carob. I emailed the company in the US some time ago, but they have not answered. I hope that you will be able to give me this information at your earliest convenience so I can place an order soon.

Elaine Hollingsworth

From: Chris [chris@thebraingarden.com.au]
Sent: Wednesday, 3 July 2002 7:45 PM
To: 'Elaine Hollingsworth'
Cc: 'jeff@thebraingarden.com'
Subject: RE: carob bits

Hello Elaine
Carob Chips are made from, Ingredients: Whole grain malted barley and corn, palm kernel oil, carob powder, soy lecithin (added as an emulsifier).
We look forward to you enjoying this and other items from our current product range.
Kind regards
Chris Neville
General manager Australia

That exchange took place over three years ago and, so far as I know, Brain Garden's labelling has not been rectified. I hope readers will take this as one more example of our need to be highly suspicious of all labels. Of course, one could always eat the pulse after sieving out the little carob/soy lecithin/malted barley and corn bits. But if they 'neglected' to include those highly allergenic ingredients, what else may they have 'neglected' in their entire range?

Energy Bars

Candy bars have a terrible reputation, and with good reason. But the food processors, ever ready to capitalise on a trend, have come to the rescue with *Energy Bars*. They are touted as healthful, but I would rather take my chances with an old-fashioned *Hershey Bar*.

The ingredients list on most bars is deliberately misleading, to say the least. They try to pull the wool over your eyes by trumpeting the fruit and nut content, but the main ingredients are food industry waste products – soy protein isolate, lecithin and whey proteins. Sugar is rarely listed because processors finally realise that health-minded people prefer to avoid it. So how do they sweeten their 'healthful' bars? High fructose corn syrup, fructose and other 'natural' sweeteners that have been proven to be worse for test animals than sugar. Some even contain artificial sweeteners like aspartame, which every manufacturer on Earth must know by now are killers.

Whey protein, a favourite of nutritionists as a protein supplement, contains a high proportion of *tryptophan*, the only amino acid that is known to cause cancer. Most people have heard of whey, but few are aware that its use stems from the 'whey problem' inherent in the cheese, butter and cream manufacturing process. Whey is a waste product that processors have to dispose of. So, with an eye on the bottom line as usual, they claim it is a health food and off-load it onto formulators of energy bars and protein powders. The manufacturers and their in-house food scientists and nutritionists know very well that this is no 'health food'. Also, beware brewer's yeast; it contains free glutamic acid (MSG), aspartic acid and phenylalanine -- ingredients in artificial sweeteners.

These poisonous little convenience foods also contain lots of soy protein isolate, which, as stated earlier, is a toxic waste product from the soy oil industry. Rather than disposing of this sludge in the hazardous waste section of the dump where it belongs, the industry found a way to make us eat it – and increase their profits.

You've probably got the message by now that my advice is to shun these nasty, enticingly-wrapped profit bars. Carry fruit and nuts when you go out so you won't be driven to them by hunger.

Deadly Powders

Protein powders, which people make into shakes, take pride of place in my food supplement hate list. They are all deadly. No exceptions. They contain soy protein isolate, whey and lots of suspicious-sounding chemicals. Some aren't even merely suspect – they are *known* to cause cancer. In the many years that I have been advising people who complain of various symptoms, hundreds have been miraculously 'cured' by simply throwing protein powders in the bin, and drinking plenty of pure water to flush out the toxins. Normal health is absolutely impossible for people who use them for any length of time.

There are also ready-made shakes. One, called *Lifestyles Dream Shakes*, has such terrible ingredients that it would be hilarious if people were not actually drinking them. Watch out for all of them. If you want a shake, try this:

Soak almonds overnight to de-activate the anti-enzymes in them (this applies to all nuts). Next day, drop them into very hot water for a few minutes. This will loosen the skin so you will be able to easily slip it off. Put them in pure water and blend well, adding any fruit that takes your fancy – frozen bananas give it a rich smoothness – and carob powder if you like a chocolate flavour. Let your imagination run wild, and stay away from food industry waste products.

Dangerous Ingredients

About dietary supplements. I apologise to any processors who are formulating a pure, effective one that I haven't mentioned. There may be one that is wonderful, but it has not yet been brought to my attention.

I do not, unfortunately, have the time or space to analyse all the popular dietary supplements, including those heavily-promoted 'sports' and 'energy' drinks. Almost all of those I have investigated have come up short. Very short. Some are so bad, in that they contain dangerous or dubious ingredients, that I feel obliged to warn my readers against them.

Even those few manufacturers that I have found to come up with acceptable products in this category let themselves down by what they put into many of their other products, so again I urge readers to study all labels and to be wary of descriptions such as 'all natural ingredients', and 'no artificial colours or flavours'. Just because something hasn't been produced in a laboratory doesn't mean it's good for you, and such generic terms as 'natural colouring' or 'natural flavouring' can be used to disguise some very dangerous ingredients.

MANNATECH is a pricey, multi-level example. When their line first appeared in Australia, I was taken in by their protestations of purity and their Ambrotose complex, which seemed to help people. I have learned since, however, that what people thought was making them more energetic was just stimulating them. Recently I saw one of their new brochures and was shocked by the ingredients in most of the products. Their sports drink, *EM-PACT*, contains some things I wouldn't touch. Their *Body Toner Revitalisant* ingredient list reads like a chemical lesson. For instance it contains: propylene glycol, dimethicone, methylparaben, propyl-paraben, etc. I was shocked to find such ingredients in a cream that could go into the body.

Herbalife's *Formula 1 Meal Replacement for Weight Control* is pretty scary stuff. It contains my old enemies, isolated soy protein, whey, fructose, lecithin, canola oil and a bunch of unpronounceable chemicals. The company certainly appears to love soy, as their *Protein Powder* contains, not surprisingly, soy protein isolate, whey protein, natural flavour (and there is a great deal of leeway permitted with this additive) and silicon dioxide. Their *Thermojetics Protein Bars* have a long ingredient list and the only one I like is water. Approach this company's wares with care.

Neways' vitamin, mineral and herbal supplements appear to be okay. They have a large range, and most of the ingredient lists pass my extremely fussy muster. A few of the formulas contain lecithin, but they can be easily avoided. However, their toothpaste, *Ultrashine*, looks as if a different company formulated it. I was shocked to find that it contains sugar and artificial sweeteners, as well as some chemicals I don't like the look of. They need to go back to the drawing board on the toothpaste and do some homework on what lecithin does to the human body. (See Page 244 for a cheap, safe toothpaste recipe you can make yourself. It will save you from poisonous commercial toothpastes and improve the health of your gums.)

Juice Plus, claimed by the American manufacturers, *NSA*, to be "the next best thing to fresh, raw fruits and vegetables," is a fruit and vegetable supplement that has good word-of-mouth, but most of it seems to come from the people who are selling it multi-level. On the surface it seems to be much better than average, but it does contain soy. An American colleague spoke at one of their seminars and they muzzled him unpleasantly when he tried to bring up the dangers of soy.

Finally, two other network-distributed brands are worth dishonourable mention. *Shaklee's* supplements have some scary ingredients, soy being the least nasty of them, as does the widely-promoted *Sunrider* range, which includes *Vitalite, Kandesen, Sunergy* and *Sunsmile*.

In fact, most dietary supplements contain soy, and it is not because the formulators think it is healthful. *It is because it is dirt cheap and plentiful.* It is up to us to vote with our wallets and refuse to be poisoned by the soy-pushers.

Amino Acids

There is so much hype about how great the proteins are in amino acids that most people have been snowed. The truth, according to Dr Peat, is that "Despite research that clearly showed that adults assimilate whole proteins more effectively than free amino-acids, much of the public has been led to believe that 'predigested' hydrolyzed protein and manufactured free amino acids are more easily assimilated than real proteins, and that they are not toxic. Even if free amino acids could be produced industrially without introducing toxins and allergens, they wouldn't be appropriate for nutritional use."

He continues, "Although several amino acids can be acutely or chronically toxic, even lethal, when too much is eaten, tryptophan is the only amino acid that is also carcinogenic... There are people who advocate the use of tryptophan supplementation to increase serotonin in the tissues as a treatment for the fibromyalgia syndrome, but the evidence increasingly suggests that excessive serotonin, interfering with muscle mitrochondria, is a major factor in the development of that syndrome."

Hans Selye, in 1965, showed that the injection of serotonin caused muscular dystrophy. Amino acids are widely sold in health stores and recommended by therapists, often for muscle building. They are not something to play around with.

Vitamins and Minerals

As readers must know by now, I am not a fan of man-made foods. My dislike applies to vitamins as well, because no test tube jockey could formulate anything that even remotely reproduces what nature intended. It takes an organic seed, sunshine, uncontaminated water and the good bacteria and worms in organic soil, plus some mysterious alchemy, for nature to produce the perfect vitamin C – a tiny rose hip or a crunchy, small green capsicum (green pepper). And I am not referring to the watery, large, flabby, supermarket capsicums, which are an insult to nature and contain nothing much but pesticides and superphosphate. There are no doubt many nutrients in that organic capsicum which work in harmony with the vitamin C, and haven't even been identified yet. So how could a processor copy what it can't fathom? Grow your own vitamin C. Plant a Brazilian Cherry Tree, and enjoy. If you don't have a garden, get a big pot and tend a capsicum lovingly on your balcony or window-sill. Give it all the organic nutrients it needs and it will reward you. Failing these measures, the only vitamin C that I consider safe and effective is listed in **Resources**.

Dr Joel Wallach sells minerals, called Majestic Earth Cheri-Mins. This product contains the very nasty excitotoxin citric acid; cherri flavours (which can mean anything); fructose, which must be avoided; and sodium benzoate and potassium sorbate which we should all shun.

David Ewins, of Moor Life International, imports the Moor Drink, a source of naturally occurring organic nutrients that I can recommend. It is easily assimilated and helps the digestive system. For more information, email: admin@moorlife.com or phone: (02) 9970-7200, or fax: (02) 9970-7120

Vitamin E is another valuable nutrient. Men badly need it for prostate health, but consider this; in the huge *Nurses' Study*, with over 120,000 participants followed for 12 – 14 years, it was found that vitamin E *from food, but not from supplements*, gave the best protection from Parkinson's Disease. Similar results were found with cognitive decline.

Supplements had little effect. A study on development of Type 2 (adult onset) diabetes at the University of South Carolina followed 895 adults over five years. They found that foods containing significant amounts of vitamin E offered protection, but supplements did not. It's just as well, because synthetic vitamin E has detrimental effects, as it is incompletely metabolised and can disrupt the metabolism of natural vitamin E in the liver. So, be wary of all multi-vitamins, because most contain this synthetic.

But don't get the idea that the "natural" E capsules are safe (see my *WARNING*). I urge you not to touch any of this dangerous rubbish, and instead derive your vitamin E only from food: soaked almonds, sunflower seeds, hazel nuts, dark green leafy vegetables such as kos (romaine) lettuce, chard, kohlrabi, pumpkin, dandelion greens and mustard greens. E is also in chicken, egg yolk, liver, turkey and salmon. Other fish contain E, but are contaminated by mercury.

If you live where you cannot get sun 12 months of the year, you will need to find other ways to get your crucial vitamins A and D. Supplements are iffy, to say the least, and I prefer to get mine from natural sources such as cream, butter and eggs from animals who have been raised organically, grazing on grass. Please see Chapters 7 and 8 for specifics.

Dr Joseph Mercola, an expert on this subject, says, "Almost all fish has mercury that will absolutely compromise your health. The one apparent exception are very small fish like sardines or anchovies that haven't been in the ocean long enough to accumulate much mercury." He explains that the *Carlson* brand of fish oil/cod liver oil goes through a molecular distillation process and is routinely tested to ensure freedom from cadmium, PCBs, lead and 28 other contaminants that are regularly found in fish and fish oil products. Dr Mercola says that he has seen substantial improvements in cholesterol levels, rheumatoid arthritis, Raynaud's and scleroderma in his patients who use Carlson's oil. It would be ideal if we could just eat fish to get these nutrients, but industry and compliant governments have so polluted our waterways that one of the healthiest foods on the planet has been devastated. But, be warned, those with compromised livers may have problems with cod liver oil. See **Chapter 8**, *Bone Health II*, for more information and **Resources** for ordering details.

Lactobacillus acidophilus is another supplement I recommend, to colonise the intestine with friendly bacteria and overcome the serious damage antibiotics do.

To compound our confusion, vitamins and minerals often interact among themselves in ways that are not fully understood by nutritionists: if you take too

> ### *WARNING*
>
> All of the so-called "natural" vitamin E capsules are derived from the dregs of soy oil processing tanks, mostly from the dreaded Archer-Daniels-Midland or Cargill conglomerates, whose nefarious practices are detailed elsewhere in this book. The vitamin E tocopherols are distilled out of this glop, and I can testify from painful personal experience that taking any vitamin E made from this semi-poison is a big mistake. The side effects creep up, but are insidious, and by the time the damage is done it is difficult to pinpoint the culprit. There are no doubt millions of people taking this misleadingly-labelled Vitamin E who are ill and/or in severe pain and have no idea why they are suffering.
>
> I have phoned every big vitamin company and learned that all their vitamin E is soy-based, and that they are not obliged by the government to disclose this on the label. If you have been taking these capsules and are in strife, quit immediately, drink lots of water, and your problems should melt away in a few days or weeks.

much of one, you may damage your ability to utilise another. But nature has it all figured out and has thoughtfully combined just the right amounts and combinations in her own brand of supplements – fresh, raw, organic vegetables and fruits.

Wheatgrass juice is an example. It contains all of the vitamins and minerals our bodies need, and it contains them in an easily-digested and assimilated form. One day, if the big pharmaceuticals have their way, you may have to rely upon this perfect supplement, because vitamin and mineral supplements will be unavailable. These evil organizations have been working on the European Parliament legislators in Brussels for years, trying to deny us our health freedom, and it is only due to huge public outrage in England and Europe that they have not succeeded – *so far*.

But they haven't given up and are now chipping away, in Australia and the US. When they go public, I hope all concerned citizens will be as outraged as I, and write to their representatives, picket and do what it takes to stop them in their tracks. If they win, I don't think they will be powerful enough to ban wheat seeds or wheatgrass juicers, and we will all have to grow our own perfect supplement. It's a nuisance, but it's cheap and it's the *best*! There are books on this subject, complete with directions (I recommend Anne Wigmore's – see **Resources**). But be wary of manufacturers of all-purpose vegetable juicers who claim their juicers will do wheatgrass. You *must* have a proper, purpose-built juicer so this precious substance will not be heated and/or oxidised by bad handling (you'll find one in **Resources**).

If you can't eat all organic, and you don't have time to grow your own wheatgrass, you would be wise to take a mineral supplement, because of our devitalised food. There have been lots of them, many sold multi-level and highly recommended (at least by their vendors). I've tried quite a few for experimental purposes and results have been patchy.

Now, finally, there is a liquid trace mineral product, (Cellyte), that I can recommend without qualification. I learnt about it from a colleague who is an experienced iridologist and Body Electronics practitioner. Her results were so positive that I experimented with the minerals myself, with the help of some willing friends, (sometimes known as my "guinea pigs"). We all had very good results, which did not surprise me, because I knew the work of the two scientists who developed Cellyte after years of experimentation – the late John Whitman Ray and Dr. Michael Halliday. I am hoping to get a supply of Cellyte from the US by the time this edition of my book is back from the printer. More details on page 334.

Folic Acid (The Synthetic form of Folate)

Folic acid is important for women – especially those who are on or have been on, oral contraceptives. It is believed that these contraceptives can cause a localised folic acid deficiency in cervix cells, making them more susceptible to cancer-causing chemicals and viruses. A deficiency of folic acid can lead to cervical dysplasia, which is an abnormal growth of tissues. Supplementing with folic acid (also known as folacin or folate) can save these women from operations for this condition. Better, of course, is to supplement before the cell division commences. Even better is to stop taking oral contraceptives!

It has been known for decades that deficiency of this vitamin in pregnancy can lead to birth defects. Certainly, it is vital for women who have been on oral contraceptives to be doubly sure that their folic acid stores are restored well before conception. The USA Public Health Service states: "In order to reduce the frequency of neural tube defects and their resulting disability, all women of childbearing age who are capable of becoming pregnant should consume .4 milligrams (400 mcg) of folic acid per day for the purpose of reducing their risk of having a pregnancy affected with spina bifida or other neural tube defects." Supplementing with B_{12} in addition to the folic acid makes it more effective. This vitamin protects people from colon cancer and cardiovascular disease, as it normalises elevated homocysteine levels.

There is a danger in folic acid supplementation. If anaemia is present, it is essential to determine if it is caused by B_{12} deficiency or folic acid deficiency. If folic acid is given to someone who is deficient in B_{12}, a dangerous B_{12} deficiency will develop. Conversely, if B_{12} is given to someone deficient in folic acid, a dangerous folic acid deficiency will result. Medical advice is essential. As always, we advise food as the best way to get minerals. Our favourites, deep green vegetables, contain this valuable mineral, but not if cooked.

Selenium

This mineral has a role to play in regulating hormonal imbalances in women, and is crucial, along with zinc, for male sperm health. It is also important in cancer prevention. Made by Nutrition Care Pharmaceuticals, it is available in Australia in a liquid form.

Selenium has been proven in American studies to hugely reduce the incidence of lung, prostate and colorectal cancers. It helps to detoxify heavy metals, fights autoimmune disorders, helps increase insulin efficiency, protects against free radical damage, activates an important tumour-suppressing gene called *p53,* and protects people from heart attacks. So, you can see that the importance of this mineral in our diets cannot be overstated.

Dietary sources of selenium come mainly from plant foods. But in places where selenium content is low, unless the food is grown organically, people will be deficient. In China, for example, the soil contains low amounts, as does the soil in the US, with the exception of the States of Colorado, Montana, Wyoming, Utah and North and South Dakota.

There is little selenium in Australian soils, and I suggest you do what I do – play it safe and take 200mcg daily. It won't hurt to add 1/3cup of soaked Brazil nuts, which are the richest source, and/or other sources, such as meat, fish, eggs, almonds, and wheatgrass. Selenium from all sources does not become toxic if kept below 2500mcg per day. Supplements are available in most countries.

The Latest Whiz-Bang Cure-All: Goji Juice

Once again, multi-level marketing hype raises its ugly head, and this time it's for a berry from the Himalayas. Possibly, eaten fresh it may have amazing curative powers. But by the time it is picked, packed, shipped, "reconstituted" and combined with lots of other juices, plus "natural goji flavour", (whatever that is), as well as the highly-suspect "natural flavours" (which can legally mean just about anything), and preserved with sodium benzoate and potassium sorbate, I'm not game to try it. Several cluey health professionals reported to me that their patients experienced quick energy, followed by sleeplessness that disappeared only days after the juice was discontinued. Further, all the kinesiology testing they did showed negative results.

Another Whiz-Bang Cure-All: Xango Whole Fruit Juice

Again, more "reconstituted" juice, this time of the mangosteen, plus lots of juice concentrates, and topped up with an acidity regulator (330), the always suspicious "natural flavour", pectin, stabiliser (415) and preservative (211). By now, you will know my opinion - you would be better off spending that money on organically grown fruit and vegies.

Maca Powder

Last, but certainly not least, is my Number One Favourite supplement, Peruvian Maca. In 1998, after reading an article in an American medical journal, I imported enough Maca to experiment on four friends and myself. We were all thrilled by its effects, so I became a reluctant pioneer and was the first person in Australia to grapple with the Therapeutic Goods Administration (TGA) in order to obtain permission to bring it in. Now many others are importing this nutrient. Some is good, but some is not properly grown (it is pale in colour and doesn't "work") and some has additives we wouldn't touch, such as guarana (caffeine) and some is in contaminated animal gelatin capsules. Regrettably, such inferior products are giving Maca a bad reputation. Please refer to **Chapter 27**, *In Other Words*, for two articles published in **Nature and Health** which explain, far better than I can, what Maca is all about, and to **Resources** for a source of guaranteed 100% pure Maca.

16

Against the Grain

The staples that are better left alone

Cutting all grain products out of your diet could prove to be the remedy for many of your ills. Yes, I know you love your pasta, rice, sandwiches, and breakfast cereals. But they don't love you! The reason is simple: mankind has not had time to adapt to these 'new fangled' components of our diet, which have only been in existence for approximately 15,000 years.

Prior to the discovery of agriculture, our primitive ancestors were hunter-gatherers, and had never been exposed to any unnatural food. If it didn't grow on trees, if it didn't spring unaided from the soil, if it couldn't be easily dug up, if it couldn't swim, or fly or run, our ancestors didn't, and couldn't, eat it. If we lived similarly, we would not be plagued by degenerative diseases. And here is the really scary part; our trillions of cells, our digestive systems, in short our entire physical makeup, is virtually the same as it was three million years ago. Our bodies have not had time to adapt to grains in the few thousand years since our ancestors learned to grow and harvest their food. Perhaps in another three million years our bodies will find a way to adapt, and we will evolve into a junk-eating species. If we survive.

Grains are pushed aggressively by most 'health' organisations, and by governments. But what do they know? Certainly governments have hopeless track records in areas of health care, and the various organisations that profess to help sick people are, for the most part, financed by the food processors they recommend. Most of these organisations wholeheartedly recommend nasties such as polyunsaturated oils, soy, and artificial sweeteners, as noted in *Chapters 6, 9* and *4* respectively. Just to be consistent, it stands to reason that they would love grains!

To compound the problem, mothers often don't breast feed and, even if they do, they frequently supplement with cereals before the baby is 12 months old.

Because a baby's digestive system is extremely delicate, and adapted to a diet of only mother's milk for the first year, this is a disaster. It leads to a permanent allergy to grains of all kinds. Unfortunately, this allergy does not necessarily take a form that is obvious, such as vomiting or hives. It can manifest as a constant mucus build-up, sometimes culminating in serious, life-threatening illnesses and premature decrepitude.

During my lectures at Hippocrates Health Centre, people who want an excuse to keep eating grains refer to the excellent health of grain-eating cultures. I point out to them, however, that there have been hundreds of studies which have proved conclusively that grain consumption is detrimental. Asians have been known for 200 years to have hypertrophy of the pancreas as well as severe tissue degeneration, due to their heavy reliance on rice.

Not Heart-friendly

Wheat causes calcium salts to be deposited in tissues, is one of the most allergenic of all foods, and causes hardening of the arteries. One of the worst aspects of grain ingestion is that grains metabolise rapidly to simple sugars and disrupt insulin levels. Those with diabetes should avoid grains (in spite of misguided medical advice), as should those with high blood pressure, high homocysteine levels, and high cholesterol.

For decades, the 'experts' have eagerly recommended grains to prevent or reverse heart disease. This is ironic, considering that grains are well known to raise triglyceride levels, and a high triglyceride level is a well-established risk factor for coronary heart disease. Twenty studies involving approximately 50,000 subjects have confirmed this: high triglyceride levels raise the probability of heart disease by 76 percent in women and 32 percent in men.

And what raises triglyceride levels? The diets pushed by the low fat, polyunsaturated, high-carb dictocrats. This is because when carbohydrates are consumed, levels of insulin are elevated, and cause triglyceride levels to rise. Now, this does not mean that triglycerides themselves cause heart attacks. What it does mean is that whatever elevates the triglycerides leads to heart attacks. And that is the low fat, high-carb diet.

The ubiquitous, grain-pushing 'food pyramid' is a crock. Instigated by the US Department of Agriculture (USDA) in the 1950s, publicised relentlessly by governments, it has brought billions to the grain-growers and has done huge damage to the health and profiles of people in Western countries. And, of course, readers of this book are by now aware that any time government endorses anything – be it food, drugs, vaccinations, war – we had all better be suspicious.

Thanks to the power and influence of the USDA, this evil pyramid is printed on many grain foods, bread wrappers, cereal boxes, etc., published in university textbooks and posted on school bulletin boards. Heavily promoted and considered almost holy writ by nutritionists, the food pyramid advises daily consumption of up to 11 servings of bread, pasta, rice and cereal, with all other foods used sparingly. Wow! People following this government-sanctioned nutritional advice are bound to end up resembling Porky Pig. And, indeed, they do: just have a look at the stomachs and backsides of the populations of developed countries who have been told for decades that their diet should be grain-based.

Being overweight is not the only negative. This is what Dr Peat has to say about grains (the italics are mine): *"Nutritional deficiency diseases probably wouldn't have been discovered if our diets hadn't been based on grains.* The starches in grains aren't their only problem, but starch is uniquely suited to activate the formation of fat, and to stimulate appetite, especially an appetite for more carbohydrate, to restore the blood glucose that has been used up in making fat. Starch also has the ability to stimulate allergic responses, to plug small blood vessels and to accelerate aging, according to the work of G.Volkheimer, and others."

Coeliac Disease

During the last 200 years the amount of cereal grains consumed has increased tremendously, and in the past four or five decades people have become more and more dependent upon fast food, which consists to a large degree of junk grains. Grain growers have exacerbated the problem, by increasing the amount of gluten in wheat by 50 percent through genetic selection. This was done to make grains easier to cultivate and harvest, and to facilitate baking. This change benefited bakeries and the USDA, but it created an epidemic of gluten intolerance and coeliac (or celiac) disease.

Coeliac Disease (CD) is a severe allergy to the gluten in wheat, rye, oats, triticale, barley, spelt and kamut. It is hard to diagnose. So hard, that people who are diagnosed as having cancer, liver disease, leukaemia, osteoporosis, autoimmune diseases, diabetes, sleep apnoea, rheumatoid arthritis, psoriasis, psychological stress, diarrhoea, lupus, spastic colon, anaemia, CFS, gall bladder disease, migraine headaches, viral gastroenteritis, irritable bowel syndrome, etc., are sometimes just coeliacs in disguise. Many would get over their life-ruining symptoms if a doctor would simply test them for CD and put them on the right diet.

Then there are the people who are gluten intolerant, or gluten sensitive, and while they will not test positive for CD, eating grains causes them serious health problems. I mean, *really* serious, like death, if they continue poisoning their bodies with grains. For example, lupus, which establishment medicine considers incurable, is often caused by gluten. The only people I've ever observed with long-term lupus who got over it were at the Gerson Institute in Mexico and at Hippocrates Health Centre. And, of course, bread is a no-no, in both places.

When Jonathan Wright, MD, was visiting Australia in the 1980s, Dr Christopher Reading, of Sydney, showed him proof that 100 of his patients who had 'incurable' lupus remained symptom-free for five years, after eliminating all gluten grains, as well as dairy, and taking oral and intravenous nutritional supplementation.

As Dr Wright said, "Even today, in 2002, just about any 'lupus specialist' in the United States will say that's impossible... and then resume writing prescriptions for *prednisone.*" Which doesn't work, of course, and causes serious problems.

One of the worst aspects of CD is that it can lead to a misdiagnosis of leukemia. This is the way it can happen:

A virus, bacteria, or anything else the body perceives as a foreign invader, can result in a raised white cell count, because the body utilises white cells in its constant efforts to protect itself and heal. To physicians, this white cell elevation can mean leukaemia. In many cases, this diagnosis is correct – after all, we are bombarded by ionising radiation, benzene and many other chemicals, all of which are known to contribute to leukaemia. There is, however, a chance for tragic misdiagnoses if the particular type of leukaemia is CLL (chronic lymphatic leukaemia). In this illness, white cells may have been elevated by the body, due to the individual having a severe intolerance to gluten.

Forever Compromised

Simply cutting all gluten-containing foods from the diet can result in cessation of all the symptoms that led to blood tests indicating leukaemia. This can mean that the patient did not have leukaemia, but coeliac disease, and if the physician prescribes conventional treatment for what he erroneously diagnosis as leukaemia, the patient's health will be forever compromised by chemotherapy, antibiotics and blood transfusions.

Gluten, as you have just learned, is in most grains, but it is also hidden in almost all manufactured foods and even vitamins. It is a cheap filler, used extensively, and usually not mentioned on the label, so effort is needed to identify and avoid it.

My suggestion is that before submitting to chemotherapy or any other drug, simply eliminate all grains, as well as dairy, which can also cause white cell proliferation, and within a few days a strong reaction should occur, as the body expels the offending substances. If the 'leukaemia' was merely an allergic reaction, the patient should feel much better after recovering from the elimination crisis, and must then maintain a strict grain-free diet permanently.

Your oncologist probably will not be that crazy about your 'miracle cure', but, hey, it's your body.

In my opinion, gluten isn't good for anyone, although many professionals say that some people do well on it. I like to remind these grain enthusiasts that when you put gluten into a Petrie dish with human internal organs, the gluten damages the tissues. That's enough to keep me away from it, and the following should be enough to make mothers' wary of infant formula:

Sweden has ten times the number of coeliacs compared with Denmark and Holland. Scientists think the reason is Sweden's infant milk formula, that has forty times more gluten than fomulas sold in Denmark and Holland.

If you know that you are a coeliac, or gluten intolerant, it is important to remember that your bones will be compromised. You will need to supplement with magnesium, zinc, vitamin D and vitamin K, and pay lots of attention to *Chapter 7*, *Bone Health I*, on osteoporosis.

According to some experts, rice, corn, amaranth, millet, buckwheat and quinoa will not adversely affect people with gluten intolerance. They do, however, have their own problems, and need to be approached with care, particularly millet, which can affect the thyroid. First, get all gluten-containing grains out of your life. After at least three weeks, you might like to try these foods, one at a time, and watch for symptoms. Your body will tell you.

If you don't have a serious illness, but just feel 'yucky', try eliminating grains from your life and see if you feel lots better. A three-week trial is needed to identify any food sensitivity, and it's worth the effort. I've never encountered anyone who did not benefit from quitting grains, but if you find it too inconvenient or too traumatic to give them up, at least cut way down. Fill the resulting void with lots of health-giving vegetables and fruits, good quality proteins and the right kind of fats. This will protect you from most illnesses, especially heart disease, the Western world's biggest killer.

When friends or health professionals say that "everyone" knows grains are healthful, remember what Bertram Russell said:

> "The fact that an opinion has been widely held, is no evidence whatever that it is not utterly absurd."

The Blood Type Diet

Hardly a day goes by without someone asking my opinion of this hyped diet plan. Simply put, **had I started following the recommendations for my blood type, I would have been pushing up daisies for the past decade, instead of having fun blowing the whistle on establishment medicine and silly diet plans**. Looking at it logically, take the example of two girls born with identical blood types.

One is breastfed for two years, and given a wonderful diet throughout her childhood by parents who never allowed anyone to smoke in her presence. This girl will be robust throughout life and will be able to eat what she likes, even "fun food", for many years without repercussions. The other girl never sees a breast, and must make do on pasteurised, homogenised, chemicalised milk, and is then given cereals at six months, long before her digestive system is ready. She will have a lifelong allergy to many things, especially to grains, because her digestive system has been so compromised by a dreadful start in life. Further, her thyroid, adrenals, lungs and entire body have been damaged, because everyone in her extended family chain-smokes. This girl is destined to be delicate all her life and will have to watch her diet carefully in order to survive. Yet, these girls, because they were born with identical blood types, are advised to eat identical food. Does this make sense to you?

I have a confession to make: I am the second girl, and my delicate constitution was a motivating factor in my lifelong study of health. It was learn or die young, and I learned that grains and soy are poisons to my body, even though they are recommended for my blood type.

17

Dental Health

Mercury, fluoride, industrial waste – are you sure your dentist isn't making both of you sick?

I strongly advise everyone to stay away from any dentist who uses mercury, even if he or she promises not to use it on you. Mercury fumes permeate surgeries of dentists who use it, and many dentists are being mentally affected in the same way as were hatmakers in Edwardian England, who used mercury in their work – hence the expression, "Mad as a hatter". One day, when everyone is aware of the truth, the expression may change to "Daft as a dentist".

In any case, old-school dentists, who do not seem concerned about the health of their patients, would be well-advised to think about their own health. Autopsies reveal that these dentists, who persist in working with one of the most toxic substances known to man, have higher brain mercury than controls, and have more suicides, spontaneous abortions, infertility, kidney damage, poisoning of the pituitary gland, and brain tumours than any other health professionals.

Shun dentists who want to paint a rat poison on your teeth (fluoride), and do not let them put glass ionomer fillings in your mouth; they exude fluoride and do continuing damage.

To make sure your oral hygiene contributes to your healthy lifestyle, I suggest you keep well away from the dental products and practices which follow.

X Root Canals

While you are choosing your alternative dentist, be sure that he or she understands that root canals are to be avoided. They have the potential to do a great deal of damage to your health. A high percentage of chronic degenerative diseases can originate from root canalled teeth; brain and nervous system diseases, arthritis, circulatory and heart diseases are common problems. Better a gap in your smile than an early death.

X Mercury Amalgam Fillings

It is impossible to achieve true health in the face of constant, low-level mercury poisoning. This is what occurs in those who have mercury amalgam fillings. From the time the mercury is put in your mouth, until the day you die (or you lose the teeth), chewing causes mercury vapour to escape. It then enters your bloodstream and is delivered to all parts of your body, including your brain. Because of the huge number of lawsuits in the US, claiming mercury-caused damages, it is only a matter of time before it is banned there. In California, dentists are required by law to inform patients of mercury risk. Several European countries have outright bans, and the German government reimburses people for mercury removal. It is commonplace for dental associations to deny the dangers, due to their fear of being broken by successful lawsuits from people they have damaged over many decades. Mercury fillings, unfortunately, are still widely used in Australia, and are still vehemently defended by many dentists. I leave you to determine their motives.

To illustrate the position taken by the 'regulators', the American Dental Association made this statement: "The ADA owes no legal duty of care to protect the public... If you are a dentist still using mercury amalgam, be careful. If you tell your patient that it is harmful, you already know that the ADA will come after you." That's their way of saying they will revoke the dentist's licence to practice. "But in light of these new findings if you don't tell your patient you might now be sued for not providing informed consent." Scary stuff, and the situation isn't any better in Australia, judging by the defensive way so many dentists deride the fears of their patients.

The California State Board of Dental Examiners published a warning that mercury is a known toxin that has been shown to escape into the body. The US Environmental Protection Agency classifies mercury filling material, once removed from the mouth, as a toxic waste that must then be carefully handled in special containers, and buried in toxic waste sites.

The World Health Organisation announced that the mercury in fillings leaks into the patient's system at the alarming rate of 3-17 micrograms a day by chewing. If your dentist pooh-poohs this, he hasn't read the research.

Prominent American researcher, Roy B. Kupsinel, MD, wrote, "The California Dental Association may be dissolved for their failure to obey a nine-year-old law to inform citizens of the dangers of the mercury-amalgam fillings at the offices of their dentist members. The State of Maine has recently passed such a law. The truth is becoming known by more and more people." These medical/dental associations are too powerful for our own good. The only way we can prevail is by refusing their dangerous procedures and finding natural dentists and doctors.

Encouraging news has come in from California. Dentists are now required to post this warning in their offices: "Dental amalgams, used in many dental fillings; causes exposure to mercury, a chemical known to the state of California to cause birth defects or other reproductive harm. Root canal treatments and restorations including fillings, crowns and bridges, use chemicals known to the state of California to cause cancer. The US Food and Drug Administration has studied the situation and approved for use all dental restorative materials. Consult your dentist to determine which materials are appropriate for your treatment."

This is the first admission by organised dentistry in the United States that amalgams pose a health risk. It has, of course, been well known in most European countries. What a shame that it is 100 years too late!

When having mercury/amalgam fillings removed, stress to the dentist that you want every speck out of your mouth. Several women have told us that their dentists drilled out just the top layer and filled over with composite to make it appear the mercury was all gone. These dentists should be taken out and shot! Their victims were unable to reverse serious health problems until the teeth were done over by ethical dentists.

In Sweden, the government actually pays citizens to have their mercury fillings removed in order to eliminate the need to spend money treating them for mercury-caused cancer in the future. And in Germany, where mercury is no longer permitted, physicians have pioneered the difficult, important work of removing the mercury from the nerves and tissues after it has been removed from the teeth. We need doctors such as these in English-speaking countries, and we could use some clued-up politicians as well.

There are bio-compatible dentistry practitioners throughout Australia who know of the mercury danger and specialise in careful removal. It takes a bit of digging to find one, but it is worth the effort and the expense (see *Resources*).

X *Toothpastes*

Toothpastes are dangerous. One of the culprits is sodium laurel sulphate (SLS), a fierce detergent used as a foaming agent. You may get the impression that your teeth are going to become sparkly clean when you see all that foam, but the truth is, SLS is officially listed as a poison, and as a primary irritant. It binds to tissues, so is not removed by simply rinsing the mouth with water. SLS also damages the friendly bacteria in the mouth, while leaving others, such as streptococci and E coli, unharmed. The worst news of all is that SLS causes periodontitis (gum disease) which is extremely painful and expensive to treat, and can lead to tooth loss.

SLS, which is common in cosmetics, shampoos, baby wash and bubble bath, has been known for years to cause brain, heart and lung damage if used long term. As well, it can cause permanent eye damage, severe skin irritation, eczema, hair loss and degradation of the immune system. There has been so much backlash because of public education about SLS that manufacturers now often list it as 'SLS, derived from coconuts'. What they neglect to mention is that it is prepared with *sulphur trioxide, chlorosulphonic acid*, and neutralised with *aqueous sodium hydroxide*. Sodium *laureth* sulphate, used in cosmetics claimed to be 'natural', is only slightly less dangerous. These chemicals, which are found in many products, must be carefully avoided.

Toxic Wastes

Further, some toothpastes are too alkaline, while others are too acid, etching the teeth and making them more vulnerable to decay. Believe it or not, *chlorhexidren, bromchlor-ophen* and even *formaldehyde* are included in some toothpastes as antibacterials – and those awful fluoride 'stripes' are made from yet another toxic waste product that manufacturers would rather sell to you than pay to dump responsibly.

As far as I know, only one government has had the sense and decency to outlaw the use of fluoride as an aid to oral health. Fluoride tablets, fluoride drops and fluoride chewing gum, for decades promoted as the crown jewels of dentistry, are to be taken off the market in Belgium because the government now agrees that they are poisonous and pose a great risk for physical and psychological health.

An example of the cavalier attitude of toothpaste manufacturers came from an American truck driver. He reported picking up a 44,000 pound load of aluminium dioxide powder in Bauxite, Arkansas. When he asked why the load was destined for a

Natural Metal Removal

There is evidence that the herb cilantro (also known as coriander and Chinese parsley) helps the body remove mercury, lead and aluminium.

While this sounds wonderful, it is not something to approach casually. First, you must be absolutely certain that there is no mercury left in your mouth. If there is, and you go on a detoxification program using cilantro, more mercury than the body can detoxify will be released, creating serious problems.

If you wish to detoxify with cilantro, once you have had the mercury removed from your teeth, it is essential to be monitored by a qualified health professional, as mercury detoxification is extremely tricky.

An Hippocrates graduate rang recently to report to me that he had been on the cilantro 'cure' for six weeks, taking three to six grams of the fresh herb daily. He was supervised by his doctor, an expert in chelation therapy, who prescribed frequent enemas, and chlorella, wheatgrass juice, extra fibre and lipoic acid to bind the metals.

He did not report unpleasant side effects and said that his urine tests showed that he was excreting mercury and lead.

Large amounts of cilantro must not be taken during pregnancy, as it stimulates uterine muscle contraction.

toothpaste manufacturer, the shipping agent told him that the aluminium mined in Arkansas is too low grade for manufacturing purposes, but that the brilliant, white aluminium powder is perfect for toothpaste. To allay the fear of Alzheimer's Disease-conscious consumers, it is concealed on the label as an "inactive" ingredient.

You can see that we must not be lulled into a false sense of security by the ingredient labels on tubes. Many are downright fraudulent, and most list only the benign-sounding ingredients. When I warn students at Hippocrates Health Centre about toothpastes, some tell me they have a 'good' one – guaranteed by a multilevel salesperson or a health food store to be safe. They bring me the tube for inspection and usually I find several ingredients I know to be dangerous. When there is nothing dangerous listed, I often fax the company requesting a complete list. Some refuse to divulge the ingredients, which makes me really nervous, and those who do, invariably fax lists that read like a poison manual. Most contain SLS, even if it's not on the label, and some contain artificial sweeteners, which you should by now know are deadly, and many actually contain sugar, which you are brushing your teeth to remove!

It is against Australian law for importers to label incorrectly. Too bad the authorities don't enforce it. When I discovered the true ingredients of several imported toothpastes, I naively wrote Carmen Lawrence, who was then the Federal Health Minister, sending proof and requesting that something be done. Years later, I am still waiting for a reply, or for the companies to be stopped.

What to Do?

The question is – what to do until a safe toothpaste is available? My dentist assured me that it is not necessary to use any toothpaste. Just brush thoroughly and floss, of course. If, after several weeks, you find that your teeth look a bit discoloured, brush with a bit of ground pumice, very gently, and they will clean up nicely. You can get it at a pharmacy or from a cooperative dentist. Do not use it too frequently, because it will remove some enamel; but then, so does toothpaste.

There is another option, and I prefer this one because I love prevention. An American dentist, Dr Paul Keyes of the International Dental Health Foundation in Reston, Virginia, claims that using baking soda (bicarbonate of soda), three percent hydrogen peroxide, and salt will clear up gum disease, as well as kill harmful bacteria. His recipe: dip your toothbrush in the peroxide, then into the bicarb and brush your teeth and go over your gums thoroughly, so the mixture can get into all the crevices.

Because the three percent hydrogen peroxide that is commonly available is stabilised with chemicals best left out of your mouth I prefer this method: get a bottle of food grade, 35 percent hydrogen peroxide from your compounding pharmacist (or order from 07 5555 7500). Because it is not stabilised with chemicals, you will need to store the excess in the freezer. **Warning: Do not use it neat, and keep it off your skin.** Dilute a very small amount (one part peroxide to nine parts water) and use it with the bicarbonate of soda, as described in the previous paragraph.

After thorough brushing, gargle with salt water. Not ordinary salt, please; use Celtic salt. Dr Keyes says that his patients have saved loose teeth, reduced gum inflammation, stopped bleeding, cured bad breath and halted other problems that were connected with gum disease. If children are started on this technique, Dr Keyes says, tooth-destroying gum disease will probably never take root. You and your children may not love the taste but, trust me, it is miles better than submitting to painful, expensive gum surgery. I've seen some wonderful results with this, but please don't neglect going to your dentist for regular cleaning as well. For those who do not wish to gargle with salt water, Epsom Salts may be used instead. But please remember never to use *Listerine* or any of the other dreadful commercial mouthwashes. They are all filled with nasty chemicals that will go straight into your body and create havoc.

Nancy Evans makes a toothpaste that I like and trust. (See page 335)

X *'Smart' Toothbrushes*

Several years ago toothbrush manufacturers came up with a new selling tool; they put a coloured stripe on toothbrush bristles that was designed to fade over the weeks, thus indicating when a new brush was needed. Duh! Without their help, you'd never have been able to work that out for yourself, would you? Either they didn't think or they didn't care what happened to that dye. All it takes is a little commonsense to figure out that the dyes are chemical, not food dyes, and that as they fade, they are absorbed through your gums into your bloodstream!

It is becoming more and more difficult to find a dye-free brush in this country. Once it becomes impossible, we may have to import them from Europe.

One Last Word About Dentists

Do not let them intimidate you! Just because dentists wear white coats, have fancy offices and superior attitudes does not mean that they are better than you are. And it certainly doesn't guarantee that they know what they are doing, or are even honest.

As an example, a periodontist told me that I had eight 'pockets' in my gums and that they all had to be treated surgically if I wanted to keep my teeth. Foolishly, I submitted to three hours of harrowing cutting, on just one 'pocket', and when she told me how many more weeks of misery I would have to endure, I was deeply depressed. It was upsetting that, in spite of my extraordinarily good diet and careful dental hygiene, my mouth could have deteriorated so badly.

I had to drive two hours for a second opinion, but it was worth it, because this periodontist assured me that the first one had advised *overtreating,* which is a euphemism for sticking it to you. Nothing needed to be done, other than a small amount of painless scraping, and no problems have surfaced in the many subsequent years. **So watch out!**

Dental horror stories abound at Hippocrates Health Centre, yet even I, with all my knowledge of dental perfidy, was victimized by a dentist who assured me he was putting white composite material into a tooth. He lied. Upon examination I discovered the substance was dark gray and when I rang him, he said it was glass ionomer, a "benign' substance.

The manufacturing data of this 'benign' substance describes it as heating glass powder with cryolite (sodium aluminium fluoride), which acts as a flux and leaks not only fluoride, but lead, arsenic and aluminium, along with aluminium fluorosilicates. According to **The Australian Fluoridation News** (Nov-Dec 2003), "The data shows that freshly cured glass ionomer releases 215ppm aluminium, 112ppm fluoride, and 100ppm of lead."

For several weeks I felt as if I had been poisoned, which I had been. It had to be replaced, by a new dentist of course, who warned me that I might lose the tooth due to the additional trauma. I suffered a great deal of pain, inconvenience and expense before the pain subsided. The tooth was not lost, and the miserable feeling of being poisoned gradually wore off.

WARNING: It is not enough to specify that you want the white composite filling material. You must tell the dentist, in no uncertain terms, that the composite must not contain any fluoride. Many do, and the dentist may have to order fluoride-free material especially. Better yet, find a dentist who works with Jenny Burke's laboratory, Australian Biologics, to find compatible dental materials for individuals.

Fayworth House 6th Floor,
383 Pitt Street Sydney, NSW 2000
Telephone: +61 2 9283 0807 **Facsimile:** +61 2 9283 0910
e-mail: austbio@mpx.com.au , jennie.burke@australianbiologics.com.au
Web: http://www.australianbiologics.com.au
This can be done by courier, throughout Australia. It's expensive, but it's for life, and very valuable knowledge to have. (See Resources).

Mercury Detox

There is a new method for ridding the body of mercury from amalgam fillings. It can even be used when some mercury fillings remain. John Sotis, (ph: 07 5526 6662), a Gold Coast dentist whose work I know and trust, first told me about this method, which mobilizes and eliminates systemic heavy metals and improves neurological and mental symptoms beyond that provided by other chelators. Some dentists who have been poisoned by working with mercury use this for their own detoxification. For information, see www.bioray2000.com and www.healthydetox.org.

Be wary of tooth-whitening processes – ingredients used have been found to cause inflammation and muscosal trauma at high concentrations. The inflammation can have unpredictable effects on tissues, and don't forget that the mucosa of the month is extremely absorptive and is a direct route to the brain.

Sydney dentist, Robert Gammal, has made a superb DVD, called QUECKSILBER -- THE STRANGE STORY OF DENTAL AMALGAM, which I highly recommend for everyone, patients and dentists alike. It explains in detail the history of mercury fillings and the compelling reasons to get them OUT -- as soon as possible -- in order to save lives. They can be purchased through his surgery individually and in bulk orders. Bio Compatible Dentistry, Suite 102, Piccadilly Court, 222 Pitt St, Sydney, NSW, 2000 Ph: 02 9264 5270 Fax: 02 9283 2230. Website: www.quecksilber.net.

Bizarre Behaviour

Give some thought to the ease with which dentists can obtain drugs, and consider the possibility that the man or woman you trust with your invaluable teeth may be addled on narcotics. People have told me of bizarre behaviour by dentists, and I have started a registry of deranged or drug-addicted dentists. The dental associations are there to protect their members, not the public, and no matter how dangerous one of their members may be, they turn a blind eye to complaints. They also do everything possible to discredit people and organizations that warn of the incredibly toxic materials blithely put into the mouths of trusting people.

Let me know about your bad experiences, so I can warn others. See page 339 for information about *ASOMAT, The Australian Society Of Oral Medicine And Toxicology*. They can guide you to a poison-free dentist in your area.

A prominent Australian dentist told me that at least half of the dentists in this country are deranged, due to years of mercury exposure. He has also been affected and is still trying to expel the stored mercury from his body.

Good dentists are out there. But a great deal of effort needs to be made to find one. Ask your friends for recommendations. Vet dentists before making appointments, and don't go to any dentist who uses mercury. Make the effort, and don't let a cowboy, masquerading as a dentist, damage you. Mercury poisoning is so serious that your life may depend upon your choice.

See the bottom of page 338 for shocking information about the cosy relationship between dentists and their insurance companies.

18

Cancer

"Statistically, life expectancy of untreated cancer patients is greater than treated ones"

You have mutating cells in your body all the time, and the only thing standing between you and full-blown cancer is your immune system. If it is strong, it acts as a scavenger and nips abnormal cells in the bud, day after day, year after year, just as long as you look after yourself properly. If you don't keep your immune system in top form, it will eventually collapse under the onslaught of junk food, drugs, tobacco and excessive alcohol.

The next step may be a diagnosis of cancer, and if the cancer industry gets hold of you, chemotherapy and radiation will polish off what is left of your immune system, and your chances of ever being well again will be slender.

In Western countries, oncologists (cancer specialists) are forbidden by law to recommend any natural therapies. Only the *Big Three* (Radiation, Chemotherapy and Surgery) are allowed; and this in spite of their dismal track record. Your best hope is to prevent this disaster from overwhelming you. If it is already too late, then the answer is thorough detoxification to allow your body to heal itself, followed by a lifetime healthful regimen. Cancer is a wake up call to alert people that, like alcoholics, they must be forever vigilant. Slip back into old habits and cancer cells will be re-activated.

When the American Cancer Society (ACS) was founded in 1913 (for the purpose of eradicating cancer) the cancer rate was one in 100 people. In spite of, or more likely because of, ACS's activities, the cancer rate is now one in three, and rising. This is not a good outcome from such a well-funded organization, and is not surprising, considering what Hardin Jones, MD, said when he resigned as its President: "If a cancer cure suddenly appeared, there would be a rash of suicides as ACS executives jumped out of windows."

Do you reckon this is the reason the ACS, aided and abetted by the US Government, pharmaceutical companies and medical associations, have devoted their vast resources and power to discredit every non-toxic cancer cure that has been discovered since then? In his speech of resignation, Dr Jones went on to say, "Statistically, life expectancy of untreated cancer patients is greater than treated ones."

Nonetheless, due to its blinkered and uncompromising policy, the ACS has effectively forced millions of Americans to seek safe therapies in Mexico, where medical freedom is permitted, and the cruel *poison-mutilate-radiate* 'cures' so beloved of conventional oncologists are not obligatory.

Lucrative Business

Healers in Mexico are not routinely jailed, as they are in the English-speaking world. Because of this, Tijuana, a California border town, has been transformed from a dusty backwater into a wall-to-wall therapy haven, some amazingly good (the Gerson Clinic has been doing phenomenal work there for thirty years that I know of), some mediocre, and some downright dreadful. Had Gerson's system, and some of the other excellent modalities, been investigated, tested and encouraged in the US, the Charlatans would have been eliminated, the effective modalities permitted, and the cancer death rate would have plummeted. But that didn't happen, of course, because as Dr Jones said, "Cancer is one of the most lucrative businesses in the world."

Take chemotherapy, for example. Most people, who have been spared up-close experience with this ghastly experiment, are not aware that the serum injected into already poisoned bodies is a potent poison. The rationale is that this poison will kill the cancer cells that have been detected. And so it does, but it also kills healthy cells, compromising, if not altogether destroying, the patient's immune system. These are a few of the side effects:

- Vomiting
- Pain
- Diarrhoea
- Fungus
- Exhaustion

- Loss of appetite
- Loss of hair, sometimes baldness
- White blood cells destroyed
- Intestinal vilii sheared off
- Death

Worse Than The Cancer

I watched as the doctors tortured my best friend to death. Her magnificent hair fell out in great chunks, her beautiful face was contorted with pain and she told me, when she was able to speak, that the chemo was infinitely worse than the cancer. In the end she begged for death, but the doctors refused to even help her with this.

How can this happen? Perhaps this will give you a clue; thanks to chemotherapy, oncology has become one of the most lucrative fields of medicine. In the US, and presumably in many other countries, patients are given chemotherapy in the offices of their oncologists. This procedure is a shortcut to riches for the doctors, because they buy the poison low and sell the poison high.

This profit-oriented treatment is referred to as 'chemotherapy concession', and it can lead to abuse. For example, even if an oncologist realises from experience that the patient is too far gone to benefit from chemotherapy, he or she may carry on regardless, making the patient's last days on Earth a living Hell, and beggaring the patient's family to boot.

"Hard to Justify"

In 2001, Ezekiel J Emanuel, MD, who is an oncologist and bio-ethicist, examined the records of nearly 8000 cancer patients. He found that when chemotherapy was administered in the last six months of life, *one-third of the patients had cancers that are known to be unresponsive to chemotherapy*! Reflecting on this, Dr Emanuel said, "Providing chemotherapy to patients with unresponsive cancers is hard to justify." I'll say!

Some of the cancers that are known to be unresponsive to chemotherapy are pancreatic, melanoma, renal cell, gallbladder and hepatocellular. So, if you or a loved one is diagnosed with any of these nasties, and your oncologist recommends a course of chemotherapy, you will know that he is either ignorant, a sadist or integrity-challenged, and that his treatment will kill the patient before the cancer does.

Government legislation continues to outlaw proven alternative natural methods of cancer treatment, while chemotherapy, a proven killer, is officially sanctioned and effectively **forced on unwilling children by the medical establishment**. Investigative journalist Eve Hillary recently uncovered yet another tragic case of a child sentenced to undergo chemotherapy – much against the wishes of her parents. Distressed by the devastating physical effects of the treatment, they carried out their own research, and discovered that:

> Chemotherapy originated from mustard gas, from which the first family of cytotoxic (cell killing) drugs were synthesised. Nitrogen mustard is still listed on schedule one of the Chemical Weapons Convention. Since then, many other equally toxic chemical agents have been developed and used as chemotherapeutic agents. Because of its high toxicity, staff must use protective clothing, goggles, boots and specialised rubber gloves when administering chemotherapy. The floor below the preparation area and intravenous stand is protected from accidental spills, as just a few drops of concentrate are so corrosive that it can damage surfaces and cause chemical burns to human skin. An accidental spill kit is located on the wall of chemotherapy rooms.

> Staff mopping up spills carefully handle the hazardous material and dispose of it as toxic waste. The chemotherapy is infused into the patient and it immediately kills

fast-dividing cells including cancer cells, but also cells forming bone marrow, immune system, digestive system, hair follicles and reproductive cells of the testes and ovary. It also kills healthy cells throughout the body, including liver, kidney and brain cells. Parents of children having chemo are cautioned to wear gloves when bathing their children or coming into contact with their urine. The chemicals saturate the body tissues, killing red blood cells, which carry oxygen to body cells. This causes fatigue, anaemia, and shortness of breath. Low white blood cell count occurs due to the death of white blood cells, the cells responsible for fighting infection. The patient develops a severely compromised immune system incapable of fighting off infection.

The immune system's natural killer cells are destroyed by the chemicals, and unable to continue seeking out and destroying cancer cells. Platelets are destroyed and with them the body's blood clotting ability. This causes nosebleeds and the potentially fatal risk of haemorrhage into lungs, intestines, brain or other organs, depending on how low the platelet count falls. Most patients retch, vomit and experience diarrhoea shortly after chemo starts. In some cases chemotherapy has to be stopped or the patient will die. Three percent of patients die from the therapy. Many others die later from longer-term complications, when the deaths are attributed to cancer and not to the treatment. Some 67% of people who do not survive the course of treatment die because of their weakened immune system's failure to overcome infection, directly attributable to the chemotherapy. Those that survive the treatment often experience longer-term sequelae.

Chemotherapy drugs are often in themselves carcinogenic chemicals that break and damage DNA. This creates a seed for a new cancer that may emerge years later as a direct effect of the treatment. The most common cancers that are caused by chemotherapy are leukaemia and lymphoma. Apart from the relatively temporary effects of hair loss, this type of therapy most often causes permanent damage to ovaries and testes causing sexual dysfunction and permanent inability to have children.

The above condemnation of this "preferred" treatment is only a small part of Eve Hillary's thorough and disturbing report. I recommend you read it and get your doctor to do the same. You will find it on the internet.

Fruitless Effort

What about surgery, to cut the darn thing out? Sure, sometimes it's successful, but slicing into an established cancerous tumour is risky, even when they 'get it all'. Unfortunately, however, they can't be certain that they've 'got it all', so they often insist upon radiation after surgery. This is usually a fruitless effort to search out and kill the billions of cancer cells the surgery disturbed and sent flooding into the patient's system.

After surgery, swarms of these wily microbes can be seen in the patient's blood under a darkfield microscope; Gaston Naessens, in Quebec, has a video illustrating this. So, the tumour may be gone, but the mutilated patient is sent home with billions of cancer cells lurking, awaiting an opportunity to proliferate and concentrate in another tumour. Then that one will have to be cut out, and then another and another, until nothing is left to remove.

As for radiation 'therapy', it is ghastly to endure, and since radiation has been known almost since inception to *cause* cancer, I'm at a loss to understand how 'Cancer, Inc.' came up with the notion that it could cure.

Dire Consequences

Alternative treatments, scoffed at by mainstream medicos, can and do work, although it takes great courage for victims of this scourge to go against the advice of well-meaning family and friends and refuse to succumb to conventional practice. One patient who did so is an Oxford University academic, Michael Gearin-Tosh, whose book, *Living Proof – a Medical Mutiny*, describes in great detail his experience in researching conventional treatment and dumping it in favour of an alternative regime. Says Michael, "I was told I had cancer and that I must expect to die soon. Almost eight years later I still do my job and enjoy life. I have not had conventional treatment. Did my cancer simply disappear? Did I do nothing? Far from it." Most of the physicians he saw encouraged him to submit to chemotherapy, warning of dire consequences when he demurred. Only one warned that the chemo itself could kill him and advised against it. He chose to deal with his cancer naturally, and his story is not only a 'warts and all' description of what he went through to beat the illness, it also serves to show how poorly the medical profession really understands the role the body can play in the treatment of cancer. His book is inspiring reading (see *Resources*) and I am happy to report that we stay in touch and that he continues to lead a very busy and healthy life.

Prevention Ignored

Prevention, the only sane way to deal with the scourge of cancer, has been ignored by the ACS, and by the medical schools. We haven't heard a peep of protest out of any of them regarding junk food, pesticides, dangerous fertilisers, preservatives, soy, artificial sweeteners, pollution, chemicalised milk, etc.

If the ACS, and its sister associations in other countries, were doing the job they were paid for, they would tell people that it is imperative to eat organic food, and they would lobby to put a stop to the Western world's catastrophic farming methods. They would encourage the addition of selenium to all soils where it is low and advise people to take supplements of this proven enemy of cancer. They would warn that excess body iron stores are cancer-causing and petition the government to make willy-nilly iron fortification of food illegal. They would have pithy words to say about parents who inflict second-hand smoke on their helpless babies. They would blow the whistle on the polyunsaturated oils pushed relentlessly by heart specialists and heart foundations. They would publicise the huge body of research proving that these oils are semi-poisonous and are so immunosuppressive that they cause cancer and are killing people by the millions. They would pay attention to the studies that prove how well-formulated progesterone protects women from all the hormone-related cancers. They would encourage people to get adequate vitamin D, citing many studies that prove this important vitamin from the sun offers amazing protection from cancer. They would publicise the use of intravenous oxygen treatment, instead of encouraging the government to jail its proponents.

But they don't do any of these things, and what exactly is it that they *are* doing to justify their salaries?

To give you an indication of how important diet is, the Native American Pueblo and Hopi tribes had a cancer incidence of one in 1000 in 1940. Then the US Government jumped in and encouraged them to eat 'good old wholesome American food'. The Pueblos agreed, and in a short time their cancer rate had increased to one in four. The Hopis didn't, and their rate remained low until, in 1982, they succumbed to the 'do-gooders'. You guessed it – their rate zoomed. Please don't follow in the footsteps of the Americans, and always bear in mind that reckless living now will lead to cancer later.

> ### *Definition of A Spontaneous Remission*
> A natural therapy the patient didn't tell the oncologist about.

My strong recommendation to all readers is: Do not support any of the so-called "health societies". They are all backed by "the bad guys" and suppress natural remedies while shilling for killer therapies. Please, starve them of funds! My donations go to ethical organisations, such as Guide Dogs, Greenpeace and many charities that assist animals.

See pages 314 - 316 for valuable information on cancer.

> If a cancer cure suddenly appeared, there would be a rash of suicides as ACS executives jumped out of windows.
>
> *- Hardin Jones, MD,*
> *Former President,*
> *American Cancer Society (ACS)*

19

Water Woes

"Tragically, we are exposing people to deadly elements of arsenic, lead and radium, all carcinogenic"

When contemplating the vast number of toxic chemicals governments permit in water supplies, one has the inescapable impression that they are out to get us. But wait – if we're all dead, who will pay the taxes needed for their salaries, cushy retirements, and fund their grandiose schemes and overseas trips? Could it be that they are simply ignorant or stupid? Or should we blame the chemical companies' lobbies – the strongest in the world? No matter the reason, once again we must think for ourselves, distrust authority, and never drink any of the stuff, especially if it is fluoridated, "for the sake of children's teeth".

In certain parts of the world *calcium fluoride* occurs naturally in the water and it causes teeth to be yellow and mottled and ugly – but extremely strong. What is dumped, willy-nilly, into the water supplies of too many English-speaking communities, however, is not calcium fluoride, but *silicofluorides*, which are 85 times more toxic than calcium fluoride.

According to an article in **The Weston A Price Foundation Magazine**, *Summer 2001*, by Anita Shattuck, "They are non-biodegradable, hazardous wastes taken from the pollution scrubbers of industries. If not dumped in the public water supplies, these silicofluorides would have to be neutralised at the highest rated hazardous waste facility at a cost of US$1.40 per gallon (or more depending on how much cadmium, lead, uranium and arsenic are also present). Cities buy these unrefined pollutants and dump them – lead, arsenic and all – into our water systems."

This has to be one of the greatest con jobs ever pulled on an unsuspecting, trusting public; in their search for a profitable way to rid themselves of their waste problem, industry came up with a brilliant idea – they decided to make us drink it! A brilliant idea for industry, but disastrous for citizens who drink and bathe in water contaminated by the uranium, arsenic, aluminium, cadmium and lead removed from the scrubbers.

If your dentist encourages you to have your teeth, and those of your children, 'protected' by sodium fluoride, just remember that in all probability he or she also considers it perfectly safe to fill your teeth with mercury, the second-most dangerous substance on Earth (see *Chapter 17*, *Dental Health*). Further, those dental associations who 'advise' governments and the general public on dental health are not scientific bodies, but trade groups that are heavily influenced by the chemical companies and drug cartels.

Somehow all of the organizations, politicians and medical people who should be looking after our health, have decided to ignore or suppress the fact that sodium fluoride was used as an insecticide, rodenticide, herbicide and fungicide, was incorporated into nerve gasses, and used in frosting and etching glass, due to its powerful scouring ability. These poisons from industrial scrubbers do not simply pass through your body – they remain there to create havoc.

For example, they are known to cause:

- Cancer
- Genetic damage
- Neurological impairment
- Lowered IQ in children
- Osteosclerosis
- Osteoporosis
- Spondylaxis
- Goitre
- Chromosomal aberration
- Dizziness
- Joint pain
- Fatigue
- Bloody vomit
- Skin rashes
- Gastroenteritis
- Hypersensitivity
- Headaches
- Urinary tract infections
- Muscular stiffness and aches

- Abdominal pains
- Depression
- Chronic fatigue
- Muscle spasms
- Eczema
- Leg swelling
- Hair loss
- High blood lead levels
- Learning disabilities
- Violence
- Sickle cell anaemia
- Down's syndrome
- SIDS
- Immune system suppression
- Dental fluorosis
- Thyroid dysfunction
- Lead uptake
- Bone fractures

Alzheimer's Disease is epidemic in heavily-fluoridated Australia and New Zealand, and in all other fluoridated communities. Decades ago the connection was discovered when doctors observed that when kidney dialysis was carried out with fluoridated water the patient, no matter the age, was quickly afflicted with Alzheimer's Disease. In heavily fluoridated areas patients died during treatment because of fluoride, and hospitals soon learned that they had to use pure water for dialysis. Governments were made aware of this, yet continued dosing water supplies.

In 1986, 1100 scientists, who worked for the Environmental Protection Agency in the US, tried to sue their own agency for ignoring important data on the dangers of fluoridation.

Even Australia's own war hero surgeon, the late 'Weary' Dunlop, came out strongly against fluoridation, labelling it "poisonous".

> ### Scientific Fraud
>
> A list of 119 scientists who oppose fluoridation was compiled by the London Anti-Fluoridation Campaign. The list includes Nobel Prize winners, and reads like a *Who's Who* of the scientific community. This is one of the statements they released to the press:
>
> **"Fluoridation is the greatest scientific fraud of this century, if not of all time."**

Despite all the authoritative and peer-reviewed research published to date, as far as I have been able to establish, only one government has had the sense and decency to outlaw the use of fluoride as an aid to oral health. Fluoride tablets, fluoride drops and fluoride chewing gum, for decades promoted as the crown jewels of dentistry, are to be taken off the market in Belgium because the government now agrees that they are poisonous and pose a great risk for physical and psychological health.

A Brave and Principled Man

Dr Hardy Limeback, BSc, PhD in Biochemistry, DDS, head of the Department of Preventive Dentistry for the University of Toronto, and president of the Canadian Association for Dental Research, is now on our side. He was formerly Canada's leading sodium fluoride authority and was the main Canadian promoter of fluoridation.

When I heard that Dr Limeback had had a dramatic change of heart, I rang him at the University. He told me that he had addressed students and faculty at his University and apologised for his former stand. He told them, "For the past 15 years I had refused to study the toxicology information that is available to everyone. Poisoning our children was the furthest thing from my mind. The truth was a bitter pill to swallow. But swallow it, I did."

A very brave and principled man, Dr Limeback is now working to stop Canadian fluoridation. "Tragically, we are exposing people to deadly elements of arsenic, lead and radium, all carcinogenic. Because of the cumulative properties of toxins, the detrimental effects on human health are catastrophic...

Residents of Canadian cities that fluoridate have double the fluoride in their hip bones, compared to the rest of the population. Even worse, we have discovered that fluoride is altering the architecture of bones." Australia and New Zealand need more dentists with integrity and courage to speak out the way Dr Limeback has done.

The bottom line: *This stuff is poisonous, in all its forms*. Tell your children's schools that you will sue them if they put it in your children's mouths. Never buy fluoride toothpaste. Shun dentists who want to paint a rat poison on your teeth, and do not allow glass ionomer fillings to be put in your mouth: they exude fluoride and do continuing damage. And please, *write letters of complaint to your political representatives*. This is the only way we can effect change.

Perhaps one day governments in English-speaking countries will come to their senses and stop allowing industry to poison us with their toxic waste. Judging from experience, it will be a long wait. Meantime, there are several alternatives to drinking tap water. Reverse osmosis filters remove the fluoride, as well as chlorine and other poisons. But the water this system produces is 'dead' and it also wastes lots of water.

Ideally, every household that uses municipal water should have efficient filters at source. Most cannot afford such luxuries and are left with little choice, other than bathing in a chemical stew which, inevitably, is absorbed by the body. For country people, when pesticides are not in the air, rain water is the obvious answer. But this is not advisable in suburbia, or in areas close to big cities, due to air pollution.

Wonderful Water

There are two bottled waters I can recommend. One, Alpha Lyte, www.alphalyte.com, comes from a 10,000-year-old deposit in Cooroy Mountain, Queensland, Australia, and it goes through a series of filtration processes. Then, ionic, crystalloid, plant-based trace minerals are added. These minerals are not produced in a laboratory, but are as nature made them, and they are crucial for health. Next, and this is important, the water goes through an energizing process, which makes it "alive". See **Resources**

Another alive water, www.grander.com.au, (07 5568-7522) is made by Grander Water Technologies (GWT). Hippocrates Health Centre has the Grander system installed at source, so all water for showers, irrigating, etc is pure. GWT has recently bottled their water and it is now available in supermarkets throughout Australia. This water also comes from a natural spring. It is called Grandoz.

An economical option is Tesla's water kit, that can be easily fitted to your water supply at source. Email: info@teslas.us. Phone 1-300-898-983.

20

Legal Drugs

Whatever happened to 'Ethical Pharmaceuticals'?

You'd better duck, because the drug barons are out to get you! *Pfizer, Merck, GlaxoSmithKline, Bristol-Myers Squibb, Novartis, Aventis* and other pharmaceutical giants (with a total market valuation in the trillions of dollars) have developed a cosy cartel to provide them with a global marketplace. This means that *they are in charge.* They own the EU, they own politicians, they own governments – and *they want to own you.* They want to make you dependent upon drugs and keep you that way for the rest of your life. If you allow them to 'hook' you, they won't care if their drugs shorten your life, because there are plenty more where you came from.

Pharmaceutical profits are immense, and growing every year, because people have come to believe, through brilliant propaganda, that there is a magic pill for every twinge, a happiness capsule if you are down in the dumps, and a miracle 'cure' for every illness. Dr Joseph Mercola recently revealed that US drug companies alone spend $15 billion per year on physician marketing, and Americans spend $1 trillion (that's *one thousand billion* US dollars) each year on drugs. Pharmaceutical companies finance the medical schools so that budding doctors learn about drugs, but not about the role of nutrition and toxaemia in illnesses. If it became public knowledge that nutrition can prevent all illnesses, and detoxifying can cure, the pharmaceuticals would be finished!

They lie and cheat and stoop to the lowest tricks to hide the toxic effects of the drugs they flog. They find the best scientific prostitutes available to falsify trials 'proving' that their drugs are safe and effective. Scientists who have the courage to bring the truth to the public are vilified. The mainstream press, largely owned by trans-national corporations, often refuses to print anything negative about drugs until the news is so hot that they have no choice. Even then, they usually drag out some tame doctor or scientist who will make a statement they can use to make the pharmaceuticals look less villainous. All

Western governments tag along with this scandalous state of affairs and the only way we citizens can protect ourselves is through word of mouth, and the internet.

The power of the bottom line rules our world. And the bottom line for the pharmaceuticals is amazing, which explains, but doesn't excuse, their immoral behaviour. You can see by the following figures, revealed by the *Life Extension Foundation Magazine*, that they have compelling motives for keeping the truth hidden from their customers:

> *Prozac:* It costs the manufacturer, Eli Lilly, eleven cents to make 100 of the 20mg tablets. This amount retails for US$247.47 – a neat 224,973 percent mark-up.

> *Xanax:* It costs the manufacturer 2½ cents to make 100 of the 1mg tablets. If you are foolish enough to buy them, they will set you back US$136.79 for the 100 tablets. A spectacular 569,958 percent profit.

These drugs will shorten your life and keep you in a confused state while you are still here. Much wiser to get your dietary act together, so you won't need to drug yourself to overcome the damage junk food does to your brain. The magazine cited many more examples, but I guess you get the idea.

To be fair, the pharmaceuticals do have heavy expenses: research, distribution, publicity, packaging, marketing, out-of-court settlements and the occasional lost lawsuit, setting up and funding quasi-legitimate 'foundations', 'institutes', 'associations' and 'advisory boards' to provide 'independent health information and advice' to the public and sponsoring influential organisations to the extent that they will never criticise the hands that feed them, bribes to politicians, scientists and government agencies such as the notoriously corrupt US Food and Drug Administration.

They are entitled to a profit, but these figures do seem a bit excessive. Of course, they couldn't do it without *your* cooperation. So, watch out, and save drug consumption for extreme, life-threatening emergencies, such as pneumonia. Remember, if you have been popping antibiotics for every sniffle, you may very well die from pneumonia, should you contract it, because your body can no longer respond to antibiotics.

The Medicines Control Agency is the drugs licensing authority in the United Kingdom. Taxpayer-funded, it is supposed to protect consumers from dangerous drugs. It is, unfortunately, one of the most secretive organizations in Britain. The *British Medical Journal, 2003; 326:119*, reported, "Its meetings are held in secret, and no minutes of proceedings, apart from revealing the names of attendees, are ever made public. Any member who would dare step out of line and reveal proceedings to the press could face two years imprisonment – if the information compromised a drug company and its work." Wow! One can't help wondering exactly what the British taxpayers are getting for their money.

Perilous Pills

If I were to devote the space necessary to really blow the whistle on the dangers of drugs, this book would expand to a thousand pages. So I will content myself with just a few examples:

BENADRYL, a popular antihistamine, can cause speech disorganization, poor attention span, delirium and unconsciousness. Studies at Yale University found that some people who were being treated for psychosis were actually suffering from Benadryl overdose. So, if your nose is running and you think you need an antihistamine, reach for your water bottle instead. Sip all day to keep hydrated, and chances are your symptoms will abate. And if your granny suddenly shows signs of Alzheimer's disease or dementia, check that the nursing home isn't doping her with Benadryl or something even more sinister, to keep her compliant.

BAYCHOL, a cholesterol-lowering drug, was removed from the market belatedly, after it was proved to cause a muscle-wasting disease.

LOTRONEX is used to treat irritable bowel syndrome (IBS), which the US Food and Drug Administration classifies as a serious condition. Because of that status, Lotronex went through an expedited approval process, which may have led FDA investigators to ignore danger signals about its safety. Some doctors say it's a great help for some people – but it's little or no help to many others, and for some it causes serious problems or even death. What's more, doctors can't tell in advance how Lotronex might affect a patient. Lotronex can cause *ischemic colitis*, a potentially fatal condition that can restrict the supply of blood to the colon and cause gangrene. This may require surgery to remove part of the colon.

Lotronex's maker GlaxoSmithKline and the FDA have been blamed for rushing the drug onto the market despite its known side effects – then, after a temporary recall, pushing the drug back into circulation without properly protecting consumers. Three months after the launch of Lotronex in February 2000, British medical journal **_The Lancet_** published a scathing editorial branding the FDA "a servant of the industry" for the way it approved the drug. The agency was compromised both by the funding it receives from drug makers and by pressure from Congress to favour the industry, author Richard Horton said. Serious side effects were known before the FDA approved Lotronex, and the agency brushed aside the safety concerns of its own scientists, he said. Patients in Lotronex studies suffered from severe constipation and from ischemic colitis, caused by restricted blood flow to the bowel. After the drug's approval, further cases of the two potentially fatal side effects forced its recall nine months later – followed by the FDA unaccountably allowing its reinstatement.

A series of class actions against the makers, and the FDA, are now being pursued in the US, and I hope the scandal will bring this corrupt organization to its knees.

TROVAN, a fluoride-based antibiotic, caused acute liver failure. Pfizer, its maker, conducted an unethical trial in Nigeria and killed and maimed many children. Of course, it's no secret the drug companies love Third World trials because they can literally get away with murder.

Four hundred drugs for colds, coughs and weight control have been removed from stores in the US because they have been linked with an increased risk of hemorrhagic strokes (brain bleeding) in young women. The offending chemical is *phenylpropanolamine*, and the products are ***ALKA-SELTZER, CONTAC, ACU-TRIM, DIMETAPP, DEXATRIM, ROBITUSSIN, TAVIST-D*** and ***TRIAMINIC***. One more reason to steer clear of all drugs, even when they are not on the above list. It's only a matter of time before that 'benign' drug you are taking will be found to cause serious illnesses, and it may be too late for you. You won't need drugs of any kind if you follow the rules in this book. But please don't get the idea I am suggesting that you quit drugs 'cold turkey'. Some are so strong that they must be phased out, with the help of an understanding doctor.

PROZAC, the huge money-maker mentioned earlier, did not get approval from the German authorities because they found that manufacturer Eli Lilly's studies showed that previously non-suicidal patients who took the drug had a fivefold higher rate of suicide than those taking placebos. A few of Prozac's side effects include agitation, manic symptoms, aggression and loss of impulse control. Hey, I thought those were the very symptoms that caused a physician to prescribe it in the first place.

The ***Boston Globe*** reported, "Using figures on Prozac both from Lilly and independent research, Dr David Healy, an expert on the brain's serotonin system and director of the North Wales Department of Psychological Medicine at the University of Wales, estimated that probably 50,000 people have committed suicide on Prozac since its launch, over and above the number who would have done so if left untreated."

According to Dr Raymond Peat, "Eli Lilly and Co. earns over US$2 billion annually on Prozac. Each suicide caused by Prozac would appear to be balanced by several hundred thousand dollars earned by the corporation. If the war on drugs were serious, this would be a good place to start."

Several years ago, the US government issued warnings about *tryptophan* supplements. According to Dr Peat, these warnings were "...widely dismissed, because the government has so often lied. Even when the public health agencies try to do something right, they fail, because they have done so much wrong." Dr Peat, in his ***Newsletter,*** *November 2000*, warns about the use of tryptophan because it is easily converted to serotonin and melatonin in the body. "The most popular kind of tranquiliser/antidepressant/phychotropic drug, the 'serotonin reuptake inhibitor' is said to act by increasing the action of serotonin in the brain. (Drugs of this type are prescribed for depression, anxiety, panic, and obsessive-compulsive disorders). ...The only amino acid that has ever been found to be carcinogenic is tryptophan. ...Serotonin research is relatively new, but it rivals estrogen research for the level of incompetence and apparent fraudulent intent that can be found in professional publications."

All antidepressants are dangerous. Banish junk food and drink, drugs and tobacco from your life and you won't need them.

The good news about the anti-inflammatory *prednisone* is that it can bring relief from pain, often within hours. The bad news, however, is very bad – pharmacologic doses suppress the adrenal glands so much that it can take years to wean a patient off of it, and the side effects include stomach ulcers, diabetes, cataracts, and many more. Another instance of the 'cure' being worse than the illness. Except, it isn't really a 'cure', because drugs cannot cure, they merely suppress illnesses. The only true cures come from detoxification.

Check The Short and Curlies!

An interesting bit of trivia came my way years ago, and I shall pass it on to you, like it or not; people who are fortunate enough to have strong adrenal glands have kinky pubic hair. In youth, of course, all healthy people have kinky pubic hair, but those with weak adrenals find that the curl lessens with age, and comes to resemble a drowned mouse by middle age, or even earlier. I wouldn't mention this somewhat touchy subject except that it is instructive; when a weak-adrenal type becomes seriously ill and takes an extremely strong drug, his or her pubic hair will suddenly become curly again. This happens because of the way the drug works. It is not, contrary to what people may surmise, because the drug is smart, and zeroes in on the cause of the illness and zaps it. It is because the drug whips the already exhausted adrenal glands, and forces them to do their job of suppressing the illness. So, the patient is not getting better, but is getting over the worst of the symptoms, because his or her adrenals have been stimulated. Once the drug is discontinued, the lank pubic hair returns, and the illness, which has been suppressed but not banished, lies in wait for the next opportunity to surface. If the patient does not get serious about diet, more drugs will be given, and eventually the poor, exhausted adrenals will simply lie down and give up. So, my advice is – have a look at your private area, and if the short and curlies are not curly, and if you want to have a long, healthy life, adopt the rules in this book.

Time to Ask Questions

Should you feel that I have gone somewhat overboard on my criticism of those multi-national drug empires who spend millions of *your* dollars on warm and fuzzy ads which portray them as caring, responsible, and philanthropic purveyors of life-enhancing products, I suggest you do a little internet research through visits to the many whistle-blowing websites (just key in 'drug companies' to your search engine), and see for yourself the depths to which these once-respected 'ethical pharmaceutical' companies have sunk in pursuit of profit. If you are a shareholder in any of them, maybe it's time for you to start asking questions. But don't expect any honest answers from your board of directors. They'd all end up in jail if they were ever to admit the truth. And so they should!

Do you still have some lingering respect for the multi-national legal drug pushers? Then consider what Dr Sherri Tenpenny sent to Betty Martini, the American aspartame activist, who sent it to me: "CellCept is a drug that they give to patients who have had **organ transplants!!** Inactive ingredients in CellCept Oral Suspension include aspartame, citric acid anhydrous, colloidal silicon dioxide, methylparaben, mixed fruit flavour, sodium citrate dihydrate, sorbitol, soybean lecithin, and xanthan gum. http://www.rxlist.com/cgi/generic3/cellcept.htm.

There is nothing in the above ingredients that isn't known to be unhealthful and much that is well known to be extremely dangerous. Yet, it is formulated for some of medicine's most vulnerable patients. I rest my case.

For harrowing testimonials about drug dangers type "quitpaxil" into your search engine and then click on "withdrawal symptoms". If, after reading this, you decide to take antidepressants, you really *do* need mental help!

Oral Care?

Throughout this book you will find explanations and descriptions of the effects of a wide variety of toxic chemicals and substances which manufacturers are permitted to put into food and other products, with disregard to the short- and long-term health effects they may have on susceptible people. With that in mind, here's a list of ingredients taken directly from the packaging of *Listerine CoolMint Pocket Pak Oral Care Strips*. The makers, Warner-Lambert, a division of Pfizer, instruct you to place a strip on your tongue and let it dissolve. Good Luck!

Pullilan	Cineole (eucalyptol)
Flavours	Methyl salicylate
Menthol	Glycerol oleate
Aspartame	Thymol
Acesulfame	Locust bean gum
Potassium	Propylene glycol
Copper gluconate	Xanthan gum
Polysorbate 80	Fast green FCF
Carrageenan	Phenylketonurics:
	Contains Phenylalanine

To be fair, they do include a warning on the pack; that the little pouch containing the strips "may present a choking hazard". That's all right, then.

Take Control of Your Health and Escape the Sickness Industry

21

Vaccinations

At best – useless;
at worst – dangerous.

Flu vaccines are nearly useless in preventing flu, and the shots weaken the immune system, making victims more predisposed to illnesses. Severe nervous system damage from the injections can take years for the body to repair, if it can be repaired at all. Side effects from the vaccines include headaches, muscle pain, fever, exhaustion and a bad case of, you guessed it, the flu, and sometimes even pneumonia. This is what Dr Joseph Mercola has to say about these medical/pharmaceutical money makers:

> "When one digs into the vaccine history (check out the Swine Flu vaccine if you want a real horror story) and scientific research (especially in Europe), it quickly becomes apparent that nobody really knows what these toxic stews of chemicals and micro-organisms do in the human body. ...I have heard some authors state that there is a direct correlation of the number of flu shots one has and the incidence of Alzheimer's. This would be due to the aluminium and mercury that is in every flu shot."

When a doctor approaches brandishing a hypodermic, bear in mind that the contents are prepared with chicken embryo fluid, which has been inoculated with the living flu strains. It is then treated with formaldehyde (embalming fluid) to inactivate the virus. Then, mercury is added to preserve the chemical stew. But that's not enough – anti-freeze (ethylene glycol) and phenol are put in to disinfect, and even animal viruses are sometimes introduced, undetected. It also contains aluminium, which contributes to Alzheimer's disease. My advice is to keep your immune system strong through strict eating habits, and sail through the flu season unvaccinated and healthy.

You still want to be vaccinated for the flu or for anything else? So be it – it's your life and your decision. It is, however, a totally different issue when helpless babies are offered up as sacrificial lambs to the inoculation industry. Let me recount just one instance of the duplicity which seems to be endemic amongst those 'caring' pharmaceutical giants. It has recently been revealed that Eli Lilly & Co. have known for decades that their mercury-based vaccine preservative *thimerosal* caused neurological injury to infants. Thimerosal is the most common preservative used in vaccines and biologics marketed in the United States and most other countries. It's widely used to help prevent a vaccine from spoiling, for inactivating bacteria used to formulate several vaccines, and in preventing bacterial contamination of the final product. However, reports have surfaced linking thimerosal to mercury poisoning in infants – often causing autism.

That Lilly have been aware of this danger for all these years has only come to light as a result of the discovery process in a series of co-ordinated US lawsuits against Lilly on behalf of injured babies. Yet they are still using it, as are other drug companies, and the company itself even put out warnings to doctors in 1999 citing:

"Primary Physical & Reproduction Effects: Nervous System and Reproduction Effects…

"Effects of exposure include fetal changes…

"Mercury poisoning may occur…

"Exposure in children may cause mild to severe mental retardation….

"Hypersensitivity to mercury is a medical condition aggravated by exposure…

"CERCLA Hazardous substance - toxic waste disposal…"

The evidence which has been uncovered comes from Lilly's own archives and shows that for some 70 years numerous well-credentialed researchers have provided the company with many papers indicating concerns about the safety of their vaccines. The documents clearly demonstrate that thimerosal was known as early as April 1930 to be dangerous. In its apparent eagerness to promote and market the product, in September 1930 Eli Lilly secretly sponsored a 'human toxicity' study on patients already known to be dying of meningococcal meningitis.

According to Andrew Waters, a senior law partner in the firm handling the lawsuits, "Lilly then cited this study repeatedly for decades as proof that thimerosal was of low toxicity and harmless to humans. They never revealed to the scientific community or the public the highly questionable nature of the original research."

Waters adds that while Eli Lilly made every effort to prevent the results of its questionable secret study appearing in medical and scientific literature, other researchers have provided Lilly with numerous articles since the 1930s indicating concerns about thimerosal and its potential hazard to humans who might be exposed or injected with the substance. The evidence clearly demonstrates that Eli Lilly was advised repeatedly that their conclusions of low toxicity were not warranted and that they failed to pass the information on to appropriate federal and public health authorities.

But they just didn't care then and they certainly don't care now. They have powerful friends to look after their interests as "a matter of national security." Just before President Bush signed the Homeland Security Bill into law (an allegedly anti-terrorism measure) an unknown member of Congress inserted a last-minute provision into the legislation, which effectively blocks lawsuits being launched against major pharmaceuticals like Lilly. The action was shrouded in mystery until House Majority Leader Dick Armey told **CBS News** he was behind it. "It's a matter of national security. We need their vaccines if the country is attacked with germ weapons," said Armey, apparently concerned that if these large companies were bankrupted through losing class actions, the US would have no defence against biological warfare!

Is it just coincidence that Lilly is a major GOP campaign donor, has a large lobbying presence in Washington, and connections to the White House that include CEO Sidney Taurel's appointment to the White House Homeland Security Advisory Council itself? Or that, having created an epidemic of infant neurological disorders, Lilly is now making more billions out of manufacturing drugs to treat those conditions?

Ask Your Doctor

What about the doctors? Are they warning mothers that vaccinations may kill or destroy their baby's health? I don't think so. Consider this bit of news from www.redflagweekly.com :

July 8, 2002

DOCS GET BONUS FOR GIVING MMR VACCINE

What next? It seems that in the UK, GPs have been getting payments for rounding up their patients for the MMR (measles, mumps, rubella) vaccine. If 90 percent are vaccinated, they receive £2,865, but the payola drops to £955 if only 70 percent are vaccinated.

It seems now that the docs are concerned that they may be wrecking their credibility with their patients. Sure, especially since the MMR has become so controversial.

Let's get this straight: they've been receiving extra money for vaccine targeting? Isn't that a CONFLICT OF INTEREST? Or are British docs too dumb to understand that?

I wonder whether this corrupt practice is occurring in Australia, in the US, in Canada, in Europe? Maybe it is, but I don't have the evidence. Why not ask your physician?

In Indiana, USA, (the State that just happens, coincidentally, to house the corporate headquarters of Eli Lilly & Co) where vaccinations against eight diseases are now *mandatory* before a child may start school, the number of autistic children grew from 116 in 1989, to 3789 in 2001. Local Congressman Dan Burton described what happened to his grandson: "Shortly after getting a round of childhood vaccinations, he became a different child. He no longer spoke. He would not look anyone in the eye. He cried endlessly, banging his head. He began running around flapping his hands. We now know he was suffering from an adverse reaction to his vaccines."

Victims of the Pharmaceuticals

Is this what you want for your child? For your grandchild? For any child, anywhere? Coulter and Fisher, in *A Shot In The Dark*, say, "The childhood vaccination program is the only possible cause of the mass epidemic of clinical and sub-clinical encephalitis." The authors provide strong evidence that DPT vaccine causes encephalitis, and state that 12,000 to 15,000 cases of severe neurological damage are caused by childhood vaccine each year in the US. But, and this is really scary, "one child in five or six is affected to some degree." This means that the millions of 'difficult' children, ADHD children, children with intractable behaviour problems who are making the lives of parents and teachers miserable, could simply be more victims of the pharmaceuticals. There are no studies to prove or disprove this hypothesis – who would fund them? But I am positive of one thing; when I was young there were no crazy children running around, teenaged murderers were unheard of, and there were no mandatory childhood injections. Sure, there were a few kids with discipline problems, but principals and fathers with straps soon sorted them out. They were not made insane by legal drugs and a polluted food supply, and were amenable to reason.

How, in a relatively short period of time, did the Western world go so far wrong? The answer is simple, of course, and we can lay the blame on the pharmaceuticals who wrested control of governments, bribed (with cushy perks) and snowed doctors, and turned formerly self-reliant Westerners into drug-dependent wimps.

What is so terrible about having measles, whooping cough and mumps? They left us with lifetime immunity and bodies that had not been severely compromised by deadly vaccinations. Of course, this approach meant that mothers, or members of the extended family that existed in those days, had to be home to look after us. Nowadays, mothers work, grandparents are languishing in nursing homes drugged out of their skulls, and daycare facilities freak out if a child shows symptoms of illness.

There are some compassionate doctors, and the Association of American Physicians and Surgeons proved it recently when they voted unanimously for a moratorium on vaccine mandates. Part of the statement read, "Vaccinations should be based on decisions made by fully informed parents, and not imposed by health officials zealous to comply with unwise vaccine laws."

Sure, and how are parents expected to become informed, and what do they do when schools ban their children?

The following letter appeared in *The Australian* in October, 2000:

Again the Australian Government is a day late and a dollar short in protecting the health of its citizens. Two years ago, New Zealand banned blood donations from people in danger of transmitting CJD. What did Australia do? Nothing! One year ago, the US withdrew from use the Hepatitis B vaccine containing mercury because it had the potential to cause brain damage in infants. What did Australia do? Worse than nothing – we introduced this very vaccine into the infant schedule! Our Government and our Minister for Health have shown time and again that when it comes to ensuring Australians have the best and safest medicines and vaccines, they are asleep at the wheel. John Howard and Dr Wooldridge, wake up while you still have a population to govern.

Meryl W. Dorey, President, The Australian Vaccination Network www.avn.org.au

Well, Dr Wooldridge no longer holds the Health portfolio, but regrettably we have seen no affirmative action from either of his recent successors.

What in the world are the pharmaceuticals thinking of, putting mercury, ammonium sulfate, beta-propiolactone, genetically modified yeast, animal, bacterial & viral DNA, latex rubber, monosodium glutamate, aluminium, formaldehyde, micro-organisms, polysorbate 80, tri (n) butylphosphate, glutaraldehyde, gelatin, gentamicin sulfate & polymyxin B, neomycin sulfate, phenol/phenoxyethanol, human & animal cells, one of the most deadly poisons on our planet, into injections?

Can no one put a brake on these profit-obsessed egomaniacs? They belong in jail, or, better yet, strung upside down in the village square as object lessons.

> A major cause of the Roman Empire's decline after six centuries of world dominance was its replacement of stone aqueducts by lead pipes for the transportation and supply of drinking water. Roman engineers, the best in the world, turned their fellow citizens into neurological cripples. Today our own "best and brightest," achieve the same end through childhood vaccination programs yielding the modern scourges of hyperactivity, learning disabilities, autism, appetite disorders, and impulsive violence.
>
> *- Harris L. Coulter, Ph.D.*

> For every complicated problem, there is a solution that is simple, direct, understandable and wrong.
>
> *- H. L. Mencken*

> Nature gave us two ends – one to sit on and one to think with!
>
> Our success depends upon which one we use the most.
>
> Heads we win –
> Tails we lose.

We Must Stick Together!

There are hundreds, if not thousands, of safe and effective natural remedies. Those in this chapter are just a few that I have found to be helpful, and I hope that readers will send me their favourites so they can be included in later editions of this book. After all, we 'health nuts' need to stick together; we are badly outnumbered by the people who think we're crazy, by governments which only support orthodox, poisonous modalities, and by those physicians who believe that the only way to 'cure' a sick body is to poison, cut or burn it.

I'm hopeful that, after reading this book, you will have decided to never touch manufactured food again. You have a choice: sacrifice yourself on the altar of bigger and better manufactured foods and pharmaceutical profits, or use the brains nature gave you to truly -

"Take Control of Your Health, and Escape the Sickness Industry".

22

Smoke Gets in Your Eyes,
your hair, your skin, your lungs,
and everyone else's

Chances are, since you're reading a book on natural health, you're not a smoker. People who are capable of sucking deadly poisons into their bodies are not likely to care much about natural health. What possible difference can it make? So, smokers, I leave you to your fate – my concern is for us passive smokers.

Second-Hand Smoke

The smoker pollutes the air you breathe in two ways: with mainstream smoke, which the smoker inhales, then exhales, and with sidestream smoke, which comes directly from the burning end of the cigarette, cigar, or pipe. A cigarette smoker spends only 24 seconds in the actual process of inhaling and exhaling mainstream smoke. But the cigarette burns for approximately 12 minutes and during that time it pollutes the air continuously with sidestream smoke. Smokers can keep cigars and pipes burning much longer. And of course all smoking pollution remains long after the smoker has stopped.

Even when a smoker inhales, researchers have calculated that two-thirds of the smoke from the burning cigarette goes into the environment. The percentage of pollution from cigar and pipe smoke is even higher. The amount of carbon monoxide generated from one cigar, in fact, is twice as high as from three cigarettes smoked simultaneously.

Insidiously, sidestream smoke contains far more of the carcinogenic tars and smoke particles and concentrations of noxious compounds than the mainstream smoke inhaled by the smoker. This exposure is deadly, because the toxic and carcinogenic chemicals released from the burning tip of the cigarette enter the atmosphere totally unfiltered by a mat of tobacco. Some studies show there is twice as much tar and nicotine in sidestream smoke compared to mainstream. And three times more of a compound called *3-4 benzopyrene*, which is a carcinogen. And five times more carbon monoxide, which robs the blood of oxygen. And 50 times more ammonia.

There is also evidence that there is even more cadmium in sidestream smoke than in mainstream. Cadmium damages the air sacs of the lungs and causes emphysema. Once cadmium gets into your lungs, you've got it. It never goes away.

An Efficient Way to Commit Suicide

Tests made in enclosed areas found that one pack of burning cigarettes produced levels of nitrosamine carcinogens ten times higher than in the inhaled smoke itself, and carbon monoxide levels of 70 parts per million. In this environment, the carboxyhemoglobin level of the non-smokers – a measure of carbon monoxide inhalation – doubled. And remember, the carbon monoxide emissions from a vehicle's exhaust in a closed garage provides an efficient way to commit suicide.

Sidestream smoke also contains free radicals and aldehydes, so the smoke delivers a double molecular-level injury by introducing pathological free radicals into the system and destroying cysteine. And, ladies, it is the free radicals and aldehydes which create wrinkles.

The Thoracic Society of Australia, in a report in the **Medical Journal of Australia**, states that an hour a day in a room with a smoker is nearly one hundred times more likely to cause lung cancer in a non-smoker than 20 years spent in a building containing asbestos. Another study shows that after only 30 minutes in a smoke-filled room the carbon monoxide level in the non-smoker's blood increases, as well as the blood pressure and heart beat.

And now for the worst news of all; it has been discovered, through autopsies, that the lungs of smokers contain radioactive particles, called radon daughters, in amounts equivalent to what would be accumulated from 300 X-rays per year. The sources of the radiation are polonium 210 and lead 210, both found in phosphate-fertilised tobacco plants and in tobacco smoke. What is most alarming is that 75 percent of the radiation in tobacco smoke enters the atmosphere and is inhaled by others. Us. You and I, our children, our aged parents, our friends. We don't *need* this additional radiation. It's bad enough that we have to have occasional medical and dental X-rays, that we are exposed to radiation from flying, from the atmosphere and from irradiated food. There is no such thing as a safe dose of radiation. It is nothing short of criminal that smokers expose us all to additional, preventable doses of this deadly poison.

The most vulnerable passive smokers are babies in the womb. If you are pregnant and still smoking, *quit now* if you have a shred of human decency. Your unborn baby cannot protect him or herself – that is *your* job. Just remember that with every puff, the amount of blood and oxygen going to the foetus is decreased. This is what creates brain damage. Five minutes after you have a cigarette, your baby's heart speeds up and breathing movements decrease. These are signs of foetal distress. Blood pressure is raised during and after smoking. This is harmful to both mother and child. Your risk of having a stillborn baby is significantly increased, and you are 80 percent more likely to have a spontaneous abortion than a non-smoker. According to Dr Samuel S. Epstein, American Professor of Occupational and Environmental Medicine at the School of Public Health in Illinois, just one cigarette per day can damage the foetus!

Assault With a Deadly Weapon

If you smoke, your baby's body and brain will weigh less at birth and its chances of mental retardation and birth defects, such as cleft palate and harelip, will be higher. There is strong evidence of development problems later in life, and your child's height may be affected. Lower IQ scores, reading disability, behavioural problems and hyperactivity are all seen in the children of smoking mothers. Nothing can excuse a woman who allows such life-threatening things to happen to her unborn child!

Babies have small lungs and very small airways, so smoke-filled air impairs their breathing. Babies and young children breathe much faster than adults, meaning they inhale more air – and more pollution – in comparison to their body weight. Infants whose parents smoke at home have a higher rate of pneumonia and bronchitis. Many researchers have found that the dreaded sudden infant death syndrome is passive smoking-related. Zinc, which is vital for healthy growth in babies, becomes deficient in babies who are forced to breathe tobacco smoke. The breast milk of smoking women contains significant amounts of nicotine.

If we lived in a decent society, people who smoke in front of babies and children would be jailed for assault with a deadly weapon. And kept there until they kicked their murderous habit.

Years ago the Surgeon General of the United States declared smoking the most important health issue of our time and urged non-smokers to avoid passive smoking. That is easier said than done. But if you don't, you'll have lots more illnesses, and you'll die prematurely. So, if you're exposed to it in the workplace, do your best to educate your boss and your fellow workers. If your friends smoke, set up new ground rules or replace your friends. And if your spouse smokes, convert him or her, or run screaming to a divorce lawyer.

> *Voltaire wrote this 250 years ago:*
>
> Section 1.02 Physicians pour drugs of which they know little, to cure diseases of which they know less, into humans of which they know nothing.
>
> *Has anything changed since?*

> The art of medicine consists in amusing the patient while nature cures the disease.
>
> *- Voltaire*

> "A lie can run around the world before the truth gets its boots on."
>
> *Mark Twain*

23

Radiation Rampage

Unfortunately it's almost inescapable, but here are some steps you can take to protect yourself

Nowadays it's virtually impossible to escape electromagnetic radiation, unless you live on a primitive island; everywhere you go, you are likely to be exposed to these dangerous and invisible rays. No matter how hard you try to limit your exposure, there are always people nearby jabbering on mobile phones, zapping themselves, and you, simultaneously. Other electronic devices like television sets, computer monitors, hand-held games, watches, household appliances, miniature batteries, overhead electricity cables, cordless phones and transmission towers which make them possible, are all around you. There's no magic shield that I can offer to protect you from the dangers inherent in this inevitable hazard of modern living; but I can offer some recommendations and aids that should at least lessen their effect on your well being and health. So, let's examine the culprits.

X *Mobile Telephones*

Some scientists say you are safe only if you are 10 metres away from a mobile phone, others say 30 metres. Not only are we 'passive smokers', we are now 'passive phoners.' My only consolation when people sit down next to me in a place from which I can't escape and start blathering, is that their brains are being deep-fried, while mine is merely being sautéed.

Our brains and eyes have never before had such concentrated exposure to microwaves such as they get from using a cellular phone, jammed close to the skull. This is unprecedented in evolutionary history, and will have, and is having, profound effects upon people who foolishly use them, and those of us who are unwillingly exposed to them. Don't be seduced by the hands-free mobiles. The earpiece concentrates the radiation even more, and zaps it straight into the head. To give an indication how serious the problem is, the Japanese buy clothes made from shielding materials.

Mobile phone use has been linked to human cancer in a scientific study, with research showing it may induce eye cancer. While most fears about mobile phones have related to brain tumours, a study of 500 people in the UK found a threefold increase in eye cancer among people who regularly use the devices.

The mechanism by which the radiation might cause cancer is uncertain, but it is known that the watery content of the eye assists the absorption of radiation.

Other research showed that cells called *malanocytes* found in the uveal layer started growing and dividing more rapidly when exposed to microwave radiation. Multibillion-pound lawsuits against Verizon Horizon – an American mobile phone company 45 percent owned by the British Vodaphone telecom provider – have been launched. Customers claim they got brain tumours and other conditions from using the devices.

And at least one concerned medical professional has come out strongly against the urge of masses of people to submit themselves to these biological hazards. *Time Magazine, February 24 2003*, reported, " 'This is the largest biological experiment in the history of the world,' shouts Leif Salford, an unusually animated neurosurgeon at Lund University, in Sweden. Salford's not talking about his own work. He's talking about the 1.3 billion people around the world who regularly chat away on their mobile phones, 'freely pressing radiological devices to their brains.' " Do you really want to be a part of that experiment, especially as the dangers are becoming more and more apparent?

If you must use a mobile, consider buying a protective case that shields the head. There is research indicating that these reduce emissions. If you use a mobile inside a car, bus, train or ferry, the radiation will be increased considerably, because in order to overcome the metal shielding the power is increased to maximum. If it's your decision to court brain tumours and all the other dangers associated with mobiles, so be it. But please, spare a thought for your fellow passengers.

In fact, much of the danger to 'passive phoners' and cell-phone users could be avoided by redesigning these communications devices; except that manufacturers refuse to incorporate technical safeguards that have long been available. The *New Zealand Herald, April 4 2003*, reported a claim by Dr Neil Cherry, associate professor in environmental health, Lincoln University, Christchurch, that, "Even though science shows that mobile phones are more dangerous than tobacco, they [*the manufacturers*] use the fact that radiation is invisible and can't be seen or smelt like smoke. There are more than 50 patents for devices or methods to make phones safer that are not being used by manufacturers."

As usual, keeping costs down and profits up are more important to manufacturers than the health of their customers. After all, there's plenty more where they came from.

In Russia, evidence that mobile phone usage can be dangerous has been taken very seriously, and the Russian National Committee on Non-Ionizing Radiation Protection (RNCNIRP) published the following in March, 2003:

RNCNIRP ADVICE ON THE SAFE USE OF MOBILE PHONES

The RNCNIRP offers the following advice on the safe use of mobile phones. These recommendations are based on the precautionary principle of the World Health Organization, published scientific and medical studies, reviews and recommendations by scientific groups and the expert opinions of RNCNIRP members.

1. Children under the age of 16 should not use mobile phones.

2. Pregnant women should not use mobile phones.

3. Those suffering from neurologic diseases such as neurasthenia, psychopathy, psychosteny, and all neurosis with asthenic, obsessional hysterical disorders and reducing of mental, physical activity, memory loss, sleep disorders, epilepsy and epileptic syndrome, epileptic predisposition should not use mobile phones.

4. The duration of calls should be limited to a maximum of three minutes, and after making a call the user should wait a minimum of 15 minutes before making another call. The use of headsets and hands-free systems is strongly encouraged. Manufacturers and retailers of mobile phones should include the following information together with the engineering specifications:
All of the above recommendations regarding use; all relevant health and epidemiological data on mobile phones, together with the radiation exposure levels associated with the phone and the name of the measurement lab.

X Cordless Telephones

Mobile phones have gotten the bad press, but portable, cordless, phones are nearly as dangerous. And the latest more sophisticated models operate on higher radio frequencies (2.4 GigaHertz), which puts them in the same category as the mobile phones.

It has long been known that medical radiation can cause baldness. Now evidence is surfacing regarding baldness behind the listening ears of heavy-to-moderate users of cordless phones. These bald patches conform exactly to the shape of the antenna's receiver. Even more disquieting, much smaller patches of baldness are showing up behind the passive ear, indicating that the phone's radiation is sailing right through the head! This information was confirmed by a hairdresser, who told me that this is a common problem among people using the 2.4 GigaHertz cordless models, that doctors are baffled (aren't they always?), and that the hair will grow back once use is discontinued. Yes, but will the brain tumour the radiation may have caused dissolve?

The **Hobart Mercury,** *July 6 1999*, reported that "Cordless telephones could pose the same threat to health as mobile phones. Scientists say radiation emitted by the handsets could interfere with the brain, causing memory loss, headaches, dizziness and even cancer."

Associate Fellow of Physics at Warwick University, Dr Gerard Hyland, an expert on electro-magnetic radiation, says cordless phones could pose a greater risk than mobile handsets because they are used frequently and for long periods. He adds, "You could say these are worse than mobiles because you have the phone and the base station, both emitting microwave radiation, sitting in the same room with you. This has got to be looked into." (Sure, and the 'study' would no doubt be funded by the very companies which manufacture the phones; care to guess what the findings might be?)

Because of the many electromagnetic devices in our office, my associates and I were extremely uncomfortable. This is understandable, considering that we were being subjected to constant electromagnetic bombardment. One attributed her daily headaches to glasses that needed to be adjusted. When I smartened up and had the office de-zapped, there was an immediate improvement; headaches gone, never to return, and a lovely, peaceful feeling.

We never thought we'd do something that 'far-out', but we all (including the entire staff at Hippocrates) are now wearing *Tesla* pendants around our necks to protect us in the outside, mobile phone-crazy world, and they really work. As well, we are protected from our own mobiles. Many of our students buy the pendants and have reported relief from pain, increases in energy, improved sleep and a feeling of calm. The devices range in size from tiny (for mobile phone protection) to large plates (for easing pain). Amazing stuff! There are many such devices on the market, but after testing we found that those made by *Tesla* (of specially treated titanium) are the best. Check **Resources** for details.

✗ *Radar Antennae*

Keep as far away as possible from radar installations. When travelling, avoid airport hotels, because many people are so disturbed by radar emissions that sleep is impossible for them.

✗ *Radio, TV and Mobile Phone Transmitters*

Don't build, buy or rent a house close to these transmitters. If the government decides to allow one to be built near you, organise your neighbours and make a huge fuss. Download scientific reports from the internet, remind the politicians that alpine forests in Europe located near large aerials are dying; threaten lawsuits, organise pickets.

The UK newspaper, *The Telegraph, April 25 2003*, reported,

Residents of a hamlet near a mobile telephone mast have recorded high levels of illness, including seven cases of cancer, raising fresh concerns over the safety of the transmitters. Among the 50 people living in Wishaw, Warwickshire, 34 people have reported medical complaints in the past two years. Five women have been diagnosed with breast cancer and two men have been told they have tumours. All live within a mile of the mast.

Regular complaints include sleeplessness, skin irritation and problems with the immune system. Now an application has been submitted to build another transmitter next to Wishaw. The Government says mobile telephone masts are no threat to public health.

Now, why does that last sentence come as no surprise? Or this, from a representative of the phone company involved, "T-Mobile is satisfied that the site meets with national and international guidelines, is safe and does not present a health risk to any member of the public."

The siting of phone masts, with the usual government acquiescence, is yet another example of corporate greed being allowed to triumph over the health of the citizens despite credible evidence of the inherent dangers involved. Dr Hyland again: "No research has been undertaken into this system and its safety. People are being used as guinea pigs. Their fears [*about masts*] are not unfounded."

X TV and Computer Screens

Keep the television as far away from viewers as the room will allow. Remember that the backs and sides of TV sets and PC monitors are even more dangerous than the screen. Limit your exposure as best you can, and be strict with children who want to sit close, as they are in even more danger than adults. There are devices for computers that offer protection, and there are screens that can be installed in front which cut radiation. Liquid Crystal Display (LCD) and Thin Film Technology (TFT) computer screens are said to be radiation-free, and plasma and back-projection television screens are safe.

X Electricity Meter Boxes

Take care that any meter boxes installed on an exterior wall of your home are well away from where your family lives and sleeps. No matter how well built, your house walls will not stop the radiation. Exposure, especially for young people, is dangerous, sometimes fatal. There have been many instances of children dying from leukemia from such exposure. These boxes can create electro-stress 50 times above normal tolerance. In Australia, Carol Fisher, from Tesla's, will make house calls to check for danger areas (see *Resources*).

On the right, Dr Mercola gives ten very good reasons for discarding this 'essential' kitchen aid. Perhaps a bit drastic for some – but, you have been warned!

There is a simple solution to this problem; eat mostly raw, and when you must cook, use an old-fashioned stove. If you decide you just can't remove your microwave, at least be sure to disconnect it, because the darn things leak radiation, even when not in use. Your health will improve, as microwaved food causes cancer-type effects in the blood, lowers haemoglobin values, causes white blood cells to decrease and leads to serious degeneration of the body.

According to *Nutrition And Healing*, *June 6, 1999,*

"Doctors Hertl and Blanc of Switzerland tested luminescent (light-emitting) bacteria by exposing them to the blood of test subjects who had eaten, or not eaten, microwaved food. They found that the luminous power of bacteria in contact with serum of test persons who consumed food prepared in the microwave oven was significantly higher than those subjects who ate food not exposed to microwave radiation. So there is a strong suggestion that some form of radiant energy may be transferred into our cells as a result of eating microwaved food."

Definitely food for thought!

Ten Reasons to Throw Out Your Microwave Oven

1 Continually eating food processed from a microwave oven causes long term, permanent, brain damage by "shorting out" electrical impulses in the brain (de-polarizing or de-magnetizing the brain tissue).

2 The human body cannot metabolise, break down, the unknown by-products created in microwaved food.

3 Male and female hormone production is shut down and/or altered by continually eating microwaved foods.

4 The effects of microwaved food by-products are residual (long term, permanent) within the human body.

5 Minerals, vitamins, and nutrients of all microwaved food are reduced or altered so that the human body gets little or no benefit, or the body absorbs altered compounds that cannot be broken down.

6 The minerals in vegetables are altered into cancerous free radicals when cooked in microwave ovens.

7 Microwaved foods cause stomach and intestinal cancerous growths (tumors). This may explain the rapidly increasing rate of colon cancer in America.

8 The prolonged eating of microwaved foods causes cancerous cells to increase in human blood.

9 Continual ingestion of microwaved food causes immune system deficiencies through lymph gland and blood serum alterations.

10 Eating microwaved food causes loss of memory, concentration, emotional instability, and a decrease of intelligence.

Joseph Mercola, MD,
writing in
The Townsend Letter for Doctors & Patients

X Wrist Watches

Battery-operated watches emit low-level radiation. Also, beware of watches which glow in the dark – they will radiate you.

X Electric Blankets

Scientists have found extremely high levels of radiation in beds using electric blankets and in heated waterbeds. If it is so cold that you must warm the bed, do so before retiring, then switch off the power. Remove the plugs also, as even when the appliance is turned off, the electricity is still flowing. Motorised beds are worse, because the spine and organs are directly above the motor.

X Bug Zappers

These devices are bad news. According to *Annals Of Internal Medicine*, *June 1, 1998*, "When a common house fly gets zapped by an electric trap, bacteria that have collected on the surface of the insect are blasted into the air. In a still air environment, a zapper can hurl bacteria as far as six feet.

"And if that zapper is near a fan or an air conditioning vent, who knows how far those bacteria will travel? Because the study shows that the bacteria covering the legs and bodies of house flies are obtained from human or animal wastes, the bug zappers may be spreading more disease than they prevent."

X Medical X-Rays

Avoid being X-rayed unless absolutely necessary. The procedure is often ordered by doctors eager to cover themselves from lawsuits, which is understandable, but hard on patients. *There is no safe level of radiation!* 'Photo opportunity' X-rays and ultra-sounds of babies should be considered child abuse. Use your common sense – why bombard a vulnerable foetus with either of these powerful energies? What might it do to the delicate mechanisms of the brain, the eyes, the ears? Do you want to be responsible for the subtle brain damage that investigators believe is caused by these unnecessary procedures?

I'd love to get my hands on the gung-ho American doctors who are condemning thousands of children to early death from radiation-induced cancers. Overused CT scans (US doctors are prescribing 2 million of these annually) are the culprits, as doses of radiation from a single procedure can be hundreds of times larger than the effective dose of radiation from a conventional radiographic procedure. What parents are not told when their doctors schedule this relatively new procedure is that these scans are calibrated for adults, so children absorb up to six times the radiation needed to produce clear images. *These doses are much larger than the doses to which the victims of Three Mile Island were subjected.* Children have more rapidly dividing cells than adults, and they are much more susceptible to radiation damage.

Look at it this way: you would want to think long and hard before subjecting your young daughter to the equivalent of up to 20 mammograms in one procedure. What did doctors do before these diabolical things were invented? Somehow we all managed to get along with the family doctor who gave us a real physical, looked at our irises, and asked pointed questions about our diets.

✗ Fluorescent Lighting and Halogen Lamps

There is a great deal of evidence that these forms of lighting are damaging. Stick, as much as possible, to natural sunlight and incandescent lighting, and if you must use fluorescent, use only the full-spectrum tubes.

✗ High-Voltage Transmission Lines

According to researchers, every fourth home in the US is built near electrical high tension wires. Cancer incidence in those homes is twice as high as it is in homes not subject to this form of radiation.

Governments, electricity providers and electronics companies are doing their utmost to falsify studies and sweep ones they can't refute under the carpet. Or just ignore them altogether.

Here in sunny Queensland (at Mudgeeraba on the Gold Coast) a large school was built a stone's throw from huge transmission towers, when it is common knowledge that 500 metres distance from these monstrosities is the absolute minimum. Hippocrates Health Centre staff joined concerned parents in protesting, and even our State MP spoke up. He said that official reports had shown the school site had magnetic field radiations in excess of two milligauss (a dangerous level.) "I find it absolutely appalling that a minister [*then Education Minister David Hamill*] would go ahead with a school on this site when he knows the dangers involved and when the community has clearly rejected it," he told the **Gold Coast Bulletin,** *September 20, 1995.* Some parents refused to enrol their children, but most went along, like sheep, when they should have been picketing.

When driving under these lines with a car radio on, there is suddenly a great deal of interference, as I'm sure most have noticed. This also happens, to a lesser degree, close to ordinary power poles, most noticeably those that support transformer boxes. This interference phenomenon also takes place in the body, with repercussions that have not even been considered by government authorities.

Certainly, we cannot live without electricity, unless we give up our 'civilised' lifestyle. What we can do, is try to limit our exposure and bear in mind the location of electricity wires when positioning our houses, and especially our bedrooms.

X Household Appliances

Switch off the electricity to any device you are not using, to reduce your exposure. Use hairdryers as little as possible. Clock radios generate electromagnetic fields and should be kept well away from people.

X Another Dangerous Invention

WHAT DOCTORS DON'T TELL YOU reported another menace to watch out for – wireless modems, with a base station that "...transmits microwaves 24 hours a day at a frequency of 2.4 GHz, extending to a radius of 150 feet." They have been found to cause heart arrhythmia, sleeplessness, abnormal fatigue, dizziness, vomiting, vertigo and oxygen deprivation in healthy people. These deadly little instruments "...are being placed in the foyers of airports, hotels, in GP's surgeries, coffee shops and students' halls of residence, so individuals can use their laptops with the minimum of fuss. From March 2004, a number of airlines will have introduced them on their planes. Following trials by BA and Lufthansa... The base station is marketed by NET GEAR and is called a Wireless ADSL Modem Gateway DG824M." This "convenience" will damage healthy people and seriously threaten the lives of delicate people, babies, children, foetuses, and those with heart problems and/or pacemakers.

Flying is miserable enough already with the extreme dryness, radiation, deep vein thrombosis and crowding. A few of these modems in so tiny an area will render flying unbearable for sensitive people. We'd better all stay home!

X Irradiated Food

Governments are pushing this technology down the throats (literally) of hapless citizens, and they are doing it without any studies of the effects it will have on our health, long-term. Short studies have been done, and some are disquieting. A group of children in India were fed irradiated wheat and they were found to have chromosomal damage after only six weeks.

Immune system damage, cardiac blood clots, testicular damage, fibroplasia and kidney disease have been indicated in several studies. Food irradiation creates radiolytic products that include formaldehyde and benzene, known cancer risks. It has been known since inception that food irradiation kills enzymes and vitamins and destroys food's nutritional value. Further, disposing, storing and transporting deadly cobalt-60 is a huge problem, aggravated by slack regulations. What are governments thinking of? Have they all gone mad? All we can do is make a fuss at the supermarket and complain to our representatives, and hope that they are not 'owned' by the multinationals. Money speaks loudly. If the supermarkets get the idea that we won't buy irradiated food, they will use their considerable clout to stop this dreadful practice.

Manufacturers and growers are already scared of a strong consumer backlash against this process, if a disturbing report I received just recently is anything to go on. In the US, Senator Tom Harkin has been largely successful in his underhanded attempts to *rename* irradiation – presumably to put the opponents off the scent. Harkin, who belongs in the nation's Hall of Shame, added an amendment to the Farm Bill that would allow irradiated foods to be labelled as 'pasteurised'. Food corporations seeking to use the 'pasteurised' label would only have to apply for permission to do so from the secretary of Health and Human Services (HHS). No checks, no balances. Moreover, Harkin's amendment also directs the HHS to revisit all the existing irradiation requirements, with no provision for public input.

> Formerly, when religion was strong and science weak, men mistook magic for medicine; now, when science is strong and religion weak, men mistake medicine for magic.
> - *Thomas Szasz*

> It's not the things you don't know what gets you into trouble. It's the things you do know that just ain't so.
> - *Will Rogers*

24

Alzheimer's Disease
On the increase – and often avoidable

There has been a staggering increase in Alzheimer's Disease (AD) in recent decades, mostly caused by Western governments. These 'authorities' have permitted and encouraged the doping of our water supplies with silicofluorides, which have been proven over and over again to cause AD (see **Chapter 19**, *Water Woes*).

The evidence against fluoridated water is compelling and has been a matter of public knowledge for nearly a century, yet we citizens in Western democracies sit back like sheep, permitting our governments to force us, through taxation, to pay for our own poison! Rather like the way the Chinese government makes family members pay for the bullet they use to execute their loved ones. Here, the middle class can afford to buy filters for their drinking water but the poor are on their own. Only the wealthy can afford the luxury of filtering their water at source so they will not have to bathe in a known neurotoxin.

I'm angry, and I don't apologise for that, and hope you agree with me that we shouldn't have to fight to keep hazardous wastes out of our water supply! We must protest, because nothing will break the government/industry stranglehold until we do.

Of course, silicofluoride is not the only cause of AD. The *December 1996* issue of *Neurology* reported on a study showing a substantially increased risk of AD in occupations that exposed workers to high levels of electromagnetic radiation. Such people will be well advised to find some way to protect themselves, as their risk is *four times higher than that of the general public* (see **Chapter 26**, *Remedies*). If on top of this risk, these workers are also exposed to fluoride, I don't like their chances.

Because we cannot see electromagnetic radiation, it is easy for governments and industry to 'pooh-pooh' concerns, and even make statements such as, "There is no peer-reviewed literature supporting these outlandish claims." But this is a bald-faced lie. *Neurology* is the official journal of the

American Academy of Neurology, and is one of the most respected scientific journals in the world.

Then there is the danger of aluminium. The investigators at *Neurology* don't like it any better than I do, and reported on a study from the University of Toronto that found a 250 percent increased risk of AD in people who drank municipal water high in aluminium for ten or more years. Researchers found that even small amounts of aluminium in the water increased AD by 70 percent.

These are scary statistics, and my advice is: shun aluminium in all its forms – cookware, foil, self-raising flours (including bread-making flours), non-dairy creamers, cake mixes, antacids, medicines, pesticides, many processed foods and drinks, certain cheeses, anti-perspirants and buffered analgesic products, all of which would be against the law if we had governments dedicated to the public good instead of the protection of industry.

Try this experiment to see what you are drinking. Boil some water in an aluminium saucepan for half an hour. When it cools, pour it into a glass and hold it up to the light. If you see a faint cloud, it is aluminium salts. Make tea with this water and, if your community water supply is fluoridated, there will be a 1000-fold increase in the aluminium. This combination will eventually lead you to a nursing home with a broken hip and/or Alzheimer's Disease.

AD, in common with other serious diseases, is much easier to prevent than to reverse, and it's never too late to start. So, to save yourself from this calamity, shun aluminium, flouridated water, toothpastes, dental fluoride and glass ionomer fillings, which exude fluoride, doing continuous damage. There's more, much more, you can do:

- Eat according to the suggestions in this book
- Drink plenty of water
- Take folic acid and vitamin B-complex, to keep your homocysteine level low
- Take hydrochloric acid, if indicated (see **Chapter 3**, *Stomach Acid*)
- Get plenty of sun without sunscreen for crucial vitamin D
- Get the mercury fillings out of your mouth
- Have no flu vaccinations – they contain mercury and aluminium and can cause AD (see **Chapter 21**, *Vaccinations*)
- Take niacin – it can actually reverse AD in certain cases
- Strictly avoid poisonous aspartame, which is hidden in many medicines and is in at least 9000 commonly-consumed products (see **Chapter 4**, *Excitotoxins*)
- Take a good quality Co-enzyme Q_{10} (Co-Q_{10})
- Keep grain consumption very low to reduce your homocysteine level
- Take as much magnesium as the bowel will tolerate.

If you have a loved one who is afflicted with this dreadful condition, don't look to the medical profession for help. All they have to offer are drugs with such adverse side effects that many countries have banned them. People who take them are often left with severe liver damage, and no improvement in their symptoms.

Many frequently-prescribed drugs contribute to our AD epidemic. L-dopa (*Senemet*) increases homocysteine levels, contributing to AD. *Bactrim* and *Septra* do the same. People who have been on *Tylenol* for two years have a 35 percent higher rate of AD. The cholesterol-lowering statin drugs are a one-way trip to a nursing home – they strip the body of essential Co-enzyme Q_{10}. The pharmaceuticals are aware of this but refuse to issue warnings. They also know that their hugely profitable, aluminium-laced, antacids are a major cause of AD, yet there are no warnings on these over-the-counter killers. I don't have the studies to hand, but my educated guess is that *all* drugs contribute to AD, and I urge everyone to get off them as soon as possible, slowly and carefully, with the help of a trained health professional. Follow the rules in this book and you won't need drugs

In 1999, research from the United Kingdom was released which detailed, in the most persuasive manner, folic acid's relationship with Alzheimer's Disease. The scientists involved in the lengthy trials proved, conclusively, that this dreadful affliction can be prevented, and even partially reversed, if caught early. There are, of course, many other factors involved with this disease, which is discussed in ***Chapter 24***.

If it all seems just too hard, take a careful look at a victim of AD.

SKIN CANCER? GENITAL WARTS?

BEWARE *ALDARA*
3M PHARMACEUTICALS' "CURE"

ALDARA CAN CAUSE:

Anaphylactic Shock
Destruction of Brain Tissue

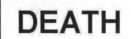
DEATH

Direct Cellular Damage
Irreversible Autoimmune Disease

Governments won't ban it, despite overwhelming evidence.
Establishment media won't publicise the obvious dangers.
WHY? Big Pharma is too powerful!

> *"In my opinion, based on my observations and research, ALDARA should be classified as a criminally dangerous material if used on any open or potentially open skin area."*
>
> Dr. Michael Tait, MB. ChB. MRCGP. MIA Coll, MAAAM, Fountain of Life Clinic, Arundel, Queensland, Australia

Victims speak about ALDARA:
"Five years ago I used ALDARA and I have been deathly ill ever since with autoimmune disease. I would have been better off had it killed me outright as my life has been a misery and my family has been wrecked."
Richard Beasley, Lindale, Texas, USA
www.aldara1.com

"I have been diagnosed with an autoimmune disorder called Graves Basedow Disease. My doctor says it's 99% sure ALDARA caused it."
S.H. Mustafa, Istanbul, Turkey

"I used ALDARA for only two days, yet continued developing sores all over my face, and every night for weeks my pillowslips were covered in blood. I was so sick I couldn't eat. I've never been so miserable, and the skin cancer didn't even go."
Gwen Ward, Southport, Queensland, Australia

"Using ALDARA on a tiny skin cancer was the worst mistake of my life. The anaphylactic shock it caused nearly killed me, and I have been left with severe, probably permanent, health problems."
Elaine Hollingsworth, Mudgeeraba, Queensland, Australia

Scientists speak about ALDARA:
"ALDARA is reasonably anticipated to be a human carcinogen, based on sufficient evidence of carcinogenicity in experimental animals."
American Cancer Society and the National Cancer Institute (USA)

Alterations of the immune system, such as those exhibited by ALDARA … "can severely impact the initiation, severity and persistence of both systemic and organ-specific autoimmunity."
United States Food and Drug Administration (FDA)

3M Pharmaceuticals speaks about ALDARA:
"Applying ALDARA directly into an open wound introduces it into the bloodstream, by what amounts to an intravenous delivery system of the drug."
A pharmacist employed by 3M who prefers that we don't use his name

"The reason to give the drug (ALDARA) intravenously to animals is to KILL them."
Dr Herbert Slade, Director of 3M's Pharmaceutical Division, under oath in US Federal Court, during a personal injury lawsuit brought by a person who was gravely injured by ALDARA.

HAVE <u>YOU</u> BEEN INJURED BY *ALDARA*?

If so, send your story to elaine@doctorsaredangerous.com or telephone +61 7 5530 2939 during business hours or fax +61 7 5569 0884. With enough complaints, governments and the media will be forced to take action. Add your voice, and help us fight back. Only PEOPLE POWER can stop Big Pharma.

For more information about ALDARA visit: **www.doctorsaredangerous.com**

This advertisement was placed as a public service by The Hippocrates Foundation, a charity recognised by the Australian Commonwealth Government. PO Box 1400, Mudgeeraba 4213, Queensland, Australia.

25

The Banned List

Stay away from these if you want to enjoy a long and healthy life

Our modern way of life is very different from that of our parents and earlier forebears. In many ways it may be considered better. But as far as the goodness of what we eat and the things we do to our bodies are concerned, it could be argued that we are at greater risk of being harmed than our ancestors ever were. Manufacturers, food processors, scientists – they all come up with "New! Improved!" delights to tempt us on a daily basis. They try to convince us that we "Can't live without them." I suggest that the truth is more likely that "You won't live long with them."

Here is my list of *Things To Avoid* if you want to give your body – and mind – a decent chance to survive to a ripe old age. It is not in any particular order, and quitting some of them may not cause any pain or inconvenience. Others may be hard for you to even consider giving up, so where possible I also list some safe alternatives that you might like to consider.

✗ *Regular Cosmetics*

During my lectures at Hippocrates, the information I give regarding cosmetics creates consternation. It's understandable, because women hate to think that they have been poisoning themselves expensively for years. I know how I felt when I discovered that those unpronounceable names on cosmetics were deadly coal-tar products that are known to cause susceptible people cancer.

Invariably, one or more of the women who attend tell me about a multi-level cosmetics company that guarantees their products are safe and pure. When I suggest that they bring the bottles and jars to the table, they *really* get depressed. Each and every label on these 'pure' and 'safe' products lists dangerous ingredients, all of which you must avoid: *propylene glycol* (a primary skin irritant), *sodium lauryl* and *laureth sulphate (SLS)*, any *parabens* and any chemical which has the word *propyl* in it – at the front of the word, in the middle, or at the end. Bear in mind too, that the ingredient *quanternium* is simply formaldehyde in disguise.

For example, when *Usana*, a high-profile vitamin producer from the US, came out with *Sense*, a cosmetic line, I was interested to see the 'natural' ingredients the salesman told me about. Their fancy brochure, which I pored over, used lovely phrases, such as "delicate soap-free formula, pure plant extracts, soothing botanicals, whole grape extracts," etc. Reality, alas, was not reassuring, and in such tiny print that I had to use a magnifying glass, the awful truth surfaced: *aminomethyl propanol, butylene glycol, phenoxyethanol, isopropylparaben, isobutylparaben, butylparaben,* just plain *propylparaben, aluminum silicate, methylparaben, sorbitol, ethylparaben*, and on and on and on, with each 'beautifier' containing between 30 and 60 ingredients, none of which I would ever allow to get anywhere near my body. Nor should you.

I'm picking on Usana because I happen to have their brochure in front of me, but most of the heavily advertised 'natural' cosmetics contain ingredients that should be avoided.

In the book, **Dangerous Beauty**, Peter Dingle, BEd, BSc Hons, PhD, a lecturer at Murdoch University in Perth with over 60 scientific publications on chemical exposure and indoor air quality to his name, says, "None of the chemicals in cosmetics and personal care products are fully tested and for most, there is only very basic information available on their health effects. The magnitude of their potential adverse effects is therefore unknown. Increasingly, there appear to be large numbers of the population affected by many of the chemicals contained in these products. Our research results indicate that between 15 and 20 percent of people are acutely affected."

And let's not forget the cruelty to animals the cosmetics companies continue to practice.

X *Shampoos and Hair Treatments*

Those warm and wonderful companies that make shampoos containing *sodium lauryl* and *laureth sulphate* (SLS) don't seem to care that these chemicals have been linked with cancer, vision disorders, dandruff, rashes, hair loss, the breakdown of cell membranes, and allergies. In industry, SLS is used in engine degreasers and floor de-waxers.

Anything that foams up is likely to contain SLS, of course, plus these dangerous chemicals. Most shampoos read like chemistry texts: *cocamido propyl betaine, peg-3 distearate, glycol distearate, polyquaternium-16, hydroxypropyl,* and on and on with a depressing list of extremely dangerous substances that belong in the toxic waste section of your local tip, not on your scalp and from there into your body.

According to biochemist Hulda Regehr Clark, PhD, ND, who has done exhaustive research, of all the chemicals contained in cosmetics and toiletries the solvent *propyl alcohol* is the worst of the lot. She has written three books (see *Resources*) on the connection between this solvent and intestinal parasites. She claims that *all* cancer patients have both the human intestinal fluke and propyl alcohol in their livers. Dr Clark says that this parasite typically lives in the intestines, where it does not do life-threatening harm. "But if it establishes itself in the liver," says Dr Clark, "it causes cancer." Fortunately, Dr. Clark claims that it only establishes itself in the livers of people whose bodies contain propyl alcohol, so wise people will avoid this solvent.

It is not enough to just avoid propyl alcohol. All of the hundreds of dangerous chemicals that are put in our cosmetics, willy-nilly, must be shunned. Some are so terrible that it would be laughable that governments permit them, if it were not deadly serious. The scope of this book does not permit long lists and explanations of the dangers of each chemical. There are already many books available if you wish to research – if not, study labels and refuse to buy anything which lists chemicals. Unfortunately, most labels don't always tell you the whole truth, as you will see elsewhere in this book.

The shampoo I use and recommend contains coconut oil, olive oil, vegetable glycerine, organic honey, spring water, yucca juice and Celtic sea salt. Good enough and pure enough to eat, and the result is infinitely better than any of the fancy, 'name' shampoos I stupidly used before learning the truth. It's made and sold by Queenslander Rebecca Kingsbury and you'll find her details in *Resources*.

Please do not fall for any of the propaganda spewed out by companies claiming to sell 'organic' cosmetics, and/or cosmetics which are 'all natural'. Most are not. Our pathetic labelling regulations make it legal to claim 'organic' status for cosmetics filled with cancer-causing chemicals, because any compound containing carbon is chemically defined as organic. Buyer Beware! All I use is the pure coconut oil we have at the Centre – definitely not the contaminated versions you're likely to find elsewhere! I use it for cleansing, moisturising and on salads, as Dr Peat so strongly recommends (more details in *Resources*).

As the late Henry Bieler, MD, who was one of the wisest doctors in the US, said to me, "Dear, if it isn't pure enough to eat, it isn't pure enough for your skin."

Hair dyes and hair sprays are extremely hazardous, as they are chock-full of evil chemicals that are easily absorbed through the scalp. Many people cannot even walk into a beauty salon without becoming ill from the toxic fumes, and hairdressers themselves are at great risk of premature illnesses and death.

✗ Fluoride

This industrial waste-product only benefits manufacturers who can actually make money out of selling it instead of paying for it to go to a toxic dump, thanks to "the greatest scientific fraud of this century" quoted in **Chapter 19**, *Water Woes*. Other reasons why all forms of fluoride should play no part in your life are detailed in **Chapters** *7* and *8* on *Bone Health*, and **Chapter 17**, *Dental Health*.

✗ Ceramic Nails

The chemicals used by beauticians to apply ceramic nails are so toxic that just being in the same salon is extremely dangerous due to the fumes they give off, to say nothing of what is ingested through the nails and skin. I urge all women to boycott the salons that permit those deadly chemicals to pollute the air. Some women describe their reactions as "feeling as if I've breathed fire."

✗ Fragrances

Scent, perfume, aftershave, some essential oils, incense and scented candles are laden with chemicals that make susceptible people ill. Those strong people who don't notice any ill-effects might give a thought to those of us who are disgusted by the strong smells and sometimes made quite ill. Fabric softeners used in laundering are especially noxious and can cause serious allergic reactions. Speaking of offensive smells, please don't buy scented paper goods – tissues, toilet paper, paper towels, etc. Remember, those strong and, to many, offensive, odours are not achieved by the addition of *Chanel Number 5*, but by dangerous petrochemicals. It is necessary to open wrappers and give these products the sniff test at the market, to be sure. Even plastic garbage bags are not immune to this nonsense, and let us remember how these chemicals pollute our environment. Further, please shun dyed and bleached paper products. Toilet paper dyes have been shown to contribute to, or even cause, cancer of the anus. And, again, think of our precious environment when buying dyed products to 'pretty up' your kitchen and bath. In a properly run society, in which the multinationals do not call the shots, these dangerous, polluting and totally unnecessary products would be outlawed.

✗ Cleaning Products

Decades ago, when I learned that all the 'tried and true' cleaning products in our house were dangerous, a light went on in my brain. It was the old "ah hah!" syndrome, and suddenly I understood why every time I washed dishes, clothes, or used any cleaning product, I sneezed and often felt slightly ill. And here I had been thinking those symptoms were due to a dislike of housework!

It was the previously-mentioned research of Dr Hulda Clark which alerted me to the carnage created by certain chemicals in household products and our food. The information in Dr Clark's book was so persuasive and horrifying that it galvanised us into action; all of our conventional household cleaning products were gathered and taken to the *Hazardous Waste* section of the tip. They were replaced by baking soda, borax and cheap white vinegar, which work adequately. I had not used air fresheners, talc, sprays or poisons of any kind since my teens, as my mother knew the dangers. Dr Clark's books are filled with photographs of common products and foods with notations underneath saying either that they are safe (precious few) or that they are contaminated with benzene, propyl alcohol, etc. She is a very brave woman, because the products she condemns are produced by huge, powerful companies that few people are courageous enough to defy. Her books are must-reading, but, like this one, may be hazardous to your emotional health.

There are at least 17,000 different chemicals in ordinary household cleaning products, most of them untested for toxicity. Interactions among them, and interactions in the body when absorbed through inhalation and skin contact, are unknown. What *is* known is that they are deadly for young children and dangerous for adults. Some people are so susceptible that they cannot even walk down a supermarket aisle where they are displayed without becoming ill.

X Gelatin

Avoid anything made with gelatin, and don't take capsules unless they are made with vegetables – 'vegie caps'. Ordinary gelatin is made from the ears and other inedible parts of animals, which are sent to rendering plants. Because of the hormones used in rearing the animals, particularly the oestrogen pellets implanted under the ears, the gelatin is contaminated by xenoestrogens.

X Camphor/Moth Balls

The fumes from moth repellents made from camphor are extremely dangerous. They are made to kill insects and do a good job. They also kill animals, children and adults, but slowly. Instead, I recommend you use essential oils to protect stored clothes from moth attack.

X Synthetic Fabrics

The only fabrics healthful to wear are the natural ones – cotton, hemp, linen, silk and wool. As reported in **Clinical Ecology, Vol 4, No 2, 1986,** A. Rashid Seyal, MD, and others observed 4000 subjects, 2000 wearing synthetic, 2000 wearing cotton next to their skin. Systolic blood pressure and heart rate were significantly higher in those wearing synthetics, and premature ventricular contractions were significantly more frequent. Synthetic fabrics are made with many dangerous, caustic substances, which have not been properly tested. Some of these chemicals interact with enzymes in the skin and are absorbed, then stored in the liver. Synthetics are particularly dangerous when worn by children, especially infants. It's an effort to avoid chemical fabrics, but it pays off, especially in hot weather when cottons are cool and allow your skin to breathe. Crinkle cotton and seersucker are great because you don't have to iron them.

X *Metal Cookware*

If you have aluminium cookware, please discard it, and never use foil. Dr Arthur Furman used to demonstrate aluminium's toxicity by putting two bowls of water on his lectern. As he explained to his audience, one bowl had been boiled in a Pyrex pan, the other in aluminium. He then placed a goldfish in each (cooled) bowl. By the end of his lecture, which only lasted one hour, the unfortunate goldfish that was in the aluminium pan water was dead. A cruel thing to do to the poor fish, but most instructive.

Never use pans lined with *polytetrafluoroetheylene* (often sold as Teflon® and Silverstone®) because the toxic fumes generated during cooking cause illness in people, and are a frequent cause of sudden death in caged birds. Stainless steel is all right, but not ideal. Copper is toxic. Titanium is safe – but very expensive. There is excellent glass cookware available, and this material is by far the best. But when it comes to food, remember, raw is better!

X *Old-fashioned Dentistry and Dental Products*

Good oral hygiene is essential for overall good health. Unfortunately, we are at the mercy of practitioners who are ignoring the well-documented dangers of mercury and amalgam fillings, and manufacturers who, among other shameful practices, have created a profitable market for the use of toxic industrial waste products in toothbrushes and toothpastes. There is so much to say on this that **Chapter 17**, *Dental Health*, is devoted to the subject, which I strongly urge you to read.

X *Mercury in Fish*

We cannot blame the dental profession for all of our mercury exposure; industrial mercury has polluted our air, soil and sea. As reported in **The Felix Letter**, *Spring 2003*, methylmercury tends to accumulate up the food chain – "with large fish at the top carrying the biggest loads. Swordfish, sea bass, halibut and ahi tuna steaks from various worldwide waters all tend to accumulate high contents of methylmercury." All it took was eating two cans of tuna a week for a woman to lose verbal skills and even forget how to tie her shoes. Her blood-mercury level was 13 parts per billion. The good news is that these dangerous levels will drop after six months on a fish-free diet, or simply switching to the sorts of fish that don't accumulate mercury. The fish with very low mercury levels are king crab, catfish and scallops. Those with non-detectable mercury levels are sardines, non-farmed salmon, sole, tilapia, clams and shrimp. Children and pregnant women should exclude tuna from their diets, according to authorities who don't go far enough. I think we all should!

X Sugar: White Death

Refined sugar is lethal. Man has crystallised and bleached the sap of cane and beet, and refined what was once a whole, balanced food into an addictive drug that contains nothing but sweet taste and calories. It is doubtful that there has ever been a greater threat to the human body since man first walked upright.

Sugar leaches the body of precious minerals and vitamins because of the heavy demands its detoxification and elimination make on the entire system. It produces an over-acid condition, and more and more minerals are required from the body in the attempt to rectify the imbalance. To protect the blood, so much calcium is leached from the teeth and bones that osteoporosis and decay, and weakening of the entire body, results.

Every organ in the body is affected. Initially, sugar is stored in the liver as glycogen. But the capacity of the liver is limited and repeated abuse will make it expand like a balloon, similar to the way alcohol causes the swelling which becomes cirrhosis of the liver. Then, when the liver is filled to its maximum capacity, the glycogen is returned to the blood, as fatty acids, and transported to the buttocks, thighs, breasts and stomach. Not a pretty sight! The next distribution in the destructive course of this deadly substance is to the organs of the body, which begin to slow down until finally their tissues degenerate and turn to fat. The entire body, of course, is affected by the inability of these organs to function properly. The lymphatic and circulatory systems are invaded, and an excess of white cells occurs, which is very dangerous. Every ounce of sugar eaten reduces the ability of the body to resist infection, because it damages the immune system, leaving the body prey to every possible illness, including arthritis, heart disease, arteriosclerosis, atherosclerosis and cancer. In fact, any health problem will improve if sugar is eliminated.

Hyperinsulinism, hypoglycemia, low blood sugar – call it what you may – has become the 'in' disease in recent years, because of the accelerated use of sugar. The symptoms are many and unpleasant: fuzzy thinking, irritability, inability to handle stress, fatigue, sometimes crippling exhaustion, eye troubles (including ocular migraine), headaches (including migraines) and, in the worst cases, blackouts, recurrent seizures, mental aberrations, including insanity, insulin shock and even coma. All this from that sparkling white stuff they put in practically everything we eat!

The insidious factor is the delayed action. If only refined sugar brought about disturbing symptoms immediately, it would have been discarded in 1500, shortly after the Dutch established the first sugar refinery in Antwerp. But the build up is slow, it tastes good, we're addicted and most people, especially children, won't listen to the many warnings about sugar destroying their health.

Hypoglycemic symptoms occur because refined sugar (in the form of glucose) pours into the blood like a torrent, causing the insulin level to soar. This makes us feel 'up' temporarily. But then the bottom drops out as the blood sugar level plummets. If sugar abuse continues, the adrenal glands become exhausted, due to the whiplash effect of the sugar level skyrocketing, then plummeting, countless times a day, year after year. As the adrenal glands are of utmost importance to the body, many illnesses (including severe allergies) result from their depletion. The next step can be diabetes, unless the diet is improved dramatically.

Most disturbing is the effect this syndrome has upon the brain. Experts in the field have found that the cells of the brain depend wholly upon the blood sugar level for nourishment, and are very susceptible to damage. Lack of concentration, inability to function mentally, temper tantrums and violence all can spring from the effect wildly oscillating sugar levels have on the brain.

Patients have been incorrectly diagnosed as manic-depressive, having psychopathic personalities and schizophrenia, when all they have is what author William Dufty calls *Sugar Blues*. Enlightened physicians are recommending that blood sugar levels be routinely checked before making any psychiatric diagnoses, as hypoglycemia is a great mimic of psychosis and neurosis. Dr John Tintera, a famous American endocrinologist, said, "It is quite possible to improve your disposition, increase your efficiency, and change your personality for the better. The way to do it is to avoid cane and beet sugar in all forms and guises." Amen.

And that includes 'raw' sugar; those delicious, appetising-looking dark sugars are nothing but refined white sugar to which molasses has been added. Honey, maple syrup and molasses are simple sugars and aggravate hypoglycemia, but at least have the saving grace of being closer to nature than refined, white sugar.

Honey and maple syrup contain minerals and vitamins, and molasses contains a great deal of calcium, iron, B vitamins, and other heat-stable vitamins, as well as pesticides, because it is a by-product of sugar refining. Further, it has been heated, so it can cause disruption to blood chemistry, as can maple syrup, which is boiled during processing. So, if you must have a concentrated sugar, unprocessed honey is the best of a poor lot. But it should be used in small quantities, and as special treats.

Refined sugar poses an even graver danger to the mental functioning of children than it does to adults. Children's brain development may be altered, or even retarded, and they may be incapable of functioning in school. How long it takes for symptoms to surface depends upon the child's genes and the strength of the glands, especially the adrenals.

✗ Artificial Sweeteners

Popular sugar substitutes, NutraSweet, Equal, Spoonful, Canderel, Benevia, E951, etc., are all forms of *aspartame*, one of the deadliest neurotoxins on Earth! Its devastating effects on health are detailed in **Chapter 4**, *Excitoxins*.

Nor is *sucralose* (sold as Splenda) any better. It has a chlorinated base like DDT and causes autoimmune disease. *Asculfame K* causes cancer and leukaemia. The herb Stevia is safe. It doesn't taste very good, but at least it won't kill you.

Xylitol is a sweetener that has been getting lots of attention lately. It is being billed as a safe sweetener to take the place of aspartame and its clones. The good news is that it tastes good and isn't the killer aspartame is. The bad news is that the studies I trust list the following side effects: weight gain similar to sucralose, diarrhoea, tumour growth, liver and kidney dysfunction. Before I had read about the side effects, I tried some and had severe stomach cramps and diarrhoea for two days after using it. I tried it a month later just to be certain and, sure enough, the bad effects came back. When I rang the manufacturer in the US, I was told, "People have to get used to it." Not this cookie!

✗ Fructose

Please don't be taken in by the fructose fans. It's easy to be led astray because people tend to associate fructose with fruit. HFCS (High Fructose Corn Syrup) is everywhere; Americans consume more of this sweetener than sugar, and Australians have a tendency to embrace America's bad habits. This additive is, unfortunately, a favourite ingredient in 'health foods'. Linda Joyce Forristal, writing in **Wise Traditions,** says HFCS has the same taste as sucrose, but "...it is obviously much more complicated to make, involving vats of murky fermenting liquid, fungus and chemical tweaking."

According to Ms Forristal, a team of investigators at the USDA, led by Dr Meira Field, compared the effects of glucose and fructose, using rats. They found that the glucose group was unaffected, but the fructose group had horrible results – their bodies fell apart! Dr Field reported, "The medical profession thinks fructose is better for diabetics than sugar, but every cell in the body can metabolise glucose. However, fructose must be metabolised in the liver. The livers of the rats on the fructose diet looked like the livers of alcoholics, plugged with fat and cirrhotic."

Dr William Campbell Douglass, in **Second Opinion**, says that HFCS significantly raises triglyceride levels, which is known to increase the risk of heart disease. And they push this stuff for diabetics and our children!

What can we do about this incredible mess civilised people have gotten into? Kicking the sugar habit is a start, of course. This is, unfortunately, a lot easier said than done, because refined sugar is highly addictive, as are smoking, alcohol, aspartame, coffee and many drugs. But kick it we must, if we are to be healthy and live out our expected lifespan with our teeth, brains and organs intact, and with a vibrant feeling of health. Yes, that *is* possible!

✗ *Soya and All Soy Products*

See **Chapter 9**, *Soy - The Abominable Bean*, and be vigilant in avoiding this dangerous non-food.

✗ *Green Ketchup*

For reasons known only to themselves (it looks like something Linda Blair spewed up in *The Exorcist*), H J Heinz has developed a green ketchup, which has now hit the Australian market. If you've succumbed, exorcise it from your home! Ketchup was bad enough already, because of the high fructose corn syrup and 'natural flavours' (a source of MSG) but in order to make it green, food dye *Yellow #5* (which can cause ADHD) is added, as well as *Blue #11*, (aka Aluminium Lake, which is associated with Alzheimer's disease and kidney problems). And, how do you reckon they remove the original red colour? Chlorine?

✗ *Processed Food*

If you eat processed food you can be sure it will be filled with potent chemicals that the human system never encountered prior to the advent of the test tube. This is yet another subject worthy of careful examination, so refer to **Chapter 5**, *Processed Foods*, for full details of what is being done to our diet.

✗ *McAnything*

For some time now I have been using a very neat visual aid in my public lectures and classes at Hippocrates, courtesy of those friendly Golden Arches people, whose contributions to the diet of young and old the world over are so well known. It is a *McMuffin*, given to me by a friend who after purchasing it, had put it in a paper box and totally forgotten about it for a series of reasons too boring to detail here.

She knew I would be interested in it because after *13 months* hidden away in its paper box she discovered this geriatric muffin to still be in pristine condition. Bugs had shunned it, the shape was unchanged and there was not a trace of mould; nor were there any other signs of what we have come to expect from the breakdown of real food.

Today, six years later, it still looks, feels and smells the same. I allow my students to examine this aged example of modern junk food marketing, but have to be watchful that none of them attempts to take a bite; it still looks 'good enough to eat.'

Once news of this venerable taste treat began to circulate, students and people who read a letter about it in **Nexus Magazine** have told me of similar experiences with McDonald's food; even a cheeseburger, pushed to the back of an office drawer and forgotten for six months, did not break down.

Several people told me they made the experiment to try to break their children of the fast food addiction. Try it yourself – it works!

And now, according to **New Vegetarian and Natural Health**, *Summer 2001/02*, McDonald's is supplying cheap cheeseburgers to primary school tuckshops, allowing the schools to tack on a profit in order to sweeten the pot. This helps the under-funded schools, but certainly does not help the health of our children.

X Epidural Anaesthesia / Spinal Injections

Let's finish this long list of no-nos with yet another 'needling' practice beloved of the medical profession. This is what **Mosby's Medical Dictionary** has to say about epidural anaesthesia (spinal anaesthetic):

> The most common adverse effects include dural membrane puncture during placement of the Touhy needle with resulting postdural puncture headache and hypotension that result from sympathetic nerve block and vascular dilation.

In other words, you get a God-awful headache that lasts for several weeks and can only be endured by constant morphine intake. And, if that is the only 'adverse effect' you get, you will be incredibly lucky. What they don't tell you is that many patients who submit to this form of anaesthetic have serious health problems for the rest of their lives.

Common sense would surely indicate that puncturing the spine, with its many nerves, is a stupid and dangerous thing to do. The whoops! factor is very much in evidence here, as the slightest deviation can lead to horrendous problems. The scar tissue that forms on the spinal column can create spinal rigidity, and cause bladder and kidney problems, muscle spasms, impotence, vertigo, migraines, allergies, thyroid conditions, and sacroiliac conditions; in fact, just about everything, depending upon the amount and position of the scar tissue. Symptoms can occur immediately, and when they do, the physicians deny any connection to the anaesthesia. Some symptoms only surface later, and are even more difficult to trace to the spinal injection. One thing is certain; no liability will ever be admitted by practitioners who refuse to accept that they should never inject or cut into the spinal column.

And it's not just the physical act of puncturing the spine that leads to countless painful problems. A dye known both as *Myodil* and *Pantopaque*, that was used between 1945 and 1987 as an injection into the spinal column to enhance the x-ray image called a myelogram, has led to thousands of Australians now having to endure chronic pain. In July 2002 the UK newspaper, **The Daily**

Telegraph, published documentary proof that many health authorities, including the Australian Federal Government, state health authorities and doctors, sanctioned the use of the dye even though they knew of its devastating effects. It contains the chemicals benzene, hydrochloric acid and sulphuric acid, and its use results in burning back pain, incontinence, loss of bladder control, visual impairment, seizures and paralysis. The condition, known as adhesive arachnoiditis, can take up to 10 years to develop.

The notorious Glaxo pharmaceutical giant, which manufactured Myodil, was well aware for at least 40 years that the procedure could result in arachnoiditis, caused by the inflammation and fusion of the nerves and membranes of the spinal cord. Doctors were even warned not to spill the chemical on rubber because it destroys it and dissolves polystyrene cups, yet apparently it was OK to inject into the spine! The Australian so-called health watchdog, the Therapeutic Drugs Administration (TGA), never even tested the product and permitted its use long after the first cases surfaced.

✗ Skin Cancer?

A skin cancer salve called **ALDARA,** made by 3M Pharmaceuticals, is in my opinion, one of the most dangerous drugs on the market today. It is so strong that it can cause irreversible autoimmune disease, and throw susceptible people into fatal anaphylactic shock. Please see page 286 for a copy of an advertisement that the Hippocrates Foundation placed in magazines in order to save lives. Our website, www.doctorsaredangerous.com has full details, and Richard Beasley's website, www.aldara1.com has a great deal of valuable information on this deadly salve, as well as a scientific monograph that should be read by any doctor before prescribing it.

Cansema, a safe plant extract that removes skin cancers safely, can be found on the internet – and it doesn't kill! (See page 308) But please do not experiment with any natural remedy if there is a chance your skin lesion could be a melanoma. This requires expert medical intervention, if you can find an ethical dermatologist.

> "The most startling fact about 2002 is that the combined profits for the ten drug companies in the Fortune 500 (US $35.9 billion) were more than the profits for all the other 490 businesses put together (US $33.7 billion). When I say this is a profitable industry, I mean *really* profitable. It is difficult to conceive of how awash in money big pharma is."
>
> *Marcia Angell, Former Editor of the*
> *New England Journal of Medicine*
>
> See her website: www.nybooks.com/articles/17244?email

Note: As of 2006, Big Pharma is now a $600 Billion-per-year mega-colossus.

26

Remedies

A simple guide to self-diagnosis, and some safe, effective and proven natural remedies

Whenever I had a health complaint, one of my first teachers, Henry Bieler, MD, always asked me the same question: "What have you been doing that's different, Dear?" This taught me an invaluable lesson, which I pass on to you. Invariably, his question led me to discover that I had caused my own problem through deviating from the strict diet I was on. So remember, if you develop symptoms, pains, etc., always think back to any changes or additions to your diet, rather than rushing to a doctor who might prescribe an inappropriate, probably dangerous, drug. First try the Dr Bieler method, and eliminate any suspicious food or beverage, drink lots of pure water, give it a fair trial and then, if symptoms haven't vanished or lessened dramatically, see a doctor. Dr Bieler said that most illnesses are self-limiting. Some, however, are so serious that only a physician can help. Don't take self-diagnosis so far that you are beyond help.

Carmen Ross-Munro wrote to tell me about her experience with gingko biloba. She said, "I was suffering terribly with an aching vein which goes from my bottom to my ankle. It was so bad that I couldn't sit for any length of time, as the pain was unbearable, and sitting seemed to put pressure on this vein."

Fortunately, Carmen's daughter happened to mention that she can't take gingko biloba because it gives her aching veins and haemorrhoids. Carmen then checked a multi-vitamin with herbs that she had been taking, and discovered that it contained gingko biloba. She quit taking it and started improving. Often the remedy for what ails us is quite close at hand – you just have to know where to look for it.

Here are some useful remedies and treatments for common health problems that will save you a lot of searching. The first section covers *specific conditions* and their treatment; the second is devoted to *treatments* or *devices* that have been found effective for treating a wide range of ailments.

CONDITIONS and THEIR TREATMENT

Exhaustion

Liquorice Root (*Glycyrrhiza glabra*) is often prescribed for tired people. It is popular because it creates a quick surge of energy. Dr Bieler used to say to me, "Beware anything that gives you energy quickly, because it is not supporting your glands, it is whipping them." After just a few weeks your glands (especially the adrenals) become so enervated that they can't function properly and you are much worse off than before. Liquorice does this, as do so many other 'quick energy' herbs and concoctions. This applies to the hyped 'miracle' pills, many of which contain contaminants.

Migraine Headaches

The Hippocrates diet, followed faithfully, has been very successful in banishing migraines, which are often caused by a buildup of toxemia. For those unprepared to eat a healthful diet, Dr Raymond Peat had this to say in one of his newsletters: "Because of my own experience in finding that eating a raw carrot daily prevented migraines, I began to suspect that the carrot fibre was having both a bowel-protective and an anti-estrogen effect. Several women who suffered from premenstrual symptoms, including migraine, had their serum estrogen measured before and after the 'carrot diet', and they found that the carrot lowered their estrogen within a few days, as it relieved their symptoms." Because it counteracts the damage done by oestrogen, progesterone is also important in preventing migraines.

There is persuasive evidence that chronic dehydration is the root cause of many migraines, so drink two litres of pure water each day (no substitutes!) and, once your water-starved body has re-hydrated, you may conquer migraines forever. Neither of these remedies will work overnight, nor are they likely to overcome consuming junk food and gluten, which is notorious for causing migraines. There is also some helpful migraine-related information in *Chapter 1*, *That "Mystery Illness"*, and *Chapter 2*, *Adrenal Insufficiency*.

Colds, Flu and Coughs

The best treatment, if possible, is to eat nothing until the cold passes, taking care to drink a great deal. The old saw, "Stuff a cold and starve a fever" is a corruption of the correct adage, which is "Stuff a cold and you will have to starve a fever". In other words, if you eat when you have a cold, chances are it will turn nasty and you will have a fever. Of course, fasting when you have to work is a problem, and that is when people get in trouble, by taking suppressing drugs so they can continue working. In the end, time is lost, because when an illness is suppressed, it is likely to turn up later, in a different, and worse, form. A cold is an elimination crisis – the method your body uses to flush out toxins. Look at a cold as a cleansing wake up call, and resolve to stop eating junk so your body will not be forced to eliminate it in an unpleasant manner. If your colds have a tendency to turn into pneumonia see Chapter 2 for help.

Zinc lozenges can offer relief, according to naturopaths I know. Dr Joseph Mercola offers the following remedy, which must be used immediately symptoms hit. Put three drops of food grade, 3 percent hydrogen peroxide into one ear canal. It will bubble and sting. In five or ten minutes, drain onto a tissue and repeat with the other ear. According to Dr Mercola, this old-fashioned remedy has an 80 percent success rate.

A remedy that works wonders on a chronic cough is a tablespoon of honey mixed with ¼ teaspoon of ground cinnamon either in tea or "neat" for as long as it takes. Drinking plenty of water can also help coughing.

Arthritis, Joint Pains, Swelling, Stiffness

All these miserable afflictions can be helped by natural methods. First, shun all soy products – they are bound to inflict joint and bone pains, sooner or later (see **Chapter 9**, *Soy – the Abominable Bean*, for more information on this non-food).

This ban includes that commercial money-spinner, lecithin, which is a by-product of soy processing, is always rancid, and gives susceptible people almost immediate gout, due to the *purines* it contains. After getting soy out of your life, flood your body with water to chase out the purines from your joints. It is important, also, to make sure your thyroid is functioning correctly. Come to Hippocrates Centre to detoxify, or go on a strict diet at home, as outlined in this book. It takes years of the wrong diet to get bad arthritis, and it will take time to flush it out of your system. Persevere and you should become pain free.

Dr Rex Newnham, world authority on arthritis and boron, told me of experiments which proved to him that people with osteoarthritis who take three tablets of boron (nine mg) per day showed marked improvement. He said that those under 60 generally got better in one month, those in their sixties took two months, while those in their 70s and 80s took three months before a cure was seen. "Those patients with rheumatoid arthritis often show an initial aggravation after about a week, and then after another week they are quite right. This is a *Herxheimer reaction*. There were no unwanted side effects, and these were sought for." He also said that juvenile arthritis can be helped in just a few days. "The youngest patient was only nine months old, with swollen joints and much pain. She was given half a tablet twice a day and was quite better in ten days. That is the dose for those under two years old." (No more than 3milligrams).

These quotes are from Dr Newnham's book, **Arthritis Without Drugs** (see **Resources**). The doses are larger than usual, so I suggest consulting a health professional.

Diet is crucial. If you are addicted to grains and sugar, get over it or learn to love your pains. Eat and drink absolutely no junk, and drink plenty of pure water. Chances are you are low on hydrochloric acid (see **Chapter 3**, *Stomach Acid*) and you may have some serious food sensitivities that can be discovered through testing. Try eliminating all nightshade vegetables for a few weeks as an experiment. They are tomatoes, potatoes, capsicums (peppers) and eggplant. A minority of arthritis sufferers are sensitive to these vegetables, and you will soon discover if you are one of them. Mandarines (tangerines) and oranges can cause severe pains in susceptible people if eaten in large quantities. You might try eating fresh ginger root, but it can take up to three months before producing results. Several people have told me that quitting vinegar made their pains fade away. If you are not able to get sunshine year-round, see Chapters 7 and 8 for vitamin D supplementation.

Many people have reported to me that they can create pains all over their bodies simply by having a meal seasoned with chili pepper. That includes the much-recommended cayenne pepper. Researchers at Harvard Medical School have recently announced that the receptor chemicals in 'hot' chili peppers are responsible for ongoing, burning pain associated with inflammation, arthritis and tissue damage. They can upset the stomach, irritate the bladder and even make urinating painful. These additives have been exempted by food labelling acts and are hard to avoid if you buy manufactured food. My suggestion: eliminate all strong seasonings for a few weeks as an experiment. Avoid passive smoking as tobacco can aggravate joint pains.

Nature didn't intend us to be afflicted with pains like these – we are doing it to ourselves by not living according to her laws.

Skin Conditions and Complexion

First, choose your parents carefully, as it is hard to overcome heredity. You can, however, go a long way toward improving your skin by following these guidelines:

- See Page 318 for an amazing curative, Wonder Balm

- Never smoke, and avoid passive smoking

- Protect your face from the sun with a hat, but not toxic sunblock

- Shun alcohol, junk food, unsaturated fats (in your diet as well as on your skin)

- Avoid fancy cosmetics and stick to pure coconut oil or olive oil for cleansing and moisturising.

Vitamin A capsules with D, pricked and spread on the face, will eliminate milia (the small, hard white lumps some people get on their faces) in one or two months of daily use. Cod liver oil may be used instead if you can't find these capsules.

Many women have reported great results using Dr Peat's Progesterone Oil (see **Resources**) on their faces. Because the oil is viscous, first spread coconut oil or olive oil on your face, then put a drop of progesterone oil on each cheek and spread. Probably most important of all is to keep your skin well hydrated by drinking plenty of pure water.

Excess Weight

Every obese or chubby person I have ever known has been on one diet or another for years, sometimes for decades. Diets do not work. Strictly-planned eating programs are inhuman. They are too complicated, tedious and hard to stick to, and lead to bingeing and depression when, inevitably, they fail to deliver. The only way to lose weight and keep it off is to establish rules and *never* deviate.

Cut polyunsaturated oils out of your life (see **Chapter 6**, *Oils and Fats*) and make your kitchen a grain and sugar-free area. Re-read **Chapter 16**, *Against the Grain* and *Sugar: White Death*, in **Chapter 25**, *The Banned List*, for details on how they create obesity and destroy health. Eat loads of vegetables, some fruit, and the healthful fats and proteins recommended in this book and your only problem will be, eventually, keeping weight on so you won't look gaunt!

Difficulty Swallowing Tablets

Some people find that tablets and capsules get caught in their throats. When this happens, simply coat the tablet or capsule first with a pure oil, and it will slip down easily when you tip back your head and swallow water.

Nausea, Vertigo, Motion Sickness

Ginger root (one gram per day), or capsules containing ginger root extract, are said to help these conditions. Ginger appears to be more effective than drugs and has no side effects.

Constipation

Magnesium (obtainable in tablet form), taken to bowel tolerance, will help the most intractable cases. A good lactobacillus is also most effective.

Asthma

Milk, grains, poor diet, passive smoking, atmospheric pollution etc., cause and contribute to this condition, and it is easily controlled with the proper diet.

Giving steroids in pharmacological doses before trying natural methods is inexcusable. Re-hydrating can cure asthma. Sip water all day.

Leg Cramps

Leg cramping which occurs in bed at night can be a sign of lack of hydrochloric acid and/or magnesium. If this is the cause, the cramps will often stop shortly after taking the tablets. Lack of potassium can also cause leg cramps – yet another good reason to eat your vegies and fruit.

Anaemia

Anaemia is a common ailment among women, especially those with heavy periods. When blood tests show low iron levels, doctors usually reach for their pads and write out prescriptions for iron tablets. If these don't help the symptoms, the next step is iron injections. These forms of iron are inorganic and badly tolerated by the body, although they do raise the iron levels and help restore energy. The bad news, aside from the damage inorganic iron can cause, is that, almost invariably, women on iron tablets get dark circles under their eyes, which are unattractive and rarely fade, even after the tablets are discontinued.

Dr Raymond Peat, in his book, **Nutrition For Women**, calls it "iron poisoning", and says, "It is known that excess iron accumulates in the liver, since there is no mechanism for excreting it. It has been noticed that infections are higher in people who are getting an iron supplement. In tests in vitro, iron damages the capacity of antibodies to destroy germs." He also says that when iron pills are taken with a normal diet, vitamin E is destroyed. This, according to Dr Peat, does not happen with natural sources of iron, such as red meat.

Without fail, every time I have talked with anaemic women, they tell me that their doctors prescribed iron tablets without asking any questions about diet and, more to the point, about hydrochloric acid (*HCl*). This really gets my back up, because of the desperate need anaemic patients have for HCl (see **Chapter 3, Stomach Acid**). Without this crucial digestive aid the body simply cannot absorb nutrients properly, and especially vitamin B_{12}, which is essential in order to avoid or reverse anaemia.

So, if you're exhausted and want to save yourself a trip to a doctor, who may get stroppy if you say you'd rather not take inorganic iron, first have a look at the insides of your lower eyelids and your fingernails. If they are white instead of a healthy looking pink, you may be anaemic. If this is the case, take vitamin C (either in food or the supplement recommended in **Resources**) with meals, as this vitamin increases absorption of iron. Eat broccoli, beetroot, peas, dried apricots, prunes and raisins, and plenty of leafy green vegetables. Eat parsley with every meal, as it is one of the finest sources of safe iron, as well as natural calcium (and is an effective breath-freshener).

Nuts and seeds help, especially pepitas and almonds. If you are not a vegetarian, recovery will probably be quicker, as red meat, fish and the dark meat of chicken are rich in iron and easily absorbed, provided you have sufficient hydrochloric acid in your digestive tract.

If, after adhering to a good diet, as recommended in this book, and following the above suggestions for correcting anaemia, you do not feel better, I strongly suggest that you get a diagnosis from a physician who is willing to take the time to examine you thoroughly and order blood tests.

Allergies

As always, look to the cause and, in this case, it is almost always low adrenal function. Concentrated proteins, eaten every three or four hours, often bring quick relief because protein supports the adrenal glands. Large amounts of pantothenic acid can bring temporary relief, but take care not to make its use habitual, as it will overbalance the other B vitamins. In an emergency, flooding the body with water will have an antihistamine effect, often stopping nose running and sneezing quickly. You might also benefit from sipping all day.

Depression

Many people are on anti-depressants, which are addictive, dangerous, and are themselves *causes* of depression. Following the rules in this book is often enough to banish this debilitating condition. Re-hydrating the body is essential. As Dr Batmanghelidj explains, "With dehydration, the level of energy generation in the brain is decreased. Many functions of the brain that depend on this type of energy become inefficient." And I don't mean taking coffee, tea, soft drinks, milk, etc. I am referring to pure, unfluoridated water. Make this a part of your life, and never deviate. Should you elect to stop taking anti-depressants, remember that this can be tricky, and should be done with the help of a qualified, understanding professional. Despite the claims of the manufacturers, who, as usual, lie shamelessly to protect their profits, these drugs *are* addictive and quitting should be done under careful supervision. Depression can often be banished by correcting an under active thyroid gland (see **Chapters 1** and **2**), but only progressive physicians are aware of this. Fasting on the liver cleanse soup in this chapter can be of great help -- depression is often caused by poor diet.

Sleep Apnoea

Try going off all grains and sugar. If the problem persists, cut out all dairy products. Give the experiment at least three weeks. Taking folic acid can help correct thyroid /adrenal problems (**Chapters 1** and **2**) which can be causes of sleep apnoea.

Diabetes

The American Diabetes Association (ADA) counsels their members to fill up on carbohydrates. They also recommend drinking as many diet soft drinks as desired, so any other advice they offer should be regarded with suspicion – if not outright disbelief (see *Chapter 4*, *Excitotoxins*).

I know why the ADA pushes diet drinks – the industry funds them and they are suitably grateful. But why such reliance on grains when it is well known that diabetics do so much better without them? Could it be that the United States Department of Agriculture is also a sponsor?

When diabetics attend the Hippocrates program they do amazingly well. They are all told not to quit their medication, because this should not be done cavalierly. Yet many feel so well that they go against instructions and stop all medicine after the first week on the program. The reason for this is simple – the toxic load of rubbish food, and particularly grains, is eliminated and many report feeling 'reborn'. Diabetics need to stay away from grains, eat loads of vegetables, good concentrated proteins, and the right kind of fat (see *Chapter 6*, *Oils and Fats*).

Diabetes expert, Diana Schwarzbein, MD, in her book, *The Schwarzbein Principle*, reports on her success with diabetics using this diet. She writes that she searched medical literature for studies that showed low-fat diets are healthful, but as she says, "I was surprised to learn that there are no long-term studies showing such results. But numerous studies concluded that fat is necessary to maintain good health."

Dr Schwarzbein believes, as do I and my colleagues, that the low-fat fad is one cause of Type II (adult onset) diabetes, the Western world's epidemic of obesity and many other serious illnesses.

Multiple Sclerosis (MS)

Contrary to what the medical profession apparently believes, and wants you to believe, this terrible affliction need *not* end in disaster. It can, in fact, be prevented and even reversed, and I have seen this happen many times. An excellent diet, of course, is absolutely essential, with special emphasis on getting enough first class protein. MS typically affects women during their reproductive years, and it is associated with hormone imbalances. Natural progesterone (not the fake ones frequently cautioned against in this book) is crucial, as is thyroid supplementation, and they will help to repair and maintain the myelin sheaths that deteriorate in MS. An early diagnosis helps – by the time a patient is wheelchair-bound, recovery is slow. Be warned – toxic dental materials and artificial sweeteners, combined with polyunsaturated fats and oils, are a major cause of MS. Quitting these can reverse symptoms, if caught early enough.

Tinea

This is a general term referring to a group of related fungal skin infections. Some pretty nasty topical drugs are recommended, but my suggestion, and please don't scream, is putting your own urine on the infection, frequently, until it is gone. Many of our patients at Hippocrates have reported better results with this cheap, plentiful remedy, than with expensive, toxic drugs.

Cataracts

Russell Blaylock, MD, wrote in his book, *Excitotoxins, The Taste That Kills*, "Cataracts are known to be related to free radical damage to the lens of the eye. Experimental studies, using chemicals that induce cataracts in rats, demonstrated that alpha-lipoic acid prevented cataract formation." Dr Blaylock said that when the supplemented animals were examined it was found that there were significant elevations of glutathion, ascorbate and vitamin E in their lenses, indicating that alpha-lipoic acid caused their bodies to make these important substances. Vitamins C, A and D, and the herb, bilberry, all protect against cataract formation. One of the best, and by far the most economical, steps you can take to protect your eyes is to never allow your body to become dehydrated.

Eye Strain, Eye Pain, Blurred Vision

Use an eye cup or an eye dropper and put your own urine into your eyes, regularly. Many have reported curing themselves of painful, incapacitating eye problems in just a few days with this simple, free remedy. (See *Resources* for reading material on this subject.) The water from inside a coconut, put in a dropper and put in the eyes several times daily offers relief. It will keep in the fridge for several days. Freeze the excess in small bottles.

Macular Degeneration (MD)

Eating your fruit and vegies will offer the best possible protection from this tragic fate. The more, the better. *Lutein* and *zeaxanthin*, which act as antioxidants, protect cells against free radicals, and free radicals are known to be a major cause of MD. These important nutrients are not made by the body, but are found in large amounts in broccoli, spinach, Brussels sprouts, kale, mustard greens, turnip greens and egg yolks. In order to facilitate absorption when you eat these foods, you will need to combine them with a bit of olive oil or coconut oil or butter. And please – no polyunsaturated oils. They are known as a major cause of MD.

Selenium, vitamins C and E, zinc, taurine and the omega-3 fats are needed to promote the health of your eyes. But be sure to remember the importance of hydrochloric acid (see *Chapter 3, Stomach Acid*). Without this all-important element, you might as well throw these minerals in the bin, for all the good they will do you. Also, be sure to watch your iron level, as too much will damage many sensitive tissues in your body, especially your eyes.

Avoid smokers and exposure to their second-hand smoke, which contributes to MD because it weakens blood capillaries, uses up your vitamin C, and increases damage to your retina.

According to Dr Stanley B Covert, of the USA, *glutathione* by injection is causing immediate and significant improvements in MD. He says that it is not yet known why the oral form doesn't work, while the injections do. He wrote in ***The Townsend Letter for Doctors and Patients***:

"The procedure is quite simple. We purchase intravenous glutathione from a compounding pharmacy in strengths of 200mg/cc. The usual starting dose is 1000 mgs, and later sometimes 1500 mgs. A 20cc syringe is used and after withdrawing the glutathione, the remainder of the syringe is filled with normal saline. This is given through a 25 gauge butterfly in the dorsum of the hand over a period of fifteen minutes. The usual cost of the glutathione is about ten dollars a gram. No adverse reactions have been seen." Please don't forget – drink at least two litres of pure water daily, and **for serious eye problems, see a qualified opthalmologist**.

Skin Cancer

Under no circumstances allow a doctor to con you into using a skin cancer "cure" made by 3M Pharmaceuticals, called "Aldara". This salve can cause autoimmune illnesses, cancer and anaphylactic shock. (For details, see www.doctorsaredangerous.com, www.aldara1.com and page 286 in this book.) In spite of overwhelming evidence that Aldara can kill, governments permit its use, yet have outlawed Cansema, a safe, natural salve that seeks out and destroys cancer cells without damaging surrounding skin. Cansema has been widely used for decades, and I have yet to hear any bad reports. Because Cansema cannot be patented, Big Pharma cannot make billions from it: consequently they have used their huge influence to pressure governments to ban it. It is still legal for use on animals, fortunately, and the ingredients and instructions remain the same. For information world-wide, email bevan@centreforce.com, or web www.centreforce.com or phone 61-(07)-4157-4262.

Water

Few of us drink sufficient water. Eight glasses per day is the absolute minimum, and will go a long way toward curing illnesses that physicians prefer to suppress with dangerous drugs. Not coffee, not tea, not juices and, emphatically, not soft drinks. If you wait until you feel thirsty, your cells have already suffered from dehydration. Amazing as it may seem, many serious illnesses can simply be due to chronic dehydration. Chronic dehydration is extremely common and dangerous to your health.

Without sufficient water, your body has no way to eliminate toxins and waste, or the histamines which cause allergies. Hydration will improve your skin amazingly, plumping it out in a youthful way. Dehydration, from which most people suffer, creates an imbalance of minerals, and disrupts hormone balance. Because of this crucial balance, and because water improves the uptake of hormones by the cells, it is important for menopausal health.

Dr Karen Coates told me about a simple, effective way to hydrate the body and the skin. Every morning, fill a two-litre bottle with pure water, and add one-quarter teaspoon of pure Celtic salt. Drink it all during the day, but not during meals, although in some instances sipping all day can be helpful. I have seen this method work extremely well with some allergies, as the water dilutes histamine and relieves symptoms. Sipping can sometimes help with chronic coughing. If your eyes become puffy or gritty, the salt should be cut down or eliminated.

Dr Coates cautions, however, that people on medications, or those with high blood pressure or kidney disease must check with their health practitioners before commencing. She warns that some drugs may change the body's biochemical response to salt and water metabolism.

Sunshine

Sunshine has long been recognised as essential for the bountiful growth of plants, yet few people realise humans need it as well, particularly for the synthesis of vital vitamin D. Despite this, governments all over the Western world have been warning us to shun the sun, when they should have been warning us to shun the junk food and oils that have caused our epidemic of skin cancers. When I was young, I never heard of skin cancer, and it wasn't because I led a sheltered life. It was because polyunsaturated oils were still only a multinational dream of avarice. Now these plastic oils are everywhere, and so is skin cancer, and it is no coincidence.

These unnatural oils, along with all the other appalling junk people are eating and drinking, come out with sweat and, combined with the sun, contribute to skin cancer. But it's not the fault of the sun – it's the fault of the people who are foolish enough to eat junk.

At the same time governments are bombarding us with horror stories about the danger of the sun, they are pushing sunscreens as if their budgets depend upon them. It makes you wonder just how much influence the manufacturers of sunscreens have on our lawmakers. Defying their edicts will mean treating government agencies and sunscreen-pushers with the contempt they deserve.

The 'authorities' should pay attention to Caryl Nowson, of Canberra's Deakin University School of Health, speaking about the value of vitamin D in preventing osteoporosis, who said, "Nursing home patients and veiled women are among high-risk groups... The main source for Australians is exposure to sunlight." And this, of course, means without sunscreen.

But bear in mind that studies comparing the abilities of 20-year-olds and 80-year-olds to synthesise vitamin D from the sun found that the 80-year-olds have fourfold less ability to make vitamin D in the skin. So, if you are not 20 any more, be careful to get enough sun, without burning. The sun is our friend if approached prudently, and it will protect us, not only from osteoporosis, but from all illnesses, including cancer. Warning: shun artificial tanning in UV beds as they dramatically increase the risk of malignant melanoma.

And, since we've mentioned sunscreens, while governments push sunscreens aggressively, they fail to mention studies that have proved them to be dangerous. For example, a study conducted by the Norwegian Radiation Protection Authority found that a weak dose of OMC (*octyl methoxycinnamate*), a chemical used in 90 percent of sunscreens, killed half the mouse cells it touched. Shining a lamp on the OMC-impregnated cells, to simulate sunshine, made the chemical even deadlier. In these tests the concentration of OMC was only five parts per million, a much lower concentration than that used in sunscreens. More than 90 percent of the cells survived in the solution without OMC. Terje Christensen, the biophysicist who ran the tests, suggests that the reactions between OMC and light are twice as toxic as OMC itself, and he believes that OMC will damage human cells if it penetrates the outer layer of dead skin. The Cosmetic, Toiletry and Perfumery Association, which represents sunscreen manufacturers in Britain, says that OMC is safe. But they would, wouldn't they?

On the other hand, *The British Medical Journal, 20 January 1996*, concurs with the Norwegians: "Scientists don't know which part of the sun's spectrum is responsible for bringing on skin cancer.... Without this knowledge, sunscreens are useless and, worse, may in fact be responsible for bringing on the cancer in the first place."

So, in the words of the song, "Let The Sunshine In".

Oxygen Therapy

In your search for health, nothing is more important than oxygen – the air that you breathe. Of all the elements your body must have, oxygen is Number One – it is in constant demand, and its absence will bring death in minutes. Low concentrations of oxygen in the blood will inevitably bring ill health.

Before industrialization and deforestation brought pollution to our world, about 35 percent of our atmosphere was composed of oxygen. Now, if we are lucky enough to live away from cities, we have only approximately 20 percent oxygen in our air. If we live in a city, or even near a city, levels can fall to as low as 10 percent. This is not the way nature intended us to live and we are suffering as a result.

Dr Kurt Donsbach, who was President of the National Health Federation in the US for 15 years, now has a clinic in Rosarita Beach, Mexico, close to the

California border (see *Resources*). Using intravenous H_2O_2, his clinic has achieved cancer remission rates exceeding 70 percent in many hundreds of patients, most of whom were told they were beyond hope. Similar results are being achieved in the many European countries that offer this therapy.

Even though Nobel Prize winner Dr Otto Warburg and famous heart surgeon Dr Christiaan Barnard were advocates of oxygen/ozone therapy, governments in English-speaking countries have contrived to demonise this safe, incredibly effective healing method. Because of this, only a handful of brave doctors are game enough to administer it to their patients. We can, however, oxygenate our bloodstreams ourselves if we wish, by absorption of oxygen water at very low concentrations. It is amazing that something so simple, and within reach of all budgets, can provide such remarkable results. So far, 'they' haven't been able to take hydrogen peroxide away from us!

It has been found in many experiments, over decades, that viruses cannot tolerate high oxygen levels in the blood. Every disease organism tested so far appears to have the same weakness, including AIDS. Even cancer growths, because they are anaerobic, contract and disappear when oxygen saturation is increased sufficiently in the surrounding fluids. Many scientific papers and books have been written about this therapy, and there are countless internet sites on the subject if you want to learn more. The intravenous therapy is more dramatic and effective, but we have been told of wonderful results with a wide variety of complaints, using the following method:

Get a bottle (you may have to place an order) of 35%, food-grade hydrogen peroxide from your pharmacy. Put a small amount into a glass dropper bottle and store the rest in your freezer, because it is not stabilised with the chemicals used on the lower percentage peroxides. It will remain in liquid form, and it is advisable to open the cap each week to allow any build-up of gasses to escape. Put a small amount in a dropper bottle, taking care not to spill any, as it is strong. *Do not under any circumstances use it neat!* On the first day, put one drop into about 150ml (5 ounces) of pure water, and drink it about 20 minutes before each meal. Do this for three days, then raise the amount to two drops for three days, and so on until you reach five or six drops. Once your complaint has eased, you may prefer to take up to 10 drops once a day as maintenance. Some extremely ill people take as many as 20 drops per day for a limited time with good results, but **please do not commence this therapy without first clearing it with a health professional.**

Bowen Therapy

This Australian-developed treatment has been successful in treating musculoskeletal problems, such as back and neck pain, scoliosis, sporting injuries, TMJ alignment, and carpal tunnel syndrome. It is also renowned for its effectiveness with internal conditions, such as migraines, digestive and elimination complaints, colic in babies, and respiratory problems, including asthma. Bowen Therapy (Bowtech) is appropriate for everyone, from the highly trained athlete to newborns, pregnant women, the elderly, and the chronically ill, as treatment given by qualified practitioners consists simply of gentle, rolling movements that activate a systematic response so powerful that a few minutes pause is observed to allow them to be integrated. My own experiences with Bowen Therapy have been remarkable, and I recommend it highly. See **Resources** for more details.

Exercise

Sensible and regular exercise will do wonders for your overall health. It is particularly beneficial for improving the cardio-vascular system, stimulating the lymphatic system to eliminate toxic waste from the body, and promoting healthy bones through the stimulation of blood flow.

You don't have to go to a gym; there are numerous activities which will keep your body in tip-top condition. Take a daily walk. If it's raining, don a raincoat and boots, or use a rebounder indoors if you have one. If not, walk smartly in place in a well-aired room, while breathing deeply. If you want to do weights, please take it easy – baby steps only, the first day. No matter what the 'gym cowboys' say, don't do more than two or three repetitions on each weight, working up in increments of two each time, provided you go regularly. And keep the weight low until your muscles are used to the workout. Ignore anyone urging you to overdo – don't become just one of many people injured, sometimes permanently, by some instructors who don't understand how muscles and bones work.

Small, lightweight dumbbells are available for those who prefer to exercise at home. You will want to get a book on the best way to use them, and be sure to follow the 'two or three reps a day until strong' rule.

Tufts University in the US did a study of nursing home patients and found that, after two months of training with light weights, the participants doubled, tripled and even quadrupled their strength. Some were even able to stop using canes. While we can't keep our bodies from ageing and dying, it's good to know that, if we keep fit with exercise, when we shuffle off this mortal coil, we can at least carry our own bags.

To illustrate what can happen to people who don't get the proper exercise, when I was in my thirties, and overwhelmed by work, I thought I didn't have time for exercise. After two sedentary years my back suddenly gave out and the pain was so excruciating that I was bedridden for two months. Friends carried me to two prominent Los Angeles orthopaedic specialists. Both assured me that I would never be out of pain unless they operated on my spine. Because of a well-earned fear of doctors, and because three friends who had submitted to such operations had been crippled by them, I preferred to remain in pain. Then my hero arrived, sent by a worried friend, and I will be indebted to both of them for the rest of my life. Mike Abrums, a brilliant exercise therapist, saved me. Under his careful tutelage I learned how to strengthen the muscles which support the spine. In six weeks he had me pain free and as soon as he judged me strong enough, he taught me to use weights. Those weights are so important to me that for decades I have carried them on long trips, even on safari through Africa.

Tonic and Rejuvenator

Wheatgrass (baby wheat) juice is an extremely important body cleanser and natural food. Since Dr Ann Wigmore rediscovered the nutritional qualities of wheatgrass juice in 1960, the juice has helped hundreds of thousands of people around the world overcome serious health problems. Chlorophyll in wheatgrass juice has been found to increase the functions of the heart, vascular system, intestines, uterus and lungs. It also disinfects, can reduce the effects of radiation, contains liquid oxygen, which promotes clearer thinking, and helps to stop cancer cells from growing because of the abscisic acid it contains. But remember: wheatgrass juice, healing as it is, will not overcome a terrible diet. Nothing will.

Liver Cleanser

Henry Bieler, MD, taught me how to make what I think is the best liver cleanse, other than adopting the Hippocrates diet. It is ideal for illnesses when fasting is not viable. Amongst Dr Bieler afficionadoes it is known as Bieler Broth, but it isn't broth – it is a purée soup, and it goes down beautifully when people need to clean themselves out. It's also a delicious and healthful all-purpose soup at any time.

All you need is an approximately equal amount of green beans, celery and zucchini, and enough pure water to cover. Cook until soft – not crunchy. The object is not to provide vitamins and minerals, but to relieve the liver of its congestion and restore it to normal function. The organic sodium and potassium in these vegetables is ideal for this purpose. Blend the cooked vegetables and the water. And if the celery is stringy, press it through a sieve. Raw parsley may be added for flavour after cooking. Dr Bieler had his patients stay on this soup exclusively for the duration of their illnesses. No seasoning is permitted, as this would negate the value of the cleansing. These vegetables should be eaten all the time - not just in soup - as they are very healing.

Olive Leaf Extract

This compound is anti-bacterial, anti-viral and anti-fungal. It is purported to destroy the bad and protect the good, as compared to antibiotics, which kill the lot and leave you weaker. I have had no experience with this natural healer, but if I had any of the above nasties, I would try it and stay away from the antibiotics. But use it only for short periods of time, as it suppresses metabolic processes the way antibiotics do, and you will need to replace the good bacteria with acidophilus after you quit taking it.

Colloidal Silver

Some people swear by this remedy, others say it didn't do a thing for them. Be aware that if you take too much it can cause argyria, a serious condition, which turns your face pale blue.

Skin Brushing

Before bathing, rub your body briskly all over with a special skin brush or a rough wash cloth. Spend at least five minutes on this and your pores will open so impurities can escape.

Magnets

These are highly recommended by Dr Earl Conroy, a New Zealand physician whose judgement I trust. When Dr Conroy's patients have serious prostate problems, he always has them buy, from a doctor in the US, a 4-inch by 6-inch by half-inch velcro-covered ceramic magnet (4000 gauss) which they can sit on for a couple of hours a day. His results with this therapy have been excellent.

He says, "The north pole of a powerful magnet will relieve inflammation of the prostate, ovaries, breasts, teeth, ankles, knees, elbows, etc. They also make a small magnet that a woman can put in her bra. This would be the first line of therapy for any breast lump or inflammation." See **Resources** for ordering, and for a book on magnet therapy.

Coffee Enemas

The first time I heard about coffee enemas I laughed. Another weirdo health fad, I thought. But then I remembered that condemning new ideas without thorough investigation is indicative of a closed, dull mind. So I did some reading and even drove all the way from my then home in Beverly Hills, California, to the Max Gerson Hospital in Tijuana, Mexico.

There, I found people in varying stages of cancer who had come for help after long, unsuccessful conventional treatments in hospitals. Most had been given up and sent away to die. Even the worst cases, after a few days on the Gerson detoxification program, were able to discontinue medication, depending instead upon several coffee enemas per day to control their pain.

Subsequently, I spent two weeks at the clinic, learning about the technique and interviewing the patients. The healing I witnessed during this short stay was amazing. Detoxification is the answer for seriously ill people, not chemotherapy that poisons healthy cells as well as cancerous cells. Not surgery that rarely gets all the cancerous cells and makes the surviving cells more virulent. And certainly not radiation. Our immune systems, crucial for all aspects of health, are irreparably damaged by chemotherapy and radiation.

This clinic is, unfortunately, very expensive, and the complex regimen must be maintained for a long time after the patient is discharged. In my experience, it takes two helpers to support one outpatient. Organic vegetables have to be sourced, thirteen juices have to be pressed each day, and a strict schedule must be adhered to. For those who can afford it, Dr Gerson's technique is superb, and I highly recommend it for seriously ill people in North America.

Coffee enemas had their genesis during a time of dire need: toward the end of World War I, Germany was blockaded and broke. Thousands of injured soldiers were in agony, due to lack of morphine, and surgeons and nurses were desperate. Somehow, with an extraordinary leap of the imagination, a nurse got the idea that an enema might help alleviate the pain of a suffering young soldier. Coffee was the only sterile solution available, and she tried it. To the amazement of everyone involved, the soldier reported great relief, the remedy was used widely from then on, and the rest is history.

Dr Max Gerson, whom Dr Albert Schweitzer called "... one of the most eminent geniuses in medical history", incorporated this unlikely remedy into his famous cancer therapy. The purpose of these enemas is not to clean the colon, but to help detoxify the liver and bring quick relief from pain of all kinds. A headache, a hangover, a yucky feeling – you name it, a properly-administered coffee enema can bring quick relief.

Dr Gerson's instructions for preparing are: "Take 3 tablespoons of ground (drip) coffee (not instant) to 1 quart of pure water; let it boil 3 minutes and then simmer 15 minutes more. Strain and use at body temperature." I recommend that you use organic coffee, which is readily available in Australia, and, I presume, in most countries.

Dr Gerson says, in his ground-breaking book, *A Cancer Therapy, Results Of 50 Cases*, "To make enemas most effective, the patient should lie on his right side, with both legs drawn close to the abdomen, and breathe deeply, in order to suck the greatest amount of fluid into all parts of the colon. The fluid should be retained 10 to 15 minutes. Our experiments have shown that after 10 to 12 minutes almost all caffeine is absorbed from the fluid. It goes through the haemorrhoidal veins directly into the portal veins and into the liver. Patients have to know that the coffee enemas are not given for the function of the intestines but for the stimulation of the liver."

The best way to administer an enema is to lie on the floor and place the enema bucket on a chair so the flow is gentle. Or simply hang your enema bag from the back of a chair.

In July of 2004, the Prince of Wales had the courage to speak out in favour of alternative cancer therapies, specifically the Gerson Therapy. He was rewarded for his opened minded honesty with an extraordinary and rude outpouring of vitriol from the entrenched medical profession. "Cancer Inc." have had things their own way for too long. They have never had to prove their chemotherapy and radiation are safe (which, of course, they are not), yet claim that the Gerson Therapy is "unproven".

Come on, doctors, it's been used since the end of World War One, with amazing success, and if you **really** want to know the truth, I have a suggestion: go to Mexico and observe, as did I, while nearly-comatose people are brought in by ambulance, on stretchers with morphine drips. They are victims of your "proven" slash/burn/radiate, and they are in agony. Watch them as they respond to the gentle therapy and replace damaging morphine with equally-effective coffee enemas. Listen to their stories of an uncaring medical profession that has stripped them of their dignity and often their life savings, and left them for dead. Follow through, as did I, and discover how many recovered completely. Then, re-think your condemnation of Prince Charles, who really cares, and is brave enough to say so.

Also, give thought to his efforts to popularize organic farming. The world could use more such as he, as well as doctors who speak out about the cancer/pesticide/superphosphate connection, just one of the many causes of our cancer epidemic.

The detoxification system used at Hippocrates Health Centre is different from Dr Gerson's, but equally successful, in my opinion. Coffee enemas are not used, but pure water enemas, followed by wheatgrass implants are encouraged. As an added advantage, the Hippocrates program costs a fraction of the Gerson therapy, and is easy to implement when students return to their homes.

Colonics, which help enormously with detoxification, are also available at Hippocrates. The Brunelle Hydrotherapy Unit stimulates all organs of the body, including the lymphatic system, via the reflex points in the colon. These units are in use, as well, at Taringa Health Centre in Southport, Queensland, Australia.

Internal Heat Treatment

Heat has been used to heal for centuries. The great Greek "Father of Medicine", Hippocrates, recommended hot water douches for pelvic pain 2500 years ago. More recently, *The Journal Of Urology*, *Volume 25, No. 6*, printed in 1936, contained a study from the James Buchanan Brady Urological Institute, Johns Hopkins Hospital, which described "striking success" using heat in the treatment of pelvic inflammatory disease and "uniformly good results in acutely inflamed prostates." The devices they used, such as the Elliott Treatment Regulator, were large, primitive hot water douches which had to be administered in hospital. Due to their success, during the 1930s anal and vaginal heating devices became available and were very popular, judging by the many new patents and articles in medical journals. During those pre-antibiotic days, surgery was avoided in 80 percent of cases, according to hospital records, certainly a better result than what we see in our knife and pill-happy age.

In recent years, fortunately, the Swiss have refined these healing devices and they are now available in a small electric unit, the *Delwa Star Rectal/Vaginal Heater,* with a battery charger that can be set to any current, and slender, comfortable probes that can be used vaginally and anally. They cost a few hundred dollars, but are infinitely less expensive than flying to a clinic in Germany for hyperthermia.

The American physicians who are pioneering use of these heat probes have spent a great deal of time in China, working alongside Traditional Chinese Medicine (TCM) physicians, who understood exactly how the probes heal. As they said, "Placement in the anus will have a powerful stimulatory effect on two meridians that run up the middle of the front and back of the body." This, according to TCM, gets the immune system to function optimally and *can trigger healing responses all over the body*. The list of conditions that can be cured, ranging from haemorrhoids to hives, is far too long to detail here. As one small example, 69 men with prostatitis, prostate enlargement or both, were treated at the Kliniken Karnan in Helsingborg, Sweden. Overall, 81.2 percent were classified as symptom-free or better, after six weekly treatments of 20 minutes each.

The Delwa Star was brought to my attention by an article in Dr Robert Jay Rowen's newsletter, **Second Opinion**. Dr Rowen wrote, "This device could spare much suffering for men prone to prostate problems. There could be significant benefit to women with vaginal, bladder, or even uterine problems... Delivering heat to this cancer-prone area of the body (lower pelvis) may also have far-reaching preventive and immune-stimulating effects against cancer-causing pathogens. But the method is too simple and unprofitable for such studies to receive funding by a profit-driven industry."

Because I have a high regard for Dr Rowen's integrity, the Hippocrates Centre bought a unit for experimental purposes, and I can testify that they are an invaluable first aid device. And, no, we do not sell them, but you can email Dr Charles McGee, head of Chee Energy, Inc, the distributor, and he will send more information. You'll find Dr McGee's contact details in **Resources**, and if you mention this book, he'll give a 10% discount.

The Bioptron

This Swiss-made light therapy device has amazing natural healing power. I have had the small and the large model for four years, and have observed amazing recoveries from pain, wound healing, burns, leg ulcers, skin irregularities, and even skin cancers. Bioptrons are used in treatment facilities, hospitals and in private homes and are my favourite first-aid device. Two quibbles – they are pricey and their colour therapy for the skin, an optional extra, is meant to be used with enclosed cosmetics that have ingredients I strongly recommend against. A write-in campaign is needed here to set this otherwise excellent company straight on chemicals in cosmetics.

The Bioptron's electromagnetic spectrum does not contain UV radiation.
Websites: www.southernlight.com.au and www.bioptron.com.
Australian distributors:

- ❖ NSW: Southern Light Therapies, Phone/Fax: 1300 650 227
  Email: sales@southernlight.com.au
- ❖ Victoria: Marlene West (MANPA)
  Homeopath and Bioptron Light Therapist and Distributor
  Ph: 03 9899 8015, 0409 159 158

Skin Problems

JAMES BAILLIE'S WONDER BALM IS JUST THAT – A REAL WONDER!

Before recommending products (precious few, as readers know) I experiment on myself. Only after I'm convinced something is safe and effective, do I call on a group of loyal friends, who have participated in many of my experiments, to have a go. In the case of Wonder Balm, we found the following:

- Ugly, dark freckles fade to nothing
- Rough skin patches become smooth
- Lumps, some thick and as large as walnuts, slowly break apart
- Keratoses (pre-cancers) slough off
- Toenail fungus improves
- Haemorrhoids disappear
- Wrinkles improve
- Scars, even very old ones, slowly fade
- Muscle aches disappear
- Sprains quickly mend
- It appears to help with skin cancers, but do not try it on melanomas

Some improvements happen quickly, others require persistence, and some problems are not affected at all. We are all different. Really dark spots can take up to two months to fade away. I LOVE this oil and recommend it to everyone. It's safe and economical.

Wonder Balm, and James Baillie's other oils, are sold only in Australia. You will find them at Castlemain Natural Store, 107 Mostyn Street; The Maldon Herbalist, 2A Main Street, and from his stall at the Daylesford Market on Sundays from 7:30 to 2:00 p.m. All in Maldon, Victoria. Or send cheques or money orders, made out to James Baillie, to P.O. Box 216, Maldon 3463, Victoria. The cost, for 270ml is $30 for one bottle, including postage, or $54 for two bottles, also including postage. For more than two bottles, add $22 for each extra bottle.

27

In Other Words...

A selection of articles of interest from other writers

Pregnenolone

by

Raymond Peat, MA, PhD (Univ. of Oregon)
Endocrine Physiologist

Pregnenolone, which is the raw material for producing many of the hormones of stress and adaptation, was known as early as 1934, but for several years it was considered to be an "inert" substance. A reason for this belief is that it was first tested on healthy young animals. Since these animals were already producing large amounts of pregnenolone (in the brain, adrenal glands, and gonads), additional pregnenolone had no effect.

In the 1940s, pregnenolone was tested in people who were sick or under stress, and it was found to have a **wide range** of beneficial actions, but the drug industry never had much interest in it. Its very generality made it seem unlike a drug, and its natural occurrence made it impossible to patent. Thus, many synthetic variants, each with a more specialised action and some serious side effects, came to be patented and promoted for use in treating specific conditions. The drug companies created an atmosphere in which many people felt that each disease should have a drug, and each drug, a disease. The side effects of some of those synthetic hormones were so awful that many people came to fear them.

Natural pregnenolone is present in young people of both sexes at a very high concentration, and one reason for the large amount produced in youth is that it is one of our basic defenses against the harmful side effects that an imbalance of even our natural hormones can produce. In excess, natural cortisone or estrogen can be dangerous, but when there is an abundance of pregnenolone, their side effects are prevented or minimised.

In a healthy young person or animal, taking even a large dose of pregnenolone has no hormone-like or drug-like action at all. It is unique in this way. But if the animal or person is under stress, and producing more cortisone than usual, taking pregnenolone causes the cortisone to come down to the normal level. After the age of 40 or 45, it seems that everyone lives in a state of continuous "stress", just as a normal part of aging. This coincides with the body's decreased ability to produce an abundance of pregnenolone.

When aging rats are given a supplement of pregnenolone, it immediately improves their memory and general performance. Human studies, as early as the 1940s, have also demonstrated improved performance of ordinary tasks. It is now known that pregnenolone is one of the major hormones in the brain. It is produced by certain brain cells, as well as being absorbed into the brain from the blood. It protects brain cells from injury caused by fatigue, and an adequate amount has a calming effect on the emotions, which is part of the reason that it protects us from the stress response that leads to an excessive production of cortisone. People feel a mood of resilience and an ability to confront challenges.

Many people have noticed that pregnenolone has a "face-lifting" action. This effect seems to be produced by improved circulation to the skin, and by an actual contraction of some muscle-like cells in the skin. A similar effect can improve joint mobility in arthritis, tissue elasticity in the lungs, and even eyesight. Many studies have shown it to be protective of "fibrous tissues" in general, and in this connection it was proven to prevent the tumors that can be caused by estrogen.

Pregnenolone is largely converted into two other "youth-associated" protective hormones, progesterone and DHEA. At the age of 30, both men and women produce roughly 30 to 50mg of pregnenolone daily. When taken orally, even in the powdered form, it is absorbed fairly well. One dose of approximately 300mg (the size of an aspirin tablet) keeps acting for about a week, as absorption continues along the intestine, and as it is "recycled" in the body. Part of this long lasting effect is because it improves the body's ability to produce its own pregnenolone. It tends to improve function of the thyroid and other glands, and this "normalizing" effect on the other glands helps to account for its wide range of beneficial effects.

Maca
Discover How This New Phytonutrient Can Ease Menopausal Symptoms
by
Amy Nancarrow
Excerpted from **Nature & Health**, *December 1999/January 2000*

Rather than hormone replacement therapy (HRT) millions of women are putting their faith in a remedy which has been used for 10,000 years, which is safe and amazingly effective: a cruciferous root vegetable from Peru called maca.

Now women have an alternative to hormone replacement therapy drugs. Maca works in an entirely different and more satisfactory way for most women than phytoestrogen herbs like black cohosh and licorice root. And men too, find that maca can counteract the difficulties they may experience in maintaining good sexual relationships as they age, due to a general slowing down in the output of the endocrine glands.

Alternative to HRT

It is important to remember that maca does not itself contain any hormones, but its action on the body jogs the pituitary into producing the precursor hormones which ultimately end up raising oestrogen, progesterone and testosterone levels, as well as helping to balance the adrenal glands, the thyroid and the pancreas. But this occurs naturally, not with time-bomb drugs which throw the entire body into a dangerous state of confusion.

Dr Jorge Malaspina, a respected cardiologist, has been using maca in his practice in Lima, Peru, for over a decade. He says, "Maca does not cause the ovaries in women to atrophy, as conventional hormone replacement therapy does." This means that maca may be discontinued at any time without danger.

He adds, "Different medicinal plants work on the ovaries by stimulating them. With maca, though, we should say that it 'regulates' the ovarian function, as well as the organs of internal secretion, such as the pituitary, the adrenal glands, and the pancreas. He has also found maca to be effective even on women who have undergone complete hysterectomies. He describes one patient who had a serum oestradiol level of 15, which is very low. After two months on maca it went up to 75. He says that a level above 60 is an adequate postmenopausal level. "Maca enables the adrenals to make sufficient hormones to avoid symptoms," he says.

Dr Malaspina adamantly prefers maca therapy to HRT. "The presence of outside hormones circulating in the system sends a message to the pituitary and the hypothalamus that there is a sufficient quantity of hormones in the body and so they stop producing them. When menopause arrives, then, the ovaries are atrophied and do not produce the oestrogen and progesterone which the body requires minimally to function. For this reason I encourage women to start with maca before menopause. It seems to help the endocrine system to stay in balance."

'Natural Viagra'

Doctors also have good news for men who are suffering age-related sexual dysfunction. They can forget expensive, possibly dangerous Viagra. Maca works extremely well, and safely.

Dr Jorge Aguila Calderon, Dean of the Faculty of Human Medicine at the National University of Federico Villareal in Lima, prescribes maca for a wide variety of conditions, including osteoporosis and the healing of bone fractures in the very elderly. He says, "Maca has a lot of easily-absorbable calcium in it, plus magnesium, and a fair amount of silica, which we are finding very useful in treating decalcification of bones in children and adults."

Dr Calderon has also helped patients overcome male impotence, male sterility, and female sterility by employing maca therapy. Additional problems he treats with maca are rickets, various forms of anaemia, menopausal symptoms such as hot flashes and night sweats, climacteric and erectile difficulties in men, premature ageing, and general states of weakness, such as chronic fatigue.

Another health professional using maca is Dr Garry F. Gordon, President of the International College of Advanced Longevity Medicine in Chicago, Illinois. He said: "Using maca myself, I experienced a significant improvement in erectile tissue response. I call it 'nature's answer to Viagra'.

"What I see in maca is a means of normalising our steroid hormones like testosterone, progesterone and oestrogen. Therefore, it has the facility to forestall the hormonal changes of ageing. It acts on men to restore them to healthy functional status in which they experience a more active libido. Lots of men and women who previously believed their sexual problems were psychological, are now clearly going to look for something physiological to improve quality of life in the area of sexuality. Of course, as someone interested in longevity, I'm aware that mortality comes on much sooner for those individuals whose sexual activity is diminished or nonexistent. I believe that people who engage in sex twice a week, or more, live longer. I've found sexual activity to be a reliable marker for overall ageing."

Maca at a Glance
What it is

Maca is a dehydrated, cruciferous root vegetable and not a drug, so it is imported without any problems. It is a benign, medicinal food which has been in use for 10,000 years, possibly more, and has had ample time to be judged effective. It is also easily affordable, costing less than $12 per month.

What's in it

Proteins, as polypeptides, make up 11 per cent of the dry maca root; calcium makes up 10 per cent and magnesium and potassium are present in significant amounts. Other minerals include iron, silica and traces of iodine, manganese, zinc, copper and sodium. Vitamins in maca are thiamine, riboflavin and ascorbic acid. The amino acid proteins in maca include aspartic acid, glutamic acid, serine, histidine, glycine, threolline, cystine, alanine, arginine, tyrosins, valine, methionine, isoleucine, lysine, hoproline and sarcosine.

Benefits

According to doctors in Peru and the USA, maca may be of benefit for:

- Menopausal symptoms: Hot flashes, tender breasts, sleeplessness and emotional upsets, "brain fog", vaginal dryness
- Osteoporosis: Significant bone rebuilding, improvement in bone density
- Energy booster: Balances the endocrine system: thyroid, pituitary and adrenal glands
- Male impotence
- Chronic Fatigue Syndrome
- Period problems: Pain, PMS, flooding and/or scant flow

Prominent health professional, Grant Woolven, says about this natural remedy: "Maca could be called a 'miracle of nature' because it has such remarkable effects on the body and mind. Because it is a food, as opposed to a medicinal herb, it can be taken every day without any negative side effects. From an Ayurvedic viewpoint, it effectively strengthens the nervous system and brain, via its effect on the kidney energy. It regulates the liver energy, resulting in a harmonising of all endocrine functions, especially the ovaries, testes and pituitary glands. Because of these effects it is excellent for catalysing emotional stability and a deep sense of psychophysical wellbeing and integration. It is no wonder some people call it the 'happiness herb'.

"Because it is 'vata-reducing' it is excellent for people who are rundown, depleted, undernourished or emaciated. It is a 'rebuilding tonic' with the added benefit of being warming energetically, which facilitates the digestive fire (agni) and good circulation. Although it is excellent for those people with endocrine imbalances, it is also excellent, when combined with rosehips, for the rejuvenation of tissue and immunity in any person at any age."

Maca
The Peruvian Powerhouse
by
Amy Nancarrow
Excerpted from *Nature & Health*, *Oct/Nov, 2001*

Since our report on the Peruvian powder, maca, many readers have written to *Nature & Health* to share the experiences they've had with this natural remedy. Limited space prevents us from printing all of them, but we want to thank everyone for writing with their individual success stories – and hope that they will inspire others in similar situations.

Heavy Periods: Cecile's Story

"I am 41 years of age and had experienced heavy menstrual bleeding since a teenager. I have had three children, and as I got older, my health has also been compromised by chronic anaemia. Each month I would feel a heaviness and pressure in my body as a build-up to my period. After the heavy flow, it would take several days to feel OK after feeling extremely tired and 'washed-out'. I started taking the herb maca five cycles (months) ago. I believe I noticed a change after three weeks, and I encourage women who take this herb to persevere through this initial phase. This is no quick pharmaceutical fix, but has been like a miracle cure for me. I can honestly say that all negative aspects and symptoms of my periods have reduced by 80 per cent, and I continue to feel more well as each month passes. The blood flow has also decreased dramatically so that I feel my energy levels and physical vitality are really very good. I would recommend this herb for any women experiencing menstrual or hormonal problems."

Hysterectomy: Melanie's Story

"After years of symptoms that kept getting worse, my doctor told me that if I didn't have a hysterectomy I would get cancer. I was really depressed because friends who have endured this operation have never fully recovered, and their marital relations were adversely affected. Then a friend told me about maca and showed me an article in your magazine. At first, I didn't really believe anything so simple could be so good, but I started feeling much better after about three weeks of taking it. For the first time in my life I'm having normal periods, and I will never have that awful operation."

Chronic Fatigue Syndrome: Peggy's Story

"Almost six years ago, I contracted Ross River Fever and was desperately ill for months. Eventually I was diagnosed with Chronic Fatigue Syndrome and nothing brought relief (I tried everything!) until I read about maca in your wonderful magazine. For the first few weeks I didn't notice any improvement.

"Then I increased my dose to one teaspoon twice a day, and after two weeks I felt human for the first time in years. I just kept getting better every month until now, a year and a half after starting maca, I am normal again. Chronic Fatigue Syndrome is a terrible affliction, and I wanted to write to you so others will know where to find help. Oh, yes, and I was able to cut my dose down to 'maintenance' after two months, so it only costs me about $10 per month. What a bargain!"

Hair and Nails: Mindy's Story

"I first learned about maca from a woman who had 'drowned mouse hair', as she called it. She had been struggling with straight, lifeless hair all her life, having to set it daily in the vain effort to give it body. One day when I was doing her hair (I have been a hairdresser for 15 years), I was amazed to discover that it is now full of pep – it's stronger, lustrous, and even has a bit of a curl. The upshot is that I've lost a client, because all she needs since maca is an occasional haircut, as she now has 'wash-and-wear hair'. She doesn't even need to dry it – a towel-rub and a fluff and she's all set! Needless to say, I started taking this 'magic powder' myself and my hair has improved out of sight, as have my fingernails. They used to be pale, and now they're a healthy pink, and growing long for the first time in my life! I've recommended maca to lots of people, and they are all having great results."

Osteoporosis: Marilyn's Story

"About a year and a half ago, when I had a bone scan, they told me I had the bones of an 80 year-old – and I'm only 52! 1 was really worried, but I certainly didn't want to take oestrogen, because of the side effects. Then I read about maca in your magazine, and I'm so grateful to you for printing that information.

"The first change I noticed was that my fingernails looked different. They were a very pale colour and they had strange white horizontal marks across them. Somebody told me that meant I had low calcium, but I don't know if that's right. It wasn't long before my nails got pink and healthy looking, and to my amazement they grew long and didn't break off the way they have all my life. I figured that meant I was assimilating my calcium (which I was getting from eating more sardines and vegetables, which I read had calcium in them). This was encouraging and I got the courage to have another bone scan, and my doctor couldn't believe it was possible to have so much improvement. He seemed pretty annoyed when I admitted that I wasn't taking calcium (he was already pretty cross that I wouldn't take oestrogen!), and when I tried to explain that the improvement was caused by a natural herb powder, he didn't want to know! I think I'm going to change doctors!

"Another thing – I don't know what maca has in it that helps the emotions, but it sure made a change in me. For years I was depressed most of the time (I also refused the Prozac the doctor suggested!), but maca has lifted my spirits. I'm happy in life, and always laughing. Thank you, *Nature & Health*, for making this big improvement in my life possible. My husband thanks you, too, because I used to be pretty hard to live with!"

Perimenopause: Susan's Story

"The perimenopausal phase began for me five and a half years ago when I was almost 41, and was characterised by irregularly spaced periods, with some continuing daily for months at a time, mood swings including depression; itchy skin; lowered libido; and the occasional hot flush. Then, nine months ago, after not having a period for six months, things became dramatically intensified. Ten searing hot flushes with accompanying sweats a day seemed difficult to endure, but they soon increased in frequency to every half hour, day and night, with the result that any significant sleep became impossible. With almost no sleep and the debilitating effects of the flushes themselves, my quality of life was dwindling and I began to wonder how long I could continue. I had previously not realised that menopause could have such a devastating effect on your body and mind. I almost felt that if life was going to be like this from now on, then it wasn't worth living.

"When I heard about maca, it seemed like an answer to a prayer, as it has in fact proven to be. Within a week the flushes had reduced significantly, and within eight weeks, they had disappeared entirely. I had to begin with quite a high dosage, and adjust it frequently during the first few months, but I am now comfortable on a quarter of a teaspoon twice daily. Also, within a week, my libido made a strong and welcome return and now the genital atrophy that had occurred has completely reversed. Sleep has become deep and uninterrupted, my energy levels have risen dramatically, my mental acuity has returned, and there have been some unexpected positive side effects, such as better-looking skin and the disappearance of an anal fistula, which had not responded to a barrage of treatments prior to this. I cannot recommended maca highly enough to other women weathering the menopausal storm."

What an Expert says:

Naturopath Anita Barry, from Ashmore, Queensland, writes: "Following are some of the experiences my patients have had on maca powder:

• A lady with severe osteoporosis was overjoyed when she told me there had been an increase in her bone density, after one year on maca.

• A patient who suffered depression, irritability and severe mood swings, making life unbearable for her family and, of course, for herself, reported incredible relief after taking maca for just a short time.

• A 20 year-old patient, whose periods had ceased two years previously, took maca and after only two months, her periods returned.

"As a natural health practitioner, I am delighted to discover a safe product that can bring health benefits to so many."

Maca: Contraindications

Because Maca regulates hormones, and because no double-blind testing has been done to prove its safety when used by those with hormone-related cancers (breast, female organs, testicular, etc) we advise extreme caution. Maca should not be taken during pregnancy, nor while breast-feeding. Also, consult your health practitioner if you have bladder or liver disease or high blood pressure. The use of fertility drugs, black cohosh, dong quai, ginseng or licorice root along with Maca is not recommended. *E.H.*

Take Control of Your Health and Escape the Sickness Industry

RESOURCES

- *Recommended Reading*
- *Products*
- *Services*

THE ESTABLISHMENT HATES THIS BOOK!

THEY HAVE MADE IT AN UNDERDOG

❖ The multinational-controlled media won't publicise it
❖ Distributors of health books say it's too far out
❖ Government-owned magazines won't accept advertising for it
❖ Publishers, owned by the multinationals, shun it
❖ The medical establishment labels us dangerous "ratbags" while they poison people with radiation, chemotherapy and other drugs with life-threatening side effects

Don't let them get away with it – join our crusade – become a
CITIZEN DISTRIBUTOR. Buy 10 books at wholesale.
You can then give away or sell at retail
For information: sales@doctorsaredangerous.com or (07) 5530-2939

PEOPLE POWER IS OUR ONLY HOPE TO OVERCOME THE TYRANTS.

Although every effort has been made to ensure that the details shown in this section are correct, the author cannot be held responsible for changes which may subsequently occur. All information is supplied in good faith, but you should also make your own enquiries, and seek professional advice if necessary, before purchasing any products and/or services, or undertaking any treatment.

Recommended Reading

The Great Thyroid Scandal and How To Survive It

Now changed to:
Your Thyroid and how to Keep it Healthy by Dr. Barry Durrant-Peatfield, MB BSc LRCP MRCS.
Sold in UK book stores and on Amazon I consider this to be one of the best books ever written on the thyroid and related problems. Highly recommended.
Published by: Hammersmith Press
www.hammersmithpress.co.uk.

Solved: The Riddle of Illness

Steven Langer MD and James F Scheer
Valuable thyroid information
Keats Publishing Inc
27 Pine Street (Box 876)
New Canaan, Connecticut
www.keats.com

Overcoming Thyroid Disorders

David Brownstein, MD
Medical Alternatives Press
4173 Fieldbrook Road
West Bloomfield
Michigan 48323
www.drbrownstein.com

Why Stomach Acid Is Good For You

Jonathan V Wright, MD, and Lane Lenard, PhD
Publisher: M Evans & Company Inc
216 E 49th Street
New York, NY 10017
Available from Tahoma Clinic Dispensary
www.tahoma-clinic.com

The No-Grain Diet

Dr Joseph Mercola
Info and Order: www.mercola.com

Tooth Truth

Frank J Jerome, DDS
Frank J Jerome
639 Washington Street
Columbus, Indiana 47201

Aspartame Disease, An Ignored Epidemic

H J Roberts, MD
Dr Roberts has alerted the world to this modern day scourge, and is recognised as a world authority on the health effects of aspartame.
Sunshine Sentinel Press
P O Box 17799
West Palm Beach, Florida 33416
USA Phone: 1800 827 7991
www.sunsentpress.com

Safe Uses of Cortisol

William McK. Jefferies, MD FACP
Every physician should be made to read this invaluable work on a little-understood topic.
Charles C Thomas Publisher Ltd
2600 South First Street
Springfield, Illinois 62794-9265
www.ccthomas.com

The Cholesterol Myths

Uffe Ravnskov, MD PhD
New Trends Publishing
Washington DC
www.NewTrendsPublishing.com

Hormonal Health: Nutritional and Hormonal Strategies for Emotional Well-being and Intellectual Longevity

Dr Michael Colgan
Apple Publishing
220 E 59th Avenue
Vancouver, British Columbia
Canada V5X 1X9

The Estrogen Alternative: Natural Hormone Therapy with Botanical Progesterone

Raquel Martin and Dr Judi Gerstung
Healing Arts Press
Rochester, Vermont
www.innertraditions.com

The Golden Fountain: The Complete Guide to Urine Therapy

Coen van der Kroon
Available through www.amazon.com and
Nexus Magazine (Australia) Ph: 07 5442 9820

Recommended Reading

Books by *Russell L Blaylock, MD*
Excitotoxins: The Taste That Kills
and **Health and Nutrition Secrets To Save Your Life**
Dr Blaylock's latest book tells what you can do to recover from aspartame poisoning.
Advanced Nutritional Concepts, LLC
PO Box 2670
Ridgeland, MS 39158-2670
USA Phone: 1 800 566 622
www.russellblaylockmd.com

Solving the MS Mystery
Hal Huggins, DDS,
5082 List Drive,
Colorado Springs,
Colorado, 80919 USA
Ph: 1 866-948-4638
www.drhuggins.com
Dr. Huggins is a world expert on toxic dental materials and explains the connection between those poisons and MS. This is an excellent book and I recommend it highly.

A Cancer Therapy: Results of Fifty Cases
Max Gerson, MD
The Gerson Institute
1572 Second Avenue
San Diego CA 92101
USA Phone: (619) 685 5353 and 888 4 GERSON
www.gerson.org

Naked at Noon, the Importance of Sunlight and Vitamin D
Krispin Sullivan, Clincal Nutritionist
Basic Health Publications, Inc
8200 Boulevard East 25G, North Bergen, New Jersey 07047
www.physicalmag.com/BasicHealth/order.html

A Shot In The Dark
Coulter & Fisher
Koren Publications
2026 Chestnut Street
Philadelphia, PA 19103

The Schwarzbein Principle
Diana Schwarzbein
www.schwarzbeinprinciple.com

Preventing and Reversing Arthritis Naturally: The Untold Story
Raquel Martin and Dr Karen Romano
Healing Arts Press
Rochester, Vermont
www.innertraditions.com

What Your Doctor May Not Tell You About Menopause
John R Lee, MD
Time-Warner Books
1271 Avenue of the Americas
New York, NY 10020
www.twbookmark.com

Natural Progesterone: The Multiple Roles Of A Remarkable Hormone
John R Lee, MD
BLL Publishing
P O Box 2068 S
Sebastopol, CA 95473

Dressed To Kill: The Link Between Breast Cancer and Bras
Sydney Ross Singer and Soma Grismaijer
Avery Publishing Group
www.penguinputnam.com

Living Proof – A Medical Mutiny
Michael Gearin-Tosh
www.simonandschuster.com

Your Body's Many Cries for Water
F Batmanghelidi, MD
Rosicrucian Books
P O Box 1087 Burwood North
NSW 2134 Australia

The Natural Way To Heal
Biochemist Walter Last
Excellent information on minerals
www.health-science-spirit.com

Dangerous Grains
James Braly, MD and Ron Hoggan, MA
www.penguinputnam.com

Recommended Reading

The Oiling Of America
Sally Fallon and Mary G Enig, PhD
www.drcranton.com
www.WestonAPrice.org

Know Your Fats: The Complete Primer For Understanding The Nutrition Of Fats, Oils And Cholesterol
Sally Fallon and Mary G Enig, PhD
Bethesda Press
Bethesda MD 2000
www.enig.com   www.WestonAPrice.org

Nutrition and Physical Degeneration
Dr Weston A Price
Every doctor and dentist should read this monumental study.
Weston A. Price Foundation
PMB 106-380, 4200 Wisconsin Avenue, NW, Washington DC 20016
Email: WestonAPrice@msn.com
www.WestonAPrice.org

Women's Health Series
Burton Goldberg
Three books containing invaluable information on women's health matters.
Future Medicine Publishing, Inc
1640 Tiburon, California 94920

Newsletters & Magazines

The Hippocrates Health Centre Newsletter
Quarterly publication summarising the latest health news.
Hippocrates Health Centre
6 Julie Way, Mudgeeraba
Queensland 4213, Ph: (07) 5530 2860
A$10 per year

Wise Traditions
A most interesting quarterly magazine. Editor, Sally Fallon (safallon@aol.com) and Scientific Editor, Mary G. Enig, PhD (marye@enig.com) are world-renowned nutritional experts.
Weston A. Price Foundation
PMB 106-380, 4200 Wisconsin Avenue, NW, Washington DC 20016
Email: WestonAPrice@msn.com
www.WestonAPrice.org

What Doctors Don't Tell You
An excellent alternative health newsletter
2 Salisbury Road
London SW19 4EZ
Email: cs@wddty.co.uk
www.wddty.co.uk

The John R Lee, MD Medical Letter
Publishers' Mgmt Corp
P O Box 84900
Phoenix, Arizona 85071

Nutrition & Healing
Dr Jonathan Wright's very valuable newsletter.
www.wrightsnewsletter.com

Nexus Magazine
Contains valuable information that mainstream publications rarely print; US,UK and New Zealand editions also published.
P.O. Box 30, Mapleton, Queensland 4560
Phone: (07) 5442 9280
Fax: (07) 5442 9381
www.nexusmagazine.com

Newsletters & Magazines

Health Freedom News
Newsletter of an organisation fighting to preserve the health freedom of America, taking on the government and stopping some of the outrageous laws it has tried, and is still trying, to enact.
255 N El Cielo Road, Suite 670
Palm Springs, CA 92262

Townsend Letter For Doctors And Patients
911 Tyler Street, Pt. Townsend
Washington 98368-6541
Email: tldp@olympus.net, www.tldp.com

Dr William Campbell Douglass' and Dr Robert J Rowen's Second Opinion Newsletters
Second Opinion Publishing
PO Box 467939
Atlanta
Georgia 31146-7939

Price-Pottenger Nutrition Foundation Health Journal
The Price-Pottenger Nutrition Foundation
PO Box 2614 La Mesa
California 91943-2614
Email: info@price-pottenger.org
www.price-pottenger.org

Informed Voice Magazine
Since 1994, Informed Choice Magazine has alerted parents and health professionals to health issues and the dangers of childhood vaccinations.
PO Box 177, Bangalow, NSW 2479
Ph: (02) 6687 2436, Fax: (02) 6687 2032
Email: info@informedchoice.com.au
www.informedchoice.com.au

The Australian Fluoridation News
You can help support this organization through their excellent newsletter, as they are fighting the deadly fluoridation/poisoning of our precious water supplies.
Box 935G, GPO Melbourne, Victoria 3001
Ph: (03) 9592 5088, Fax: (03) 9592 4544

The Thyroid Revolution
Highly recommended.
www.thyroidrevolution.com

Products

Pure Maca Powder
In my opinion, Maca is the finest food supplement ever discovered, but beware of cheap, pale-coloured, strange-tasting powders now flooding the market. Many contain Guarana and the animal capsules are not recommended. Hippocrates Health Centre was the first to import Maca into Australia and we guarantee our powder to be 100% pure and effective. Read more about its properties and how to use it, on page 320
Empowerment Products
Ph: (07) 5530 2939
Fax: (07) 5569 0884
Email: sales@doctorsaredangerous.com
Online: Secure Order Form available on
www.doctorsaredangerous.com

Thyroid and Other Natural Hormones
(Prescriptions are necessary)
Queensland compounding chemist Jerrv Loizou manufactures hormone creams without the use of dangerous preservatives. He supplies porcine thyroid in vegetable capsules and will ship his products throughout Australia. Overseas orders must be accompanied by a prescription from a registered Australian doctor. When ordering, please mention that you want the products I recommend.
Australian Bio-Identical Hormone Laboratories
PO Box 2522, Southport, QLD 4225
Australian & Overseas orders:
Ph: +61 7 5555 7505, Fax: (07) 5555 7506
Email: orders@compoundingchemist.com.au

Products

Thyroid Supply
(Prescriptions are necessary)
North American readers with thyroid problems can obtain *Armour Laboratory Desiccated Thyroid (porcine)* from Will Tomkins at Pine Pharmacy. He will also fill overseas orders.
Pine Pharmacy
2316 Pine Avenue, Niagara Falls
New York 14301
USA Ph: 1 716282 1112
USA Fax: 1 7162820654

Coconut Scraper With Vacuum Base
This inexpensive ($20) gadget is perfect for removing the hard white meat from coconuts.
Available in Indian stores worldwide
Shree Kangaroo Enterprises
Gotatewadi
Goregaon(E)
Mumbai, India 400 062

Vitamin C
Rose Hip Organic Granules provide large amounts of vitamin C as well as vitamins A, B and E. Taken as a tea, this product is good for cleansing the kidneys and gallbladder, and acts as a diuretic. Sprinkled over food, or simply taken by spoon, the granules taste delicious and are the finest source of vitamin C we have found. The Rose Hips are grown in Chile's Southern Andes,one of the few remaining unpolluted regions on Earth.
Hippocrates Health Centre
Australian orders:
Ph: (07) 5530 2860
Overseas orders:
Ph: +61 7 5530 2860

Vitamin K
i-HerbInc
USA Phone: 1 626 358 5678
USA Fax: 1 626 303 7275
www.iherb.com
These products are cheaper if ordered online.

Source Naturals 500 mcg vitamin K
Available from the US

D-Mannose
(for urinary tract infections)
This drug-free cystitis cure is sold in health stores in the US, through Dr Jonathan V Wright's Tahoma Clinic Dispensary and one Australian representative.

Australia

Ian Christenson Ph: (07) 4954-5348

US

Tahoma Clinic Dispensary
515 W Harrison, Suite 150
Kent, Washington
USA Phone: 1 888 893 6878
www.tahoma-clinic.com
Overseas buyers may also order D-Mannose from Bio-Tech-Pharmacal (see address below).

Armour Thyroid and Hydrocortisone without prescriptions:
(Not allowed into some countries)

International Pharmaceutical Services

www.internationalpharmacy.com

US Ph: 1 650 573 6200
US fax: 1 650 573 6400

3 West 37th Avenue, #23,
San Mateo, CA
94403 USA

Boron, Selenium, Nicotinic Acid
Borax can be used instead of Boron.
Takapuna Health Store
Attn: Andrew Jones, Takapuna, New Zealand
NZ Phone/Fax: 64 9 486 1245.
Email: nzhealthstore@yahoo.com

BioSalt
Large crystals of Himalayan salt from the Hunza region.
BioNatural
1 Overland Drive, Vermont South, Victoria
3133, Ph: 1 300 555 686
www.BioNatural.com.au

Take Control of Your Health and Escape the Sickness Industry

Products

Coconut Oil

The coconut oils in Australian shops are refined, bleached and deodorised (RBD) oils and are *not recommended*. The food grade coconut oil imported by Hippocrates Health Centre has been approved by the TGA, is organic, virgin, cold pressed, unrefined, unbleached, undeodorised, and is not hydrogenated. Coconut oil hardens in cold weather, so place bottle in warm water or the sun.

Hippocrates Health Centre
Australian orders:
Ph: (07) 5530 2860
Overseas orders:
Ph: +61 7 5530 2860
USA:
Penner's Pantry
8567 50 E Street
Putnam, Illinois 61560
USA Ph: 1 815 646 4449
Email: penners@starband.net

Cod Liver Oil

For reasons explained in **Chapter 8***, Bone Health II, Carlson's* is the only cod liver oil we, and expert nutritionists, recommend.

Carlson Labs, Inc
15 College Drive, Arlington Heights
Illinois 60004-1985
USA Ph: 1 800 323 4141 (toll-free) or
USA Ph: 1 847255 1600
USA Fax: 1 847255 1605
Email: carlson@carlsonlabs.com
www.carlsonlabs.com

Hydrochloric Acid with Pepsin

Some Australian brands were taken off the market, so we asked a New Zealand firm to make one to our specifications - in a vegetable glycerine capsule, without preservatives. It is the best we've used.

Hippocrates Health Centre
Australian orders:
Ph: (07) 5530 2860
Overseas orders:
Ph: +61 7 5530 2860

Silica

NTP	**Flora Sil**
Ph: 1 800 225 500	Burnaby
Ph: (02) 4997 2530	British Columbia
Fax: (02) 4997 0199	V5J-B9
14 Winta Road	Ph: 1 888 436 6697
Tea Gardens, NSW 2324	

www.NTPhealthproducts.com

The Champion Juicer

This is the only juicer we can recommend. It has been used at Hippocrates Health Centre for over 18 years, and we consider it the best in the world.

Hippocrates Health Centre
Australian orders:
Ph: (07) 5530 2860
Overseas orders:
Ph: +61 7 5530 2860

Magnets

Please refer to **Chapter 26***, Remedies*, for details of the therapeutic benefits of magnets. *Lothrop* supplies a range of effective devices. More information is contained in William Philpott, MD's, *Biomagnetic Handbook*.

Lothrop Industries
17171 SE 29th Street
Choctaw
Oklahoma 73020
USA Fax: 1 405 390 2968

Bottled Water

Alpha Lyte
Australian orders:
Phone/Fax: (07) 3287-4644
Email: info@alphalyte.com
www.alphalyte.com provides addresses of local suppliers

Bottled Water

Grander Water Technologies
Ph: 1800 675 771
Gold Coast Area: 07 55 68-7522
www.grander.com.au
Available in supermarkets

Products

Cellyte Mineral Supplement

Cellyte is an extract of a pure form of the organic mineral complex found in nature, derived mainly from plant matter, using a unique patented technology. It is the result of years of research by a team of natural health specialists, including Dr. Michael Halliday and the late Dr. John Whitman Ray.

Cellyte contrains over 72 key minerals in a crystalloid electrolyte form, which is the most efficient way to deliver minerals to the body. The small particle size and unique micro-electrical charge of the mineral complex in cellyte allows it to be rapidly absorbed and utilised by the cells of the body. Moreover, the complex also contains various beneficial phytonutrients, including amino acids, co-enzymes and vitamins, and sugnificant quantities of oxygen.

(This is the mineral supplement that Elaine, after years of trial and error, takes herself.)

Empowerment Products
Australian orders: Ph: (07) 5530 2939 Fax: (07) 5569-0884
Overseas orders: Ph: +61 7 5530 2939 Fax: 61 7 5569-0884
Internet orders: www.doctorsaredangerous.com

Protection from Radiation and Geopathic Stress

Electromagnetic frequencies from mobile phones, mobile phone towers, electrical transformers, computers, radar, satellites, the high voltage power lines that dot landscapes, etc. etc., are damaging to our health. These non-ionizing electromagnetic fields do not exist in nature, and our bodies do not know how to deal with them. As Nicola Tesla, who invented AC electricity said, "The alternating current I have invented will prove to be the most dangerous thing on Earth, and I must find an alternative." Tesla's understnading of frequencies led him to create the resonance that was necessary to counteract the biological effects of radiation for which his inventions were responsible. The company which now bears his name manufactures pendants and plates for personal and environmental protection, and I have had a great deal of experience with the work they are doing. Many people (those of us at Hippocrates Health Centre included) have reported amazing improvements in health and wellbeing after having Tesla's products installed.

This company also tests for and neutralises geopathic stress, which has been found to be a common factor in many serious illnesses, sleeplessness and psychological conditions. I have observed amazing recoveries: as just one example, a friend moved into a new home and was unable to sleep well for five years. Gold Coast Tesla practitioners, Cheryl and Walter, tested her bedroom and found underground water that carries electromagnetic frequencies. Once Tesla products were installed, the woman returned to her normal sleep patterns and felt well again. She was thrilled!

I recommended this testing and these products without qualification. To find a local practitioner, see below.

Tesla's Innovational Technologies
136/199 Toorak Road, South Yarra, Victoria 3141. Ph: (03) 9644 4595
Gold Coast Office: Ph: 0418 990 539 and 1-300-898-983
Email: info@teslas.us   www.teslas.us

Delwa-Star Rectal/Vaginal Heater	***Wheatgrass Juicer***
Please refer to ***Chapter 26***, *Remedies*, for details of the internal heat therapy facilitated by this product.	The only juicer on the market that properly juices wheatgrass.
Charles T McGee, MD	**Hippocrates Health Centre**
P O Box 5154 Coeur d'Alene	Australian orders:
Idaho 83814	Ph: (07) 5530 2860
USA Ph: 1 888 263 9214	Overseas orders:
www.cheeenergy.com	Ph: +61 7 5530 2860

Food Enzymes

The food enzymes Hippocrates Health Centre imports from the USA are formulated to the specifications of famed enzyme expert, Edward Howell. They are plant-based and contain no fillers (such as rice bran or rice powder), no preservatives, and are encapsulated in vegie-caps. See **Chapter 8,** *Bone Health II.*

Hippocrates Health Centre
Australian orders:
Ph: (07) 5530 2860
Overseas orders:
Ph: +61 7 5530 2860

Rebounder

We recommend the *RH48 Lymphaciser*, rather than ordinary mini-trampolines, because it is enormously superior. Manufactured from the highest-quality materials, sprung for the Southern Hemisphere. It features right and left-hand springing. Comes in a range of colours, with a one-hour demonstration video.

Hippocrates Health Centre
Australian orders:
Ph: (07) 5530 2860
Overseas orders:
Ph: +61 7 5530 2860

Arbor Test Microscope

A scientific product which readers may find useful in helping to observe and understand their natural ovulation cycle better, this precision-made optical microscope uses a saliva sample to display and interpret hormonal changes taking place. The makers suggest that analysing your saliva on a regular basis will allow correct determination of the phases of the menstrual cycle and a timely recognition of any deviations.

Advanced Health Technologies
Suite 102 Piccadilly Court
222 Pitt Street, Sydney, NSW 2000
Ph: 0415 370 269
Fax: (02) 9283 2230
www.arbormicroscope.com

Miessence Certified Organic Skincare / Cosmetics

The entire range is tested by Australian Certified Organic (ACO) that guarantees they are organic, and of food grade quality and completely free of synthetic chemicals. A few of their products contain small amounts of soy lecithin. You may wish to specify, when you order, that you want to avoid these particular products.

Pip Rose, Independent Representative
Ph: (07) 5533 0367
Email: piprose4@bigpond.com
www.onegrp.com/Piprose

The "Immaculate" Range

Great safe complexion care product range includes the shampoo I use and recommend highly. Reasonably priced, too.
Rebecca Kingsbury
Ph: 1300 720 937
www.immaculateorganics.com

Organic Rosehip Skin Care Products

Nancy Evans imports her ingredients from the unpolluted Andes, and formulates her products from the best, purest ingredients. She has an extensive line of skin care products, too numerous to list here, an oil that causes scars to fade, the only safe sunscreen I know, moisturisers, and a pure bar soap that can be used as a shampoo.

Organic Rosehip Skin Care Pty Ltd
Retail sales:
2/23 Entrerprise Ave,
Tweed Heads South NSW 2486
Ph: (07) 552 3910 Fax: (07) 5523 9155
Email: nancyevans@rosehipskincare.com
www.rosehipskincare.com

Services – Therapeutic

The Bowen Therapy (Bowtech)

This is a unique form of neuromuscular re-patterning, which works primarily through the nervous system on both structural and energetic levels. The technique is gentle and non-invasive, and can be performed through clothing. Since 1986, when Oswald and Elaine Rentsch established the Bowen Therapy Academy of Australia, over 14,000 people have taken Bowtech training worldwide, with 70 registered instructors in 16 countries. There are 12 countries with Bowen associations affiliated to the Bowen Therapy Academy of Australia.

Bowen Therapy is appropriate for everyone, from the highly trained athlete to newborns, pregnant women, elderly, and the chronically ill. Bowen has been successful in treating musculoskeletal problems, such as back and neck pain, scoliosis, sporting injuries, TMJ alignment, and carpal tunnel syndrome. It is also renowned for its effectiveness with internal conditions, such as migraines, digestive and elimination complaints, colic in babies, and respiratory problems, including asthma. A Bowen treatment consists of gentle, rolling movements. These stimulations activate a systematic response so powerful that a few minutes pause is observed to allow them to be integrated. A pattern of movements and pauses continues throughout the treatment. The rhythm is soothing and most patients fall asleep at least once during the session. Benefits are usually apparent within two sessions, even when longstanding conditions are being treated. Bowen results are lasting and profound.

Bowen Therapy Academy of Australia International Head Office
PO Box 733, Hamilton VIC 3300, Australia
Phone: (03) 5572 3000 Fax: (03) 5572 3144   Email: bowtech@h140.aone.net.au
Gold Coast residents should contact **Pip Rose** (Ph: (07) 5533 0367, Email: piprose4@bigpond.com), whom I know from personal experience to be an expert practitioner and of great help.

Services – Medical, Diagnostic

Expert Thyroid/Adrenal Help In The UK

Dr. Barry Durrant-Peatfield, MB BS LRCP MRCS
The Peatfield Clinic of Nutritional Medicine,
The Old Bakery, Rotham Road, Meopham, Kent, UK DA130QB
Ph: 44-1474-815-793   info@drpeatfield.com
For information on the internet, type into your search engine: **Dr. Barry Durrant-Peatfield**

See Chapter 2 for Dr. Durrant-Peatfield's life-saving information on the thyroid and adrenals glands.

Highly Recommended Australian Naturopath
Leisa Wheeler, N.D.
Hippocrates Health Centre,
6 Julie Way, Mudgeeraba, Qld. 4213
0413-143-707   info@leisawheeler.com.au   www.leisawheeler.com.au

Thyroid Regeneration (as described in *Chapter 1, That "Mystery Illness"*)

Dr Earl W Conroy, BSc, DC, ND, NZNMA
The protocol developed by New Zealand medical practitioner Dr Earl Conroy has proved successful in restoring proper function to both hypothyroids and hyperthyroids. Please enclose a $5 note for the data.

Waiora Mara Clinic
212 Graham Valley Road
RD 1, Motueka, New Zealand 7161
Email: waiorama@ihug.co.nz

Digital Infrared Thermal Imaging (DITI)

This non-radiating diagnosis system is described in *Chapter 12, Breast Health*. DITI is used throughout Australia, but we have been unable to get a list of practitioners. We suggest writing or ringing the Southport office for information in your area. For data, please enclose $5.00.

DITI
P O Box 243, Southport
Queensland 4215
Ph: (07) 5591 3878
Fax: (07) 5591 4559

Thermography Breast Diagnoses (as described in *Chapter 12, Breast Health*)

Practitioners:

Jenny Burke
Australian Biologics
Fayworth House
383 Pitt Street
Sydney, NSW 2000
Ph: (02) 9283-0807
Fax (02) 9283-0910

Paul Alexander
Tara Centre
384 Oxford Street
Mt Hawthorne, WA 6016
Ph: (08) 9444 4190   Fax: (08) 9444 4192
www.taracentre.com.au

Dr Donsbach's Clinic
(Dr Kurt Donsbach, DC, ND, PhD)
Hospital Santa Monica
880 Canarios Court
Chula Vista, California 91910
USA Phone: 1 800 359 6547 and 619 428 1146
Hospital Avenida Mazatlan O/N
Rosarito Beach BC Mexico
Treatments include ozone and hydrogen peroxide, nutrition, biomagnetics, colonics, chelation, etc.

Glen Rees
Warragul Natural Health
16 Queen Street
Warragul, Victoria 3820

Medical Infrared Digital Imaging
Jean Koek (0413 627 577)
Unit 6, Southern Cross House

9 McKay Street
Turner, ACT 2602
Ph: (02) 6262 5252
Fax: (02) 6262 5510
Email: info@medicalinfrared.com.au
www.medicalinfrared.com.au

The Gerson Institute
1572 Second Avenue
San Diego, CA 92101
USA Phone: (619) 685 5353 and 888 4 GERSON
www.gerson.org

Founded by Charlotte Gerson, daughter of Max Gerson, MD, the Institute's affiliated clinic, located in Tijuana, Mexico, treats a variety of chronic illnesses; in particular, all forms of cancer.

Services – Medical, Diagnostic

A Better Method for Testing Your Thyroid

Thyroid serum testing is inexact and leaves patients in limbo, because physicians refuse to prescribe needed medication unless serum tests of TSH show a markedly low result. ARL is now offering a test kit that is more accurate because the blood is dried on filter paper, either at the patient's home or in the physician's office. The result is an indication of the hormone level present in the blood at that moment, and it is not influenced by a time or temperature delay. Further, it is more accurate, because using this technique the lab is able to get an accurate measure of TSH, free T3 and free T4. Usually, serum testing is done only for TSH.

Analytical Reference Laboratories,

Third Floor, 568 St. Kilda Road
Melbourne, VIC 3004, Australia
1 300 554 480
Ph: (0) 3 9539 5411
Fax: (0) 3 9527 7277
E-mail: info@arlaus.com.au
www.arlaus.com.au

This test is called **The Thyroid Profile Blood Spot** and the kit can be ordered by your doctor.

Services – Dental

The Australasian Society of Oral Medicine and Toxicology

ASOMAT is a non-profit professional organisation of dentists and doctors, whose purpose is to promote concepts of bio-compatible dentistry which are supported by scientific, peer reviewed research. These concepts encompass a more holistic view of dentistry than does the traditional model. ASOMAT promotes mercury-free dentistry, as well as other safe methods of restoration. Some of the Australian members are listed on this page. For further enquiries contact: *ASOMAT* P O Box A860, Sydney South, NSW 1235 Ph: (02) 9867-1111 Fax: (02) 9283-2230 www.asomat.org

ASOMAT Members:

Robert Gammal	**John Sotis**	**Eric Davis**
Suite 102, Piccadilly Court	Suite 10, Mermaid Central	40 Duffield Road
222 Pitt Street	2431 Gold Coast Highway	Margate Beach
Sydney	Mermaid Beach	Queensland 4014
NSW 2000	Queensland 4218	Ph: (07) 3284 5755
Ph: (02) 9264 5195	Ph: (07) 5526 6662	
www.bcd.com.au		

Roman Lohyn	**Wally Hassoun**	**Andrew Taylor**
(President of ASOMAT)	707 Malvern Rd	Newrybar (Near Byron Bay)
8th Floor, 175 Collins Street	Toorak	Northern NSW
Melbourne Victoria 3000	Victoria 3142	02 6687 2552
		agtaylor@bigpond.net.au

Overseas, the equivalent of ASOMAT is the International Academy of Oral Medicine and Toxicology - IAOMT - with branches in many countries: To find a qualified natural dentist search the internet.

The world's foremost authority on the dangers of toxic dental materials is Colorado dentist, Dr. Hal Huggins, who developed all the protocols for the safe removal of these toxins. He has campaigned tirelessly for the past thirty years to make people aware of the serious health risks from materials such as mercury, nickel and root canal treatments. A growing number of dentists world-wide are now practicing bio-compatible dentistry based on the Huggins protocol.

Finding a dentist who can remove amalgam (mercury) fillings and root canals and replace them with safe, biocompatable materials is a real challenge. Many do 'half a job' but few do it properly. Dr. Huggins says that over 60% of people who have amalgam fillings removed without following the correct protocol become sicker. It's vitally important that you educate yourself so you can choose the right dentist. The Huggins **Protocol for Amalgam Removal and Dental Revision** can be downloaded as an inexpensive e-booklet from www.drhuggins.com, together with comprehensive information about toxic dental materials and how to avoid them. (Dr. Hal Huggins, 5082 List Drive, Colorado Springs, CO 80919 USA 1-866-948-4638.)

Sydney bio-compatible dentist Rob Gammal has produced two excellent DVDs, titled **Quecksilber** and **Rooted,** that graphically describe the dangers of amalgam fillings and root canal treatments. These DVDs can be purchased online at www.bcd.com.au.

Because of thousands of complaints about damage done to our readers by dentists, we have recently formed an Association called D.I.V.A (Dental Incompetence Victims Association). It costs nothing to join – all we ask from members is to tell your story, name the offending dentists (they cannot harm you any more than they already have) and give us details of what has happened to you. We will take steps to stop these outrages, and need a large membership to counteract the Australian Dental Association, which exists only to protect dentists against people they have damaged. Also, we need to bring out the truth about dental insurance companies. **Or company.** Shockingly, there is just one insurance company for dentists, and if a dentist dares testify against an incompetent dentist, his insurance company will take away his insurance. Worse, the insurance company sometimes pressures dentists to perjure themselves in court to protect another dentist. What chance do we have? Only by organizing. Please see the website, www.dentistsaredangerous.com JOIN US AND FIGHT BACK!

Services – Information & Action

Roy B Kupsinel, MD
PO Box 620550
Oviedo, Florida 32762-0660
USA Phone: 1 407 365 6681 Fax: 1 407 3651834
Email: rkupsinel@aol.com
Prominent American medical researcher.

Rex E Newnham, PhD, DO, ND
Cracoe House Cottage,
Cracoe, Nr. Skipton
North Yorkshire BD23 6LB, England
UK Phone: 44 1767 30240
Boron expert, international nutritional consultant, research specialist in trace minerals and nutrition.

Aspartame Consumer Network
Mary Stoddard
P O Box 780634
Dallas, Texas 75378
USA Ph: 1 214 352 4268
Email: marystod@airmail.net

Mission Possible
Betty Martini MPNC
P O Box 220102
Chantilly, Virginia 20153
Email: bettym19@mindspring.com
www.aspartame.com
International anti-aspartame campaign.
Related sites:
www.dorway.com
www.aspartamekills.com
www.holisticmed.com/aspartame
Victims support group:
www.presidiotex.com/aspartame
Email: info@avn.org.au
www.avn.org.au

Judy Kitchen
3637 Serra Road
Malibu, CA 90265
USA Phone and Fax: 1 10 456 6837
Hydrochloric acid expert.

New Zealand Soy Action Group
Valerie and Richard James
PO Box 3285
Onerahi, Whangarei, New Zealand
Email: divulge@xtra.co.nz
www.soyonlineservice.co.nz
Leading campaigners and activists against the use of all forms of soy.

Australian Vaccination Network
Meryl Dorey
PO Box 177
Bangalow, NSW 2479
Ph: (02) 6687 1699
Fax: (02) 6687 2032

National Pure Water Association
Croft End, Lowick Bridge, Cumbria LA12 8EE
United Kingdom
Email: jane@npwa.freeserve.co.uk
www.npwa.freeserve.co.uk
This not-for-profit organization, founded in 1960 by Lord Douglas of Barloch, KCMG, to campaign for safe drinking water, is at the forefront of a worldwide campaign against the fluoridation of public water.

> You just need to be a flea against injustice.
> Enough committed fleas biting
> strategically can make even the biggest dog
> uncomfortable and transform
> even the biggest nation
> - *Marian Wright Edelman*

> If you are as angry as I about what has
> happened to our world, please join me
> and become a biting flea on the
> backsides of the multi-nationals
>
> - *Elaine Hollingsworth*

Important Warning...
Acid Supplementation

During the years this book has been widely circulated, I have received hundreds of comments from people whose digestive and other health problems have been significantly helped by taking Hydrochloric Acid, *HCl*, as recommended in **Chapter 3**, *Stomach Acid.*

One woman, however, told me that she couldn't get the "burn signal", even though she took 12 capsules. I was very concerned and advised her not to take any at all before finding out why so much acid had no noticeable effect in her stomach.

After doing some digging I found that if acid supplementation in large amounts is not felt, it can be due to nerve blockage in the spinal column. Fortunately, there is a simple test to ascertain if there is such a blockage in your spine: get a bottle of *Nicotinic Acid* (**not** just Niacin or Niacinimide) tablets from your health food store. You may have to send to New Zealand. (see Resources).

Then, play it safe and first thing in the morning take only half a tablet before eating. If this does not produce the expected "niacin flush" on your skin (refer to page 112 for more details), try a whole tablet. Once the flush starts, observe to see if it extends to your fingers and toes. If it does not, chances are you have a spinal nerve blockage and will need an adjustment by a qualified osteopath or chiropractor. Dr John Whitman Ray, of *Body Electronics* fame, advised that the first cervical vertebrae should be adjusted first.

Some people, when they initially try HCl, are so deficient in stomach acid that it can take many capsules before they feel a slight burning in the stomach. My suggestion, if seven capsules do not produce a burn, is **not to take HCl without the nicotinic test**, and to review **Chapter 3,** *Stomach Acid.*

This is not something to play around with, and a nutritionist who understands our desperate need for an acid environment in the digestive system would be a great help. Also, Dr Jonathan Wright and Lane Lenard's book, *Why Stomach Acid Is Good For You* (see **Resources**), is a valuable tool for anyone with digestive problems.

Yes, But What <u>Can</u> I Eat?

Simple, But Not Easy

The solution to adopting a healthful, life-lengthening diet lies not in having shelves of recipe books, but in adopting principles and sticking to them for the rest of your life. Strict rules need to be followed: they are simple to understand, but not easy to implement, because temptation is everywhere.

Your Mother Was Right

Vegetables are the foundation of a great diet. Throughout this book I have quoted studies proving how important they are to every facet of health, including cancer prevention. A recent, 15-month study of 2000 subjects found that those with the highest vegetable and fruit intake had a 70% reduced risk of heart attack and other cardiac problems. (This was reported in Health Sciences Institute's e-alert, which sends out free emails I highly recommend.)

Raw is preferable, of course. Bear in mind that we were not evolved to eat cooked food, and that our primitive forbears lived on a diet of raw food for millions of years. If you are not prepared to eat all raw, at least be sure to eat a salad before eating cooked food. This will get your enzymes perking so that they can cope better with the cooked food that follows.

There are many different salad combinations. A wide variety should be eaten – dark green lettuces (not head lettuce), cucumbers, tomatoes, carrots, beet root (beets), capsicums of all colours (peppers to Americans), red onions and any other vegetables that take your fancy. Chop, shred or dice them in various combinations. Rocket, coriander (cilantro), parsley and any number of green herbs in pots make great additions, and provide calcium your body can assimilate, other valuable minerals and great flavour.

Every day I have a large salad with most of these vegetables and herbs. Because they give an appealing texture, I add a cut-up avocado and a small amount of virgin olive oil as well as a squeeze of lemon. Then, and this really makes it yummy and crunchy, I sprinkle two tablespoons of seeds over the salad. The result is so filling that it keeps me going all day. (Instructions for preparing the seeds are below.) Please do the best you can to use organic vegetables for their life-saving minerals and vitamins. If a seasoning is desired, the only ones I have found that don't contain HVP and other poisons are A. Vogel's Trocomare and Herbamare.

My favourite way to get lots of raw veggies down is by drinking a glass of freshly squeezed carrot, celery, beet root, parsley, cucumber, etc., as well as any greens that are available. Organically raised raw egg is delicious, blended with the juice. I add Maca, minerals and RoseHip granules, and blend it all for a nourishing, filling meal.

Most people are not prepared to go the all-raw route. For those, I recommend eating a wide variety of steamed vegetables, with particular emphasis on zucchini, celery and string beans, the three liver-cleansing vegetables that are in the Dr. Bieler soup described on page 313. Potatoes, steamed or baked, and seasoned with herbs and butter, chives, shallots, or chopped red onions (raw or cooked), are a delicious and filling addition to a vegetable meal. For those few who are allergic to the nightshade vegetables (potatoes, capsicum, tomatoes and eggplant) special care is needed. And, don't forget Dr. Bieler's soup if you or a family member are feeling toxic.

Nature's Treat

Fresh, raw fruit can be prepared in so many ways: you are only limited by your imagination. Fruit salads are lovely, especially if bananas are included for thickness. Sauces can be made of fruit to drizzle over the salad, by blending several fruits with avocado and/or frozen bananas. The addition of dried fruit, especially dates, creates a rich sauce. I sometimes sprinkle nuts on fruit salads, even though nuts and fruit are not an ideal combination. But, hey, I'm not perfect!

Fruit smoothies are great on warm days and are a lovely treat for children. Use fruit juice or make almond milk (directions below) and put in the blender with frozen banana and any other frozen or fresh fruit you like. Just remember – when freezing fruit, it should be very ripe, and hard skins must be removed first. Cut frozen fruit in chunks before blending. For variety you might like to add a raw egg before blending, but be sure of the purity of the eggs you buy. Frozen mango and banana, blended 'til smooth, makes a delicious ice cream, and it won't shorten your life!

One of my favourite treats is fruit I have dried myself. Each season I get cases of ripe mango, banana and pineapple, taking care that they are extremely sweet. I have a dehydrator, which makes it easy, but they can also be dried on cookie sheets in an ordinary oven, turned to ON, but no higher, in order to preserve the enzymes. The great advantage of this is that the sulphur and possibly dirty conditions used during commercial drying are eliminated. Dehydrators must be set at 40 degrees Celsius or below, or

100 degrees Fahrenheit or below, so enzymes are not killed. If you use an oven, take care that the fruit does not go mouldy.

Dehydrators can be used to make delightful treats. As just one example, soaked, ground almonds can be blended with soaked (and drained) dates and orange juice to form a paste that can then be spread on a dehydrator tray, using a blank. In order to keep it from sticking, a tiny amount of coconut oil should be spread on the blank first. Dry until it reaches the desired consistency – crunchy or soft. Let your imagination create other treats, or refer to the many available recipe books for dehydrating food.

Don't Neglect Your Protein

If you are vegetarian you will need to learn to prepare nuts so that the anti-enzyme factor is eliminated. When selecting nuts, make sure they are not rancid, and use as wide a variety as possible. Do not, however, use cashews or peanuts, as they are not healthful. Put all the nuts in a large container and add more than enough water to cover, so that when they swell they will still be covered. Put enough good quality sea salt in the water to make it taste noticeably salty. Soak them overnight, or longer. Drain in a colander, then put in a dehydrator until they are dry and crunchy. Keep the temperature low to preserve enzymes – it will take about two days before they are ready, depending upon the room temperature and humidity. If you do not have a dehydrator, nuts can be dried on cookie sheets in an oven at the ON setting, no higher, and will need to be stirred occasionally.

Almonds should be handled separately. Soak them over night and next day drop them in extremely warm water to loosen the skin, which can then be easily removed. The skin has oxalic acid in it, which is to be avoided. They can then be added to the dryer, along with the other nuts. If you wish to make almond milk, simply blend with juice or water 'til smooth. Almonds contain easily assimilated calcium, and should be used frequently.

When drying seeds you may prefer to keep them separate from nuts, as they are tiny and tend to get "lost". The salad addition mentioned earlier is comprised of pepitas (pumpkin seeds), sunflower seeds and pine nuts. Dry them using the nut drying technique, draining through a sieve instead of a colander, and sprinkle them over vegetable salads or cooked vegetables, or use them in other creative ways of your own.

Before our oceans became so polluted, fish were an excellent form of protein and healthful oils. No more – they are now contaminated with mercury. Farmed fish are the worst of the lot, as mentioned earlier in this book, so don't trust them. Because they are tiny, sardines are thought to be free of mercury, and if you use only those packed in water they can be a tasty addition to salads and other dishes, as well as a safe way to get calcium, protein and the good oils sardines contain.

If you eat red meat, roast, grille or sauté it lightly. Absolutely never barbecue meat, or anything else: charred foods are the most cancer-causing thing you can eat. And, please, never eat meat that has been injected and fed grains. Grass fed is the only safe meat.

The same rules apply to chickens. If you don't like to roast or grill, chicken pieces cooked slowly in coconut oil are delicious. Do not be phobic about the skin, which should be kept on.

Eggs are a fine protein, especially when eaten raw. Again, they must be from free-range birds and they must be fresh.

It is impossible to be healthy if you eat the wrong fats and oils, so please review Chapter 6 and follow the instructions. If you fancy stir-fry, use coconut oil. It is healthful and delicious. But remember, it's essential to take good quality food enzymes when eating cooked food.

Once you have established the above rules, and have stuck to them for a while, you will see that eating healthfully is easier than it seems. The secret is to KEEP IT SIMPLE. You will discover such improvements in wellbeing that your efforts will be rewarded. The trick here is to forget about fancy recipes and stick to the principles of safe food preparation. And don't forget these inviolable rules:

- No soy
- No sugar
- No grains
- No fried food
- No barbecued food
- No dairy
- No polyunsaturated oils
- No artificial sweeteners
- No processed foods
- No poisoned water
- No recreational eating

Yes, I know it's hard and your social life will suffer. But YOU won't. You will be infinitely stronger and healthier and you will live decades longer. I've been living this way for nearly fifty years, and if I can do it, you can do it. Remember – some of us are stuck down quickly due to bad food choices, while others are able to defy the odds for years because they were born tough. But no one can get away with ignoring the laws of nature, long-term.

My Recovery From Thyroid & Adrenal Exhaustion
By Marisue Venables

I have no medical degree, yet there is little anyone could tell me about living with low thyroid and adrenal problems that I haven't experienced.

I had thyroid surgery before I was twenty because I had nodules on my thyroid. In removing the cysts, they took out half of my thyroid gland but didn't put me on medication because my blood panels registered normal. Had anyone bothered to ask, even at that age, I had the well-developed classic symptoms of hypothyroidism, or in my case, Hashimoto's Autoimmune Thyroiditis. The signs are easy to spot, the patterns are so distinctive you may as well carry a banner, and the downward spiral, if not treated, is absolutely predictable.

Like a flashing red light, low body temperature tops the list of signals that all is not right. Granted, if you grow up in Florida, the warm weather makes the discrepancy less apparent, but no one seemed to think it was odd that in winter I slept under an electric blanket topped with a huge pile of comforters.

I've learned that if you are sick enough to run a fever, doctors simply decide it's very mild and you're being dramatic. While I was in college, I had to be carried to the infirmary in the dead of winter because I couldn't get out of bed. My temperature was high enough that they kept me, but 100°F flagged me as a malingerer. Once it dropped, they wanted me out of there—and I could barely walk.

Over twenty years later, I discovered the significance of that incident. After reading Broda Barnes book, **Hypothyroidism: The Unsuspected Illness**, I began to track my daily temperature. At the time, I had a history of throwing out thermometers because when I would shake them down, the mercury wouldn't rise. What an eye-opening new perspective! My average temperature was in the 91.6°F to 92.6°F range— over six degrees below normal. When I finally got a doctor to listen, he said, "Don't be ridiculous! There are millions of people out there who have low temperatures, and there's nothing wrong with them."

The medical community would quickly mobilize if a patient were carried into any Emergency Room running a fever seven or more degrees above normal. With the growing epidemic of thyroid problems, it's possible they see that more often than they think, but simply don't recognize it. The starting point matters.

It never occurred to me that I had any option other than to cope with whatever life brought. By the time I realized how serious my problems were, heavy periods with severe cramps had turned into fibroids, ovarian cysts, and an emergency hysterectomy. Foggy brain progressed to more than just a little slow to get started in the mornings. My digestion all but came to a halt. My thick hair was falling out in great gobs. I lost the outer third of my eyebrows. I had no Achilles reflex response. My antibody levels were off the charts. Though the ratio of men to women with Hashimoto's is one in a hundred, I passed it on to my youngest son.

I had totally changed my way of life when I was in my twenties, scrupulously diligent about nutrition. I was the unhealthiest person I knew.

Because I was so focused on my thyroid, it didn't occur to me that I was missing an equally important puzzle piece in my overall problems. My health suddenly deteriorated to the point that my skin was drying up and I was losing muscle mass. Nights brought rampant insomnia punctuated with panic attacks; days were foggy with heavy fatigue. I made a final concerted search for a doctor to help with new, mystifying symptoms. Thousands of dollars bought no relief at all. A chance look at a saliva test told me what my doctor should have noticed. My adrenals had finally run out of cortisol—I had adrenal exhaustion. Less than a week on a trial of 20mg of Cortef a day, in divided doses, proved I was correct. I was determined to find a natural solution, which turned out to be Adrenal Cortex to supply the cortisol I needed, plus Whole Adrenal to support my glands as they recovered. Five tablets of each, twice a day, put me back on track.

I finally made it, but it was all so unnecessary.

There is nothing obscure about the signs and symptoms. They tell a story. But most doctors tout the blood tests as being the final word. Nothing else is admissible. We are so used to hearing ourselves broken down into blood values, we often forget there are other questions to be asked. "How do you feel?" should top the list. "What would you like to see changed?" can give you some clues. Ultimately, results are what is important. Who cares what the tests say if you still feel lousy?

Excellent desiccated glandulars, available from Nutri-Meds, in ideal doses that support health, can provide valuable help. I took over the company in 2003 when I realized the products were significant to my own recovery. I want to offer those options to others struggling to achieve health.

The natural glandulars are offered as nutritional supplements only, so they are available without prescriptions. The range of products include thyroid in 130mg tablets or capsules that include 1 grain of active factors; whole adrenal provides important support to stressed glands; adrenal cortex that supplies 2mg of cortisol per tablet; the best form of progesterone available, pregnenolone, and **DHEA**.

The company focuses on thyroid and adrenal health, and ships worldwide. You can find them online at www.nutri-meds.com

Marisue Venables
Nutri-Meds
PO Box 751206, Petaluma, CA 94975-1206
Ph: 1-888-265-3353 Email: support@nutri-meds.com

INDEX: *To Key Subjects*